Exercise Electrocardiography

Stanley P. Brown | LeeAnn Joe | Cameron S. Huxford

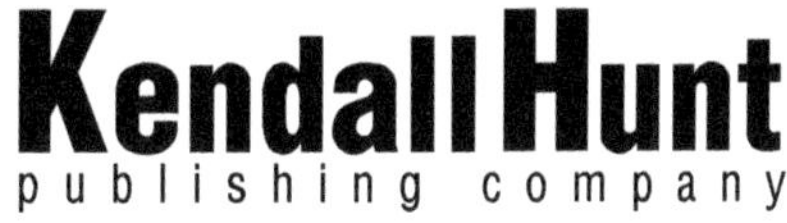

Cover image © Shutterstock.com

Kendall Hunt
publishing company

www.kendallhunt.com
Send all inquiries to:
4050 Westmark Drive
Dubuque, IA 52004-1840

ISBN: 978-1-5249-8297-3

Published in the United States of America

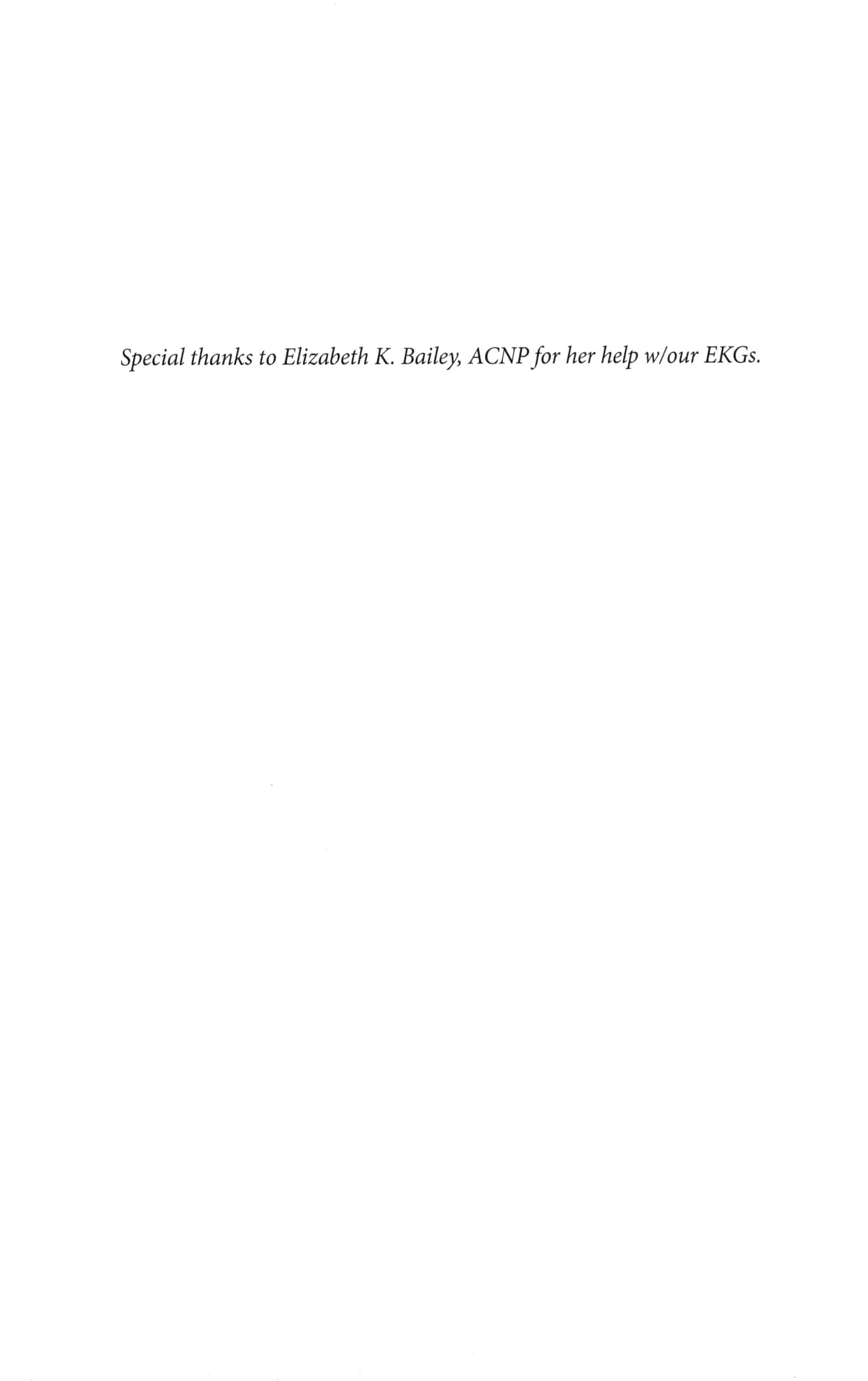

Special thanks to Elizabeth K. Bailey, ACNP for her help w/our EKGs.

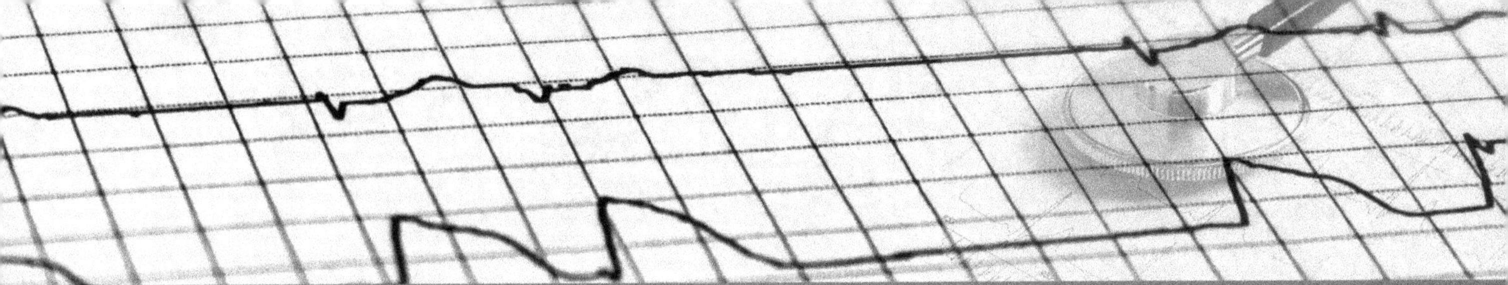

Table of Contents

PART ONE

CARDIOVASCULAR BASICS

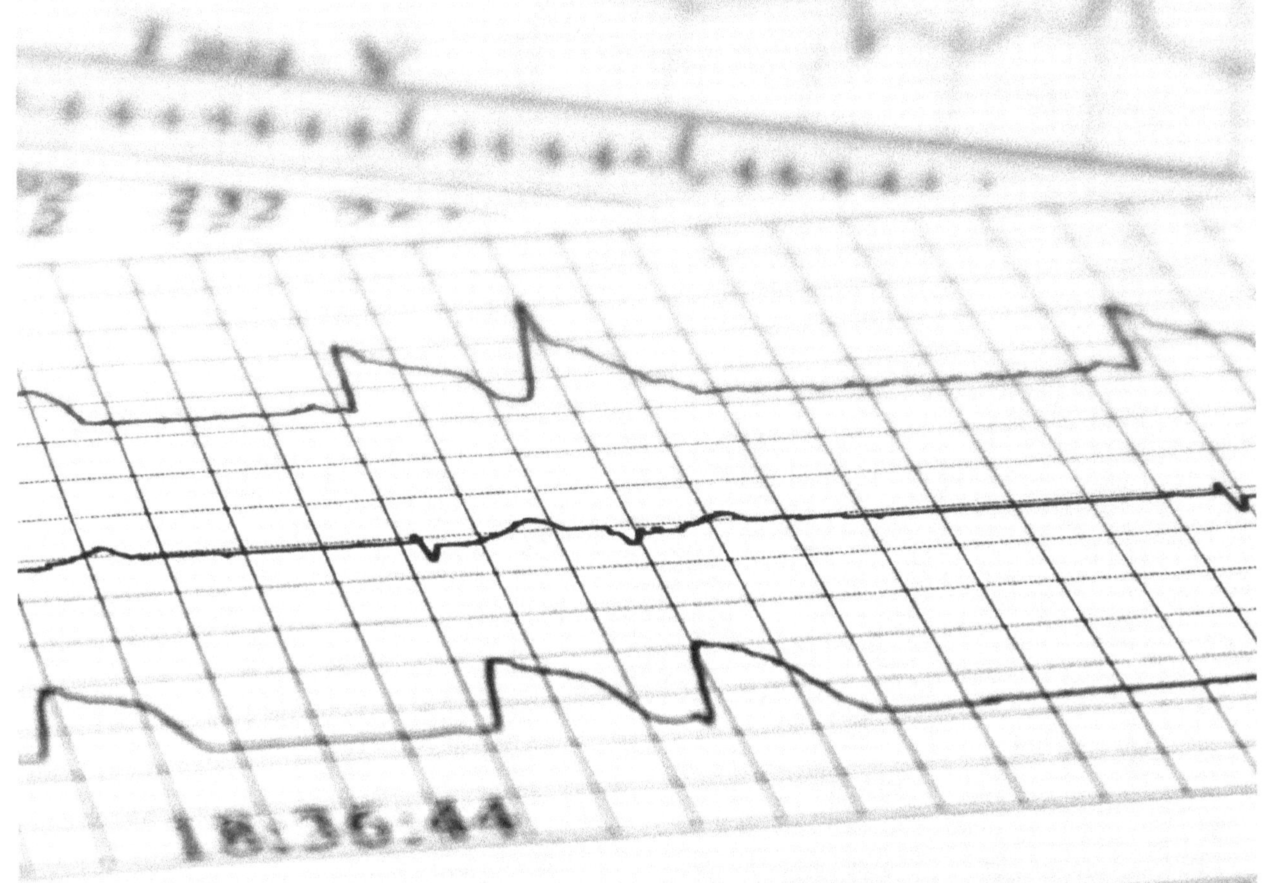

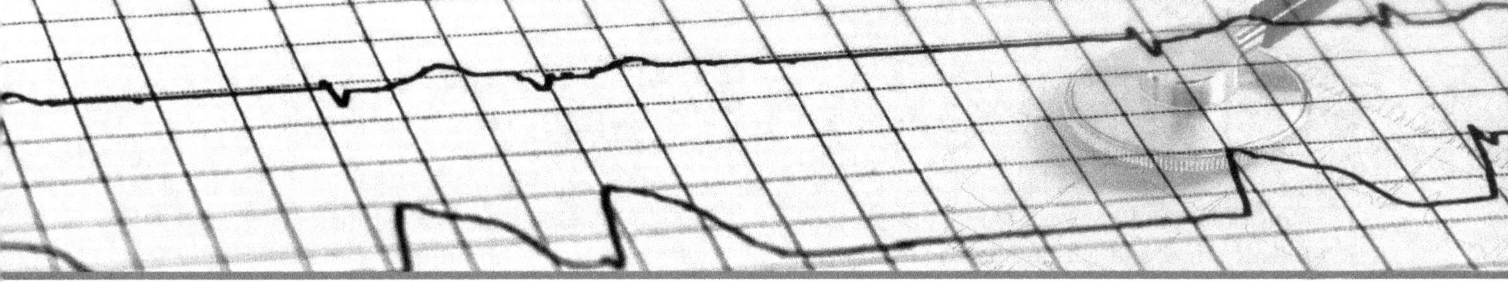

CHAPTER 1

Concepts of Cardiovascular Function

The cardiovascular system experiences the largest disruptions to homeostasis during exercise of any other organ system besides the pulmonary system.

CONTENT OUTLINE

- Cardiac Electrical Activity
- Cardiac Cycle
- Cardiac Output
- Heart Rate
- Stroke Volume
- Vascular Function
- Myocardial Oxygen Consumption
- Chapter Questions

The heart weighs about 300 g and consists of four hollow chambers that function as pumps and four valves that maintain unidirectional blood flow. As shown in Figure 1.1, the orientation of the anatomy creates both side-to-side (right and left pumps, each with its own circuit) and top-to-bottom (top pumps act as primers for the lower, main pumps) pumping function. As shown, this arrangement dictates a dual pumping action through circuits that, while continuous, are, nevertheless, functionally separate. The right pump transports blood through the pulmonary artery to the lungs (pulmonary circuit), whereas the left pump transports blood through the systemic arteries to the rest of the body (systemic circuit). Each side is composed of an upper atrium and a lower ventricle. The right atrium receives blood from the systemic veins, and the right ventricle pumps blood to the lungs for oxygenation. The left atrium receives oxygenated blood from the lungs, through the pulmonary veins and the left ventricle pumps blood out to the systemic arteries.

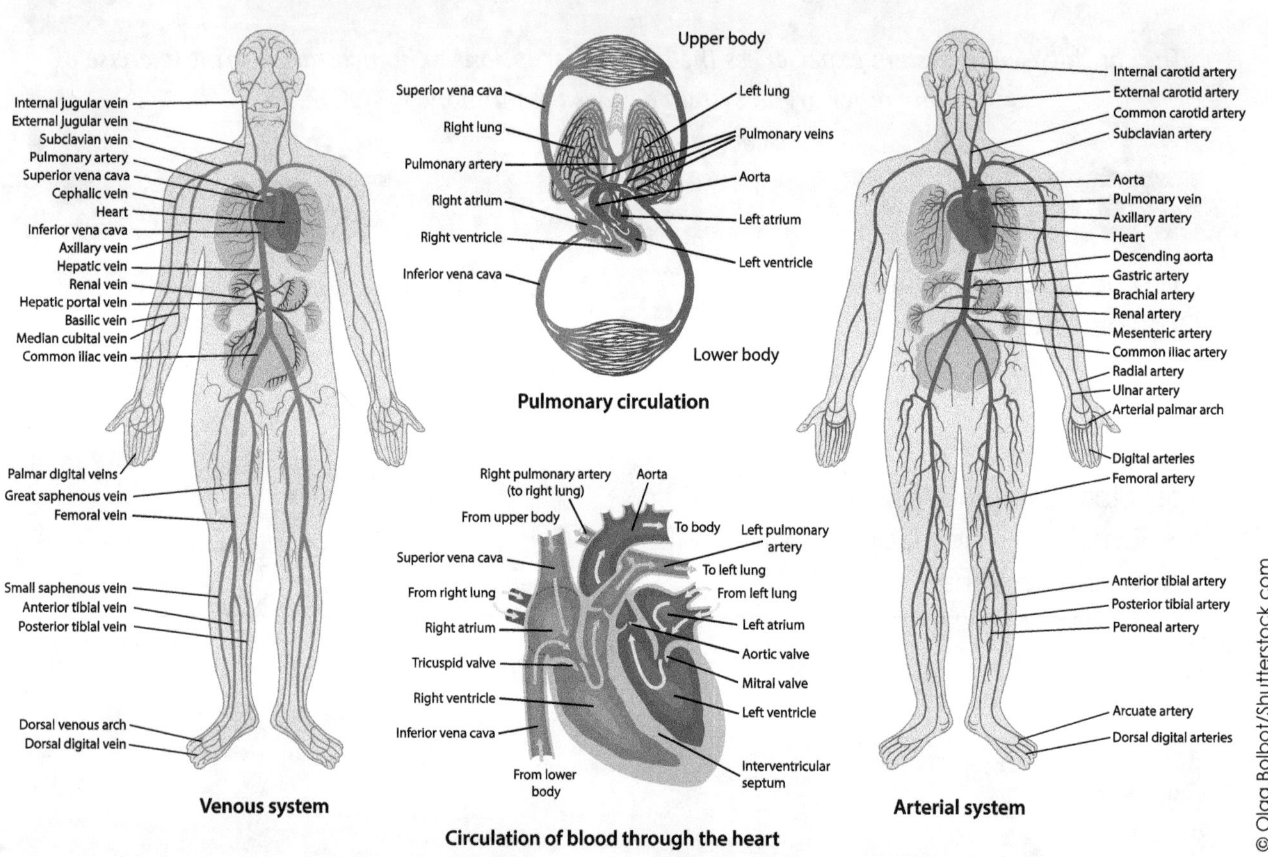

FIGURE 1.1 Diagram of the circulatory system. The right side (blue) of the heart is the pulmonary circuit, and the left side (red) of the heart is the systemic circuit.

Atria are low-pressure, thin-walled chambers that primarily serve as reservoirs to receive and store blood during ventricular contraction. Approximately 70% of the blood in the atria passively enters the ventricles before atrial contraction forces the remaining blood (30%) into the ventricles. Soon thereafter, the ventricles contract, forcing blood into the systemic and pulmonary arteries. Ventricular walls are thicker than atrial walls, whereas the left ventricular walls are thicker than those of the right ventricle. The larger muscle mass of the left ventricle is necessary to move blood against the higher pressures of the systemic arterial tree (i.e., overcome higher **afterload** forces).

Two sets of valves exist within the heart: the **atrioventricular (AV) valves** and the **semilunar valves**. These one-way valves help ensure unidirectional blood flow. The AV valves are located between each atrium and ventricle, on the right the *tricuspid* and on the left the *mitral* (bicuspid). The cusps of the valves are larger than their valvular openings, causing them to overlap in the closed position. Attached to the free edges of the valve cusps are tendinous cords, called **chordae tendinae**, arising from **papillary muscles** that protrude into the chamber from each ventricular wall. Subsequent to AV valve closure, ventricular contraction begins and concurrently stimulates papillary muscle contraction, causing the chordae tendinae to become taut, thereby pulling down on the cusps of the AV valves and preventing eversion of the valves (opening of the valves upward into the atria) during ventricular **systole**. In certain disease processes, these valves can be damaged, allowing blood to flow from the ventricle to the atrium. When this happens on the left side, the resulting condition is **mitral regurgitation**. Case Study 1.1 explains the unique hemodynamic responses of a patient with mitral regurgitation.

CASE STUDY 1.1: MITRAL VALVE REGURGITATION

Jan is a 42-year-old woman who was seen for complaints of chest pain and lightheadedness. She described her chest pain as sharp sensations in the left upper chest lasting several seconds but did not involve shortness of breath, diaphoresis, or nausea and was not associated with exertion. Jan has a history of palpitations and was diagnosed previously with premature ventricular contractions. Jan also notes isolated extra beats of her heart but has not had any syncope events. Jan has smoked 2 packs of cigarettes per day for 24 years and drinks alcohol occasionally. She is not on any medications and denies a history of hypertension, myocardial infarction, rheumatic heart disease, diabetes mellitus, elevated cholesterol, and allergies. Her family history is unremarkable. Her electrocardiogram (ECG) evaluation was normal, but the echocardiogram revealed the following: left ventricular size at upper limits of normal with normal left ventricular wall motion; normal left ventricular ejection fraction; moderate systolic superior displacement of anterior mitral valve leaflet is evident and in the presence of minimal mitral regurgitation may represent moderate mitral valve prolapse; normal trileaflet aortic valve was visualized with good opening and a normal left atrial size. An examination using pulsed doppler with color flow imaging confirmed the presence of mild to moderate mitral valve regurgitation.

Description

Mitral valve regurgitation (valvular insufficiency) is the result of either congenital or acquired disorders affecting the mitral valve. With mitral valve regurgitation, the mitral valve leaflets do not close properly during ejection of the blood from the left ventricle into the aorta. As a result, when the left ventricle contracts, blood is ejected through the aortic valve but is also regurgitated through the mitral valve to the left atrium. One common cause of mitral valve regurgitation is rheumatic fever. Other causes include systemic lupus erythematosus, infectious endocarditis, and age-related degenerative changes to the mitral valve. Patients in the early stages of mitral insufficiency may not have any symptoms and may have a normal exercise capacity. Progression of the problem may result in symptoms such as fatigue, shortness of breath, fluid retention, and cardiac arrhythmias. The most common arrhythmia seen in these patients is atrial fibrillation. In later stages, exercise capacity may be reduced because of reduced maximal cardiac output.

Intervention

Mitral regurgitation is generally treated surgically; however, physical therapists or exercise physiologists may see patients who are being medically managed. With surgical intervention, a prosthetic valve is used to replace the defective mitral valve. Following surgery, these patients usually progress well with recovery.

The most common reasons to provide medical management of mitral regurgitation instead of surgical management are either that the defect is not very severe or the patient does not want or cannot have surgery. Regarding the medical management of patients with mitral regurgitation, the primary goal of therapy is to optimize the extraction of O_2 by the working muscles. This goal can be accomplished by judicious exercise prescription that improves O_2 delivery to the tissues but that does not exacerbate cardiac symptoms. During exercise, it is important to closely monitor these patients for signs of dyspnea, fatigue, dizziness, coughing, or lightheadedness. ECG use during exercise will be helpful in monitoring the dynamic stability of these patients. Should patients exhibit untoward signs or symptoms, they should be referred back to their physicians for further examination. Examples of exercises that may be helpful in patients with mitral regurgitation include aerobic activities using large muscle groups, strengthening exercises, relaxation, and energy conservation techniques. To complement the exercise program, these patients should also be educated in smoking cessation, cardiac risk factors, dietary modifications, stress management, disease progression, and the ability to recognize physical signs of overexertion.

The semilunar valves consist of the pulmonary valve separating the pulmonary artery from the right ventricle and the aortic valve separating the aorta from the left ventricle. Each of these valves has cuplike cusps attached to its valve rings. The semilunar valves are thicker than the AV valves because they are exposed to greater mechanical abrasion forces.

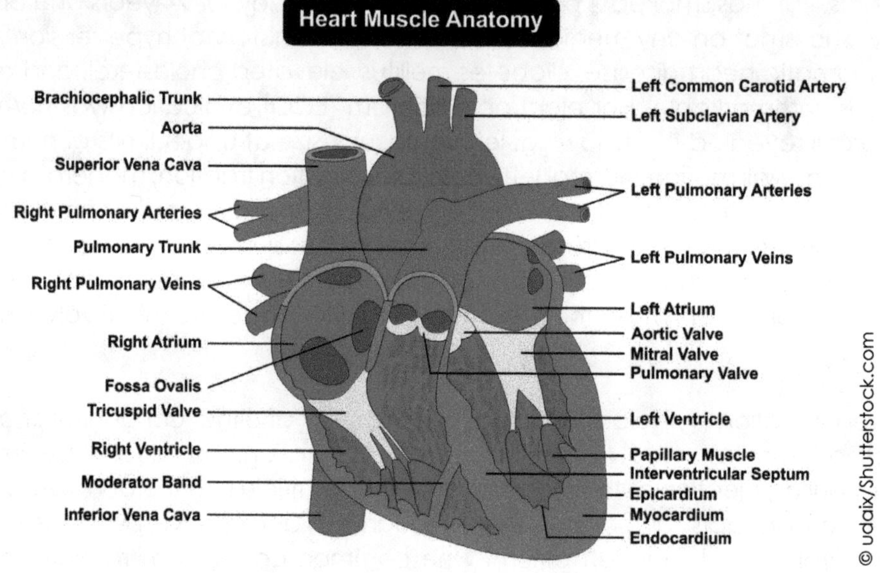

FIGURE 1.2 Frontal section of the heart showing interior chambers, structures, and valves.

The wall of the heart is composed of three layers. The outermost layer is a thin connective layer, known as the **epicardium**; the thick, middle, muscular layer is the **myocardium**, whereas the innermost layer consists of thin endothelial cells, called the **endocardium** (Fig. 1.2). The endocardium makes contact with the blood in the chambers and is watertight, preventing blood in the chambers from leaking through to the other layers. However, the myocardium is the focal point because it is responsible for contracting and creating a driving force (pressure) to eject blood from the ventricles. **Intercalated discs** link individual muscle fibers to one another so that when the heart is electrically stimulated, the impulse quickly spreads throughout the myocardial **syncytium** (Fig. 1.3). The intercalated discs contain **gap junctions** that allow a wave of **depolarization** to pass very quickly from one cell to another, allowing all of the cardiac muscle in the atrial syncytium or ventricular syncytium to contract synchronously.

The heart is a highly vascularized organ, receiving its blood supply via the right and left main coronary arteries, which originate from the base of the aorta and wrap around the heart to ensure blood flow to all areas of the myocardium. The coronary veins lie adjacent to the coronary arteries and drain blood into the right atrium via the coronary sinus (the major venous blood-collecting vessel of the coronary circulation) on the posterior aspect of the right atrium. The left and right main coronary arteries branch extensively to supply blood to the entire myocardium (Fig. 1.4). Article 1.1 contains a discussion of the coronary circulation and myocardial O_2 demand during exercise.

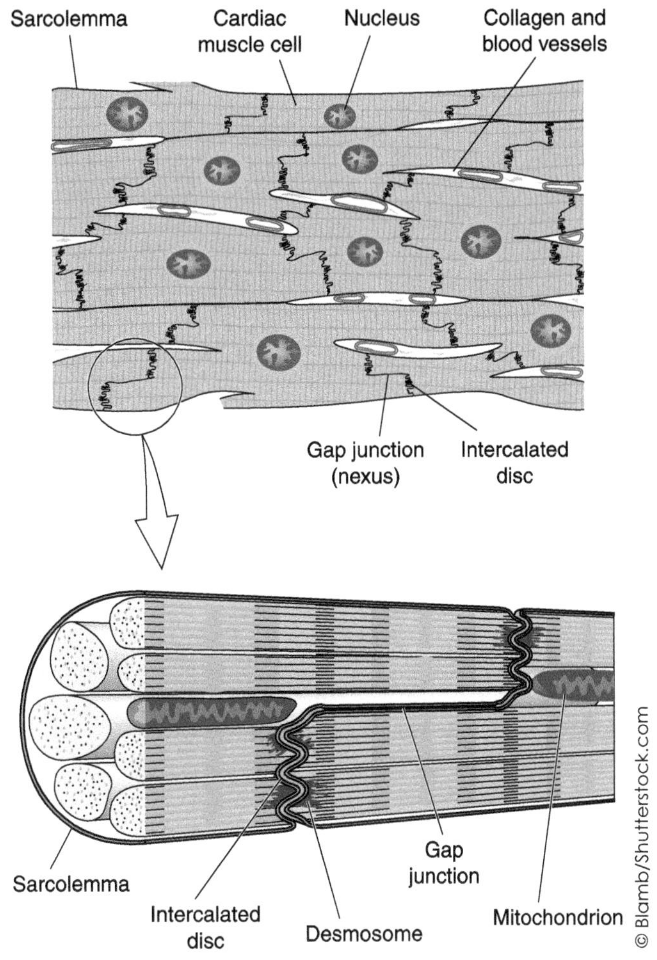

FIGURE 1.3 Schematic of myocardial fiber.

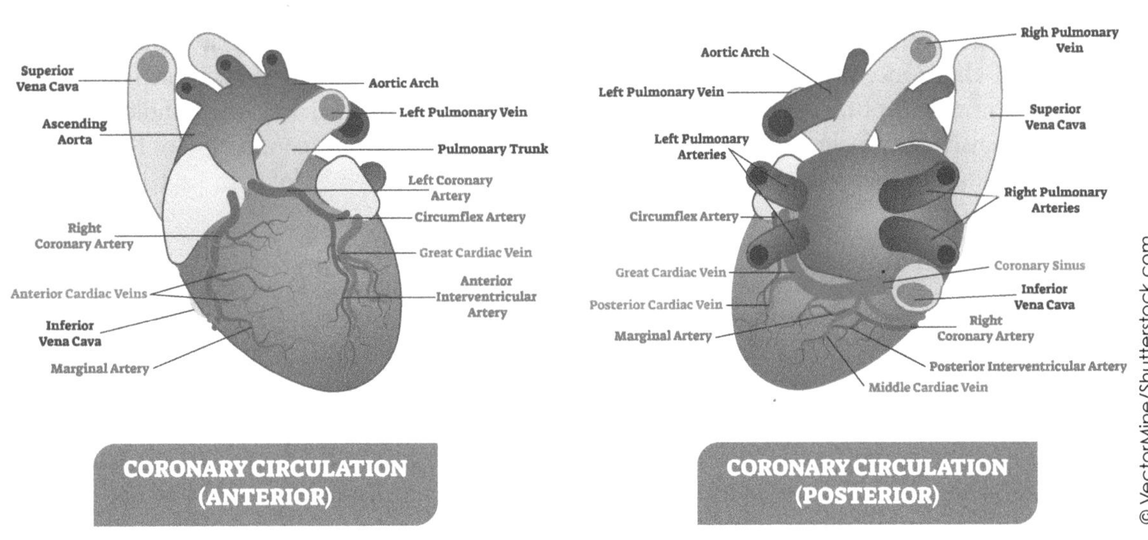

FIGURE 1.4 Cardiac arteries and veins. Left (anterior view). Right (posterior view).

ARTICLE 1.1: CORONARY CIRCULATION AND MYOCARDIAL O_2 DEMAND

The right coronary artery (RCA) is the principal supplier of blood to the right ventricle and atrium, whereas the left coronary artery (LCA) is the principal supplier of blood to the left ventricle and atrium. Although this arrangement, termed *coronary flow dominance*, is generally true, there is some overlap. For instance, the RCA in humans is dominant in 50% of individuals, the LCA is dominant in another 20%, and the remaining 30% of individuals receive an equal supply from both main arteries. An individual difference in blood flow dominance is the reason why some individuals with blockages in the RCA have left ventricular infarctions and others have right ventricular infarctions.

Regardless of the pattern of flow dominance, the heart requires a large O_2 supply per minute. Under resting condition, myocardial oxygen consumption ($M\dot{V}O_2$) equals about 10 $mL \cdot min^{-1} \cdot 100\ g^{-1}$ of the myocardium. In order not to exceed the normal coronary blood flow rate of about 80 $mL \cdot min^{-1} \cdot 100\ g^{-1}$ of myocardium, the heart must extract about 70% of the O_2 carried by the coronary blood supply. This resting level of O_2 extraction by the myocardium is equal to the maximal amount of O_2 extracted by skeletal muscle under heavy exercise. This means that during exercise, when the heart has an increased demand for O_2, the supply is met through increased blood flow to the heart and not by increased extraction. This also means that there is a direct relationship between coronary blood flow and $M\dot{V}O_2$. During maximal exercise, the myocardium requires as much as 50 mL O_2 per 100 g of myocardium. Flow must increase to about 350 $mL \cdot min^{-1} \cdot 100\ g^{-1}$ of tissue to deliver this much O_2.

Cardiac Electrical Activity

Some myocardial fibers are specialized conductive fibers (pacemaker fibers) that can spontaneously generate cardiac electrical activity (**automaticity**). These cardiac fibers have little contractile ability and exhibit varying conduction speeds. In the extreme upper and posterior portion of the right atrium, cells of the sinoatrial (SA) node normally control the overall rate of cardiac depolarization (Fig. 1.5). The SA node has the fastest depolarization rate (approximately 60–80 times every minute) and is referred to as the cardiac pacemaker. All other conductive cells of the heart can potentially serve as the cardiac pacemaker, but because their intrinsic rates are slower, they do not normally fulfill this role.

Once the SA node depolarizes, the electrical activity spreads across both atria and to the atrioventricular node (AV node). Here, the impulse is delayed approximately 0.13 seconds to provide time for atrial contraction to pump the remaining blood (~30%) into the ventricles and for AV valve closure. The impulse then travels to the AV bundle (**bundle of His**). Once the impulse reaches the AV bundle, it rapidly spreads down each bundle branch, which continue down the septum towards the apex and then through the ventricles. The bundle branches then subdivide into extensively branching Purkinje fibers. The organization and fast conduction of these specialized conductive fibers allow for the near simultaneous depolarization and contraction of both ventricles.

The heart's electrical activity is measured by surface electrodes that can then be traced on the electrocardiogram (ECG) or by direct application of electrodes into cardiac tissue that trace the cardiac **action potential** (AP) (Fig. 1.6). At rest, excitable cardiac cells are polarized, with a negatively charged inside and positively charged outside. This charge difference across the membrane is created and maintained by the movements of sodium (Na^+) and potassium (K^+) ions across the cell membrane through both diffusion and active transport mechanisms, similar to other excitable tissues. Table 1.1 displays important concentration gradients inside and outside the cardiomyocytes.

The resting membrane potential (RMP) of nonpacemaker cardiac muscle fibers (i.e., typical contractile fibers) is approximately –90 mV (phase 4). With depolarization (phase 0), a reversal potential occurs, bringing the cell to about +20 mV at the peak of depolarization owing to the opening of Na^+ channels, producing a rapid influx of Na^+ ions. As **repolarization** begins, Na^+ channels close, whereas K^+ channels open. The result is a brief

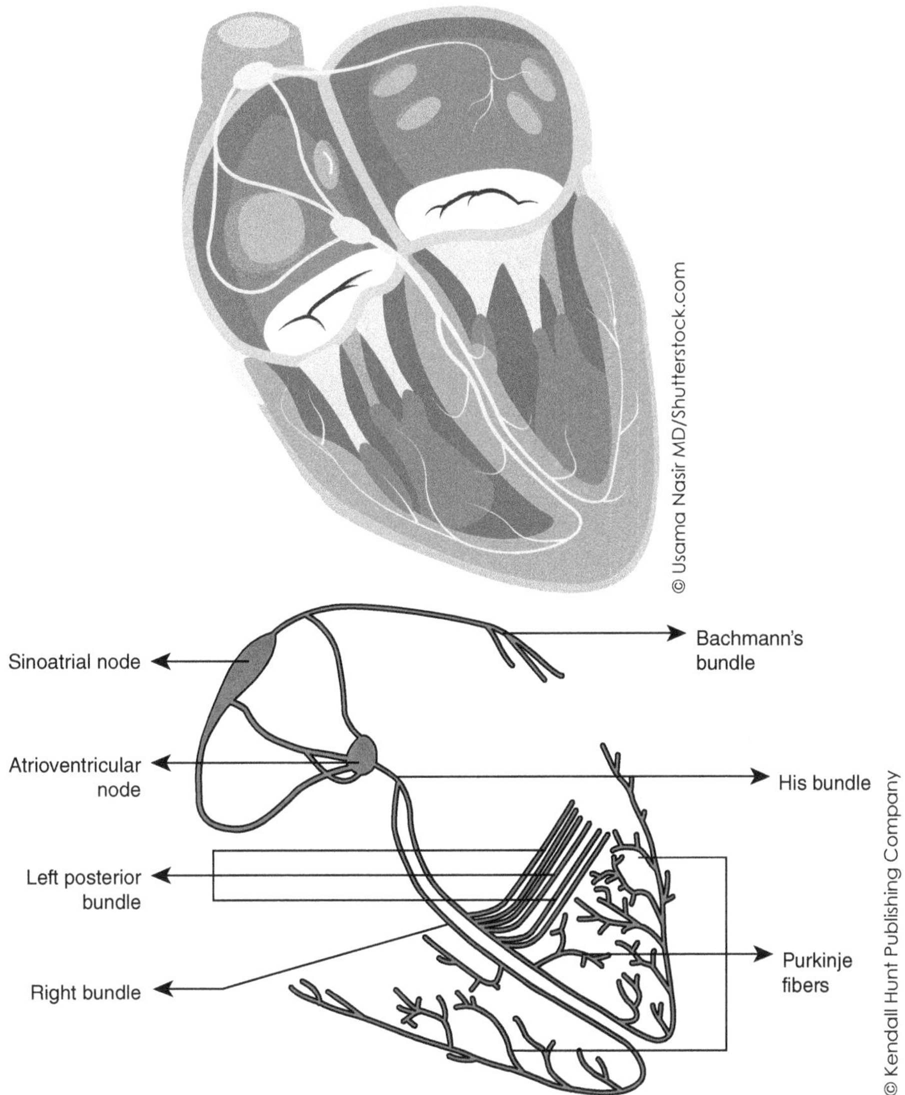

FIGURE 1.5 The intrinsic electrical conduction pathway of the heart showing the SA and AV nodes and the internodal pathways. The smaller image shows the heart's electrical conduction pathways separated from the myocardium.

K^+ efflux, often called the "notch" (phase 1). Subsequently, L Type Calcium (Ca^{++}) channels open, concurrently decreasing K^+ membrane permeability. While the L Type Ca^{++} channels are open, simultaneous influx of Ca^{++} and efflux of K^+ produce the "plateau" phase (phase 2). As Ca^{++} channels close, K^+ permeability again increases and repolarization (phase 3) resumes, returning the action potential to the RMP.

For specialized conductive fibers (pacemaker fibers), **autorhythmicity** occurs because the cell membranes of these fibers are primarily "leaky" to Na^+ ions. Increased negativity at the end of one AP instigates the opening of Na^+ channels. Na^+ "leaks" in until a **threshold potential** (TP) is reached. Thus, pacemaker fibers exhibit a slowly rising phase 4 from a level of about −70 mV (compared with −90 mV for nonpacemaker fibers) to a TP of about −55 mV, which triggers the start of depolarization (Fig. 1.6). Once the TP is reached, Ca^{++} channels open to create a Ca^{++} influx and depolarization (phase 0), as opposed to Na^+ channel opening in nonpacemaker cells. At the peak of depolarization, Ca^{++} channels will close, whereas K^+ channels open, leading to repolarization (phase 3). Note that pacemaker fibers do not exhibit phases 1 or 2 seen in nonpacemaker cells.

If the SA node becomes diseased and fails, the AV node can step in to fulfill the role as cardiac pacemaker at a rate of about 40 to 60 depolarizations per minute. *If an individual presented to you with this rate, on viewing the ECG, would you be able to tell whether this slow rate was a result of exercise training or the result of their heart being paced by the AV node?* The answer rests partly (perhaps largely) in the appearance of the ECG.

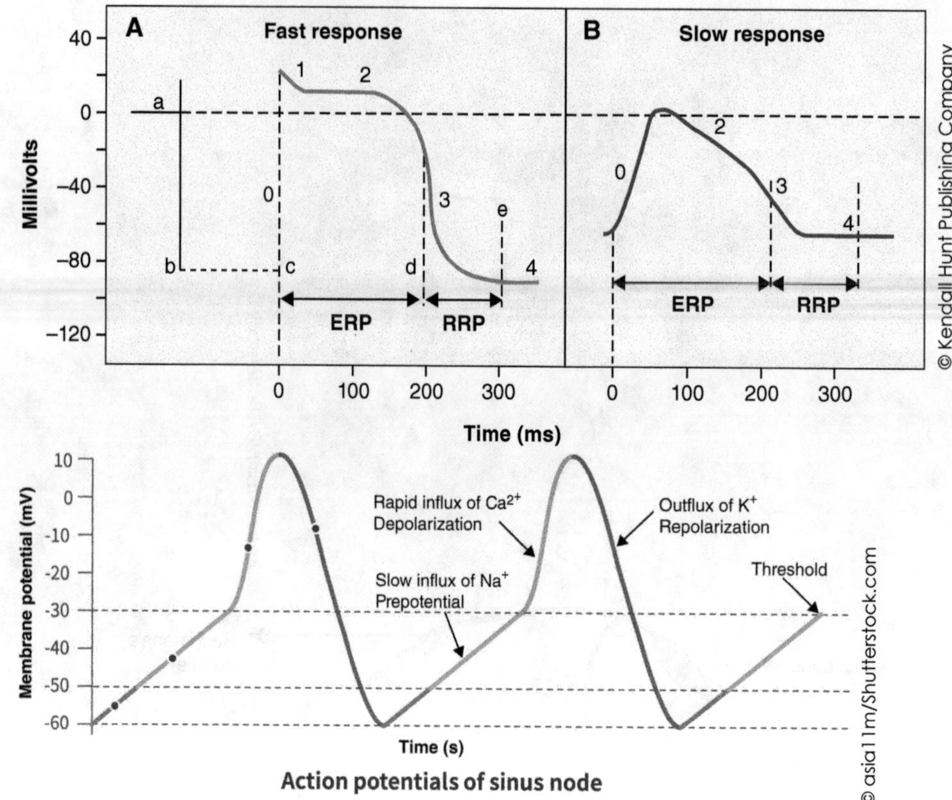

FIGURE 1.6 Cardiac action potentials are shown in **A** (fast response cells) as contrasted with **B** (slow response cells). The ERP is the effective refractory period and the RRP is the relative refractory period. The bottom illustration shows two consecutive SA node (pacemaker) potentials detailing the main ion movements at each phase. The action potentials from slow response cardiac tissue have a resting potential less negative (~55 mV), a phase 0 upstroke that is less steep, a smaller amplitude, the absence of a phase 1, and a phase 2 plateau that is less evident.

TABLE 1.1 Ion Concentrations Inside and Outside Cardiac Muscle Cells

Ion	*Extracellular Concentrations (mM)*	*Intracellular Concentrations (mM)*
Na^+	145.0	10.0
K^+	4.0	135.0
Cl^-	140.0	30.0
Ca^{++}	2.0	0.0001

Ventricular conductive fibers, such as Purkinje fibers, can also serve as cardiac pacemakers, usually producing a cardiac rate of 20 to 40 beats·min^{-1}.

Cardiac electrical activity is measured by electrodes placed at specific sites on the surface of the body. This process is called **electrocardiography**, a technique that has proven to be a very important clinical tool. Physicians use the ECG to diagnose heart abnormalities, such as electrical disturbances, to determine how well the heart is receiving its own blood supply and to assess tissue damage associated with heart attacks. The exercise physiologist can use the ECG to monitor heart rate (HR), rhythm, and ischemic responses while a patient is exercising.

For myocardial cells to contract (mechanical activity), they must first depolarize (electrical activity). Therefore, the electrical impulses captured on the ECG occur prior to the mechanical events of the heart. The different parts of the ECG waveform represent specific electrical events in the heart (Fig. 1.7). The P wave occurs prior to atrial contraction and results from the spread of depolarization throughout the atria (atrial depolarization). The QRS complex follows the P wave and represents depolarization of the ventricles. Because atrial mass is smaller in relation to that of the ventricles, the electrical activity associated with atrial repolarization is obscured by the QRS complex. The T wave represents repolarization of the ventricles. There is a **refractory** period following the depolarization of different areas of the heart. During this period, any stimulation of the heart will result in a less forceful contraction or no contraction at all. The effective refractory period (ERP) for cardiac contractile muscle lasts approximately 200 ms, and the relative refractory period (RRP) lasts between 50-100 ms, for a total of about 250-300 ms (Fig. 1.6 A & B). This extended period is critical, since the heart muscle must contract to pump blood effectively and contractions must follow the electrical events. Without extended electrical refractory periods, premature contractions would occur in the heart and would not be compatible with life.

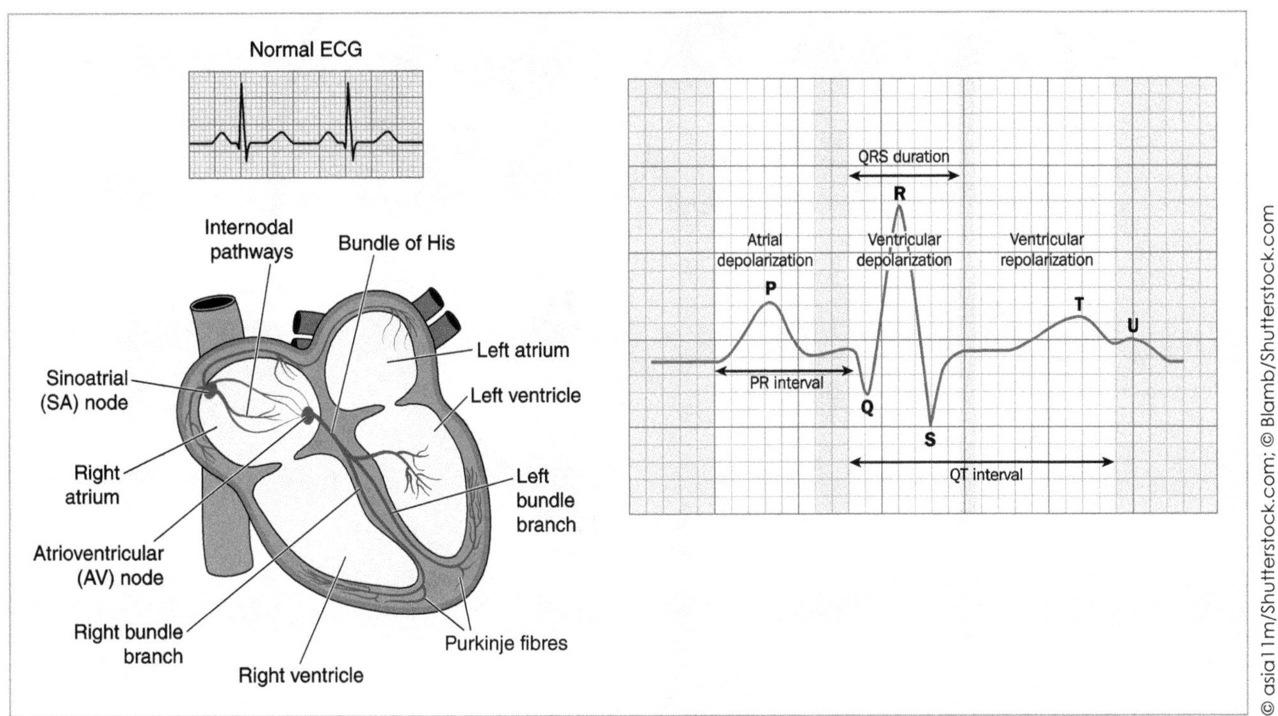

FIGURE 1.7 Conduction system of the heart and its relationship to the electrocardiogram.

The ECG describes each **cardiac cycle** as a cluster of three distinct waveforms: P, QRS, and T wave. For the heart that is beating rhythmically, these three waveforms appear together and are easily discernible as one cardiac cycle. Electrical and cardiac blood flow pathology may upset the appearance of the ECG, allowing the ECG to become a valuable tool in the diagnosis of cardiac problems. Therapists should be familiar enough with electrocardiography to correctly recognize ECG waveforms during their patients' monitored exercise therapy. In this way, the exercise session may be discontinued if abnormalities are noted.

Cardiac Cycle

The cardiac cycle comprises the electrical, mechanical, and audio events that repeat in cyclic fashion many times each minute. Cardiac mechanical events refer to the changes in pressure and volume that ensue in response to myocardial contraction. Mechanical events also encompass the operation of the cardiac valves, which open and close owing to pressure differentials between the two sides of the valves, which are a result of changes in cardiac contraction and blood flow. The cyclic functioning of the cardiac valves produces the major heart sounds detected during each cardiac cycle. In normal function, cardiac mechanical events follow electrical stimulation of the heart.

The cardiac cycle is divided into two phases (Fig. 1.8). The active phase of systole occurs immediately after cardiac depolarization, and the passive phase of **diastole** begins with cardiac repolarization. These mechanical, electrical, and audio events are shown in Figure 1.9.

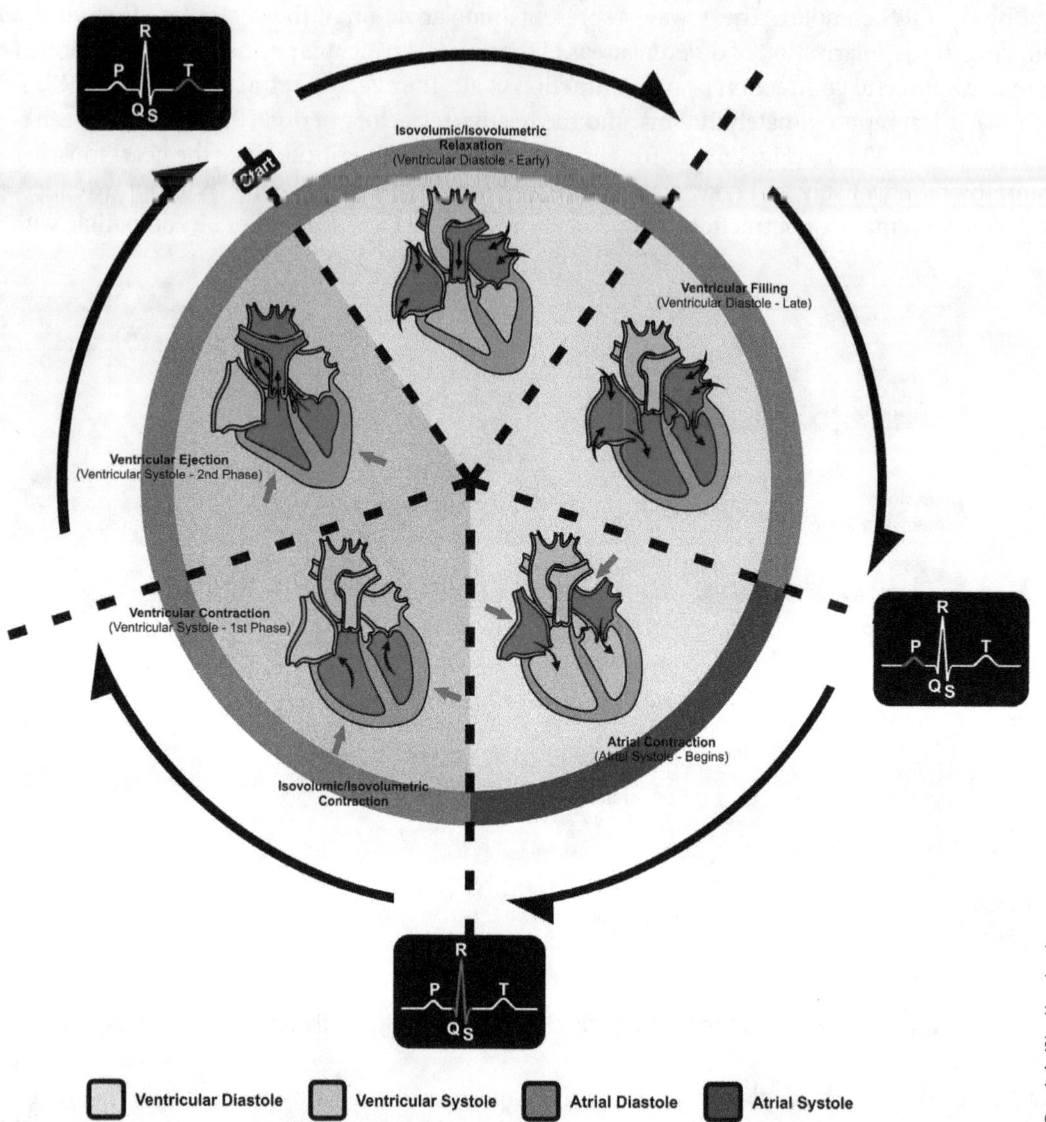

FIGURE 1.8 The cardiac cycle.

Ventricular Diastole

When the heart is in diastole, the ventricles are relaxed and fill with blood. During diastole most of the blood (70%) flows passively from the atria to the ventricles through open AV valves. At the end of the diastolic period, aortic pressure attains the diastolic blood pressure (DBP, approximately 80 mmHg), the lowest point recorded on the aortic pressure curve (shown on Figure 1.9 at the point coinciding with the opening of the aortic valve).

Diastole begins as systole ends and is marked by the closure of the semilunar valves. When the aortic valve closes, a dicrotic notch, called the incisura, is produced on the aortic pressure curve. This is shown as a small spike in pressure in Figure 1.9 (aortic pressure curve). The closure of the semilunar valves produces the second heart sound (phonocardiogram in Fig. 1.9). The beginning of ventricular diastole starts with a phenomenon called **isovolumic relaxation**, measured as the time period between closure of the semilunar valves (pulmonary and aortic) and opening of the AV valves (tricuspid and mitral). Because both sets of valves are closed at this time, isovolumic relaxation is characterized as a rapid drop in ventricular pressure without a change in ventricular volume. Note the stable volume curve during this time period (ventricular volume curve in Fig. 1.9). Isovolumic relaxation ends when the AV valves open, at which point blood begins to enter the ventricles during a period called rapid ventricular filling. These events generate the third heart sound.

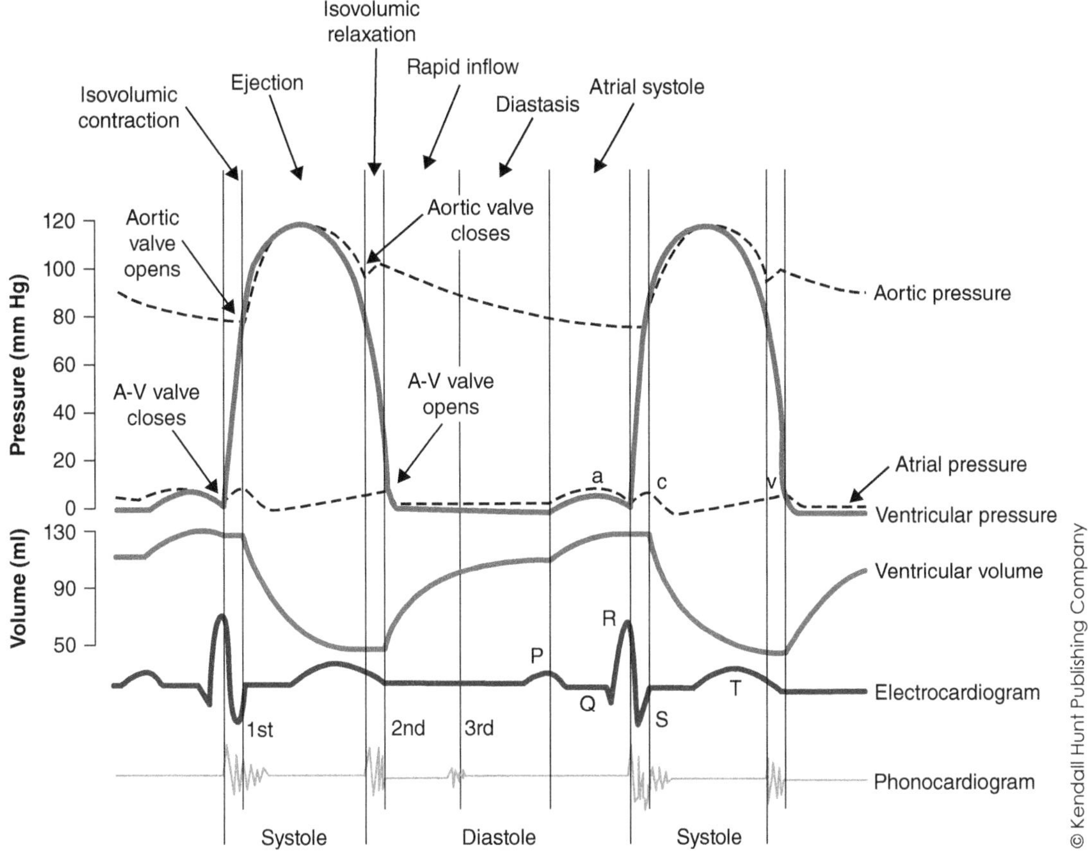

FIGURE 1.9 Left atrial, aortic, and left ventricular pressure pulses correlated in time with ventricular volume, heart sounds, and the electrocardiogram for two complete cardiac cycles.

A slow ventricular filling phase, called **diastasis**, signals the coming end of diastole. This small, slow addition to ventricular filling is indicated by a gradual rise in atrial, ventricular, and venous pressures (venous pressure curve not included), and in ventricular volume. Toward the end of this passive flow of blood, the atria depolarize (P wave on the ECG) and then contract (atrial systole), forcing blood remaining in the atria into the ventricles. This completes the period of ventricular filling. The extra amount of blood (~30%) provided to the ventricles by atrial contraction is referred to as the atrial "kick."

As the amount of blood in the ventricles increases over time during diastole, intraventricular pressure gradually increases because of the increase in ventricular volume. Because there are no valves at the opening of the venae cavae and the right atrium or at the junctions of the pulmonary veins and the left atrium, atrial contraction can force blood in both directions. However, because there is inertia generated by the flow of blood into the atria, little blood is pumped back into the venous tributaries during the brief and not very powerful atrial contraction.

Ventricular Systole

During systole, the ventricles contract and eject blood into the pulmonary and systemic circuits, producing the systolic blood pressure, shown as the high point on the aorta pressure curve in Figure 1.9. Right ventricular and pulmonary artery pressures (not shown) are much lower (about 1/6 less) than the corresponding pressures on the left side. The onset of ventricular contraction coincides with the peak of the R wave of the ECG (Fig. 1.9) and the initial vibration of the first heart sound. At this time, the venous pulse curve (jugular vein pressure not shown) closely follows the atrial pressure curve (Fig. 1.9). The "a" wave is caused by atrial contraction, which immediately precedes ventricular contraction. The "c" wave is caused by transmission of a pressure wave produced by the abrupt closure of the tricuspid valve (right heart) in early ventricular systole. The "v" wave is caused by the pressure of blood returning from the peripheral vessels and the abrupt opening of the tricuspid valve.

Ventricular contraction commences immediately after atrial contraction. As ventricular pressures continue to rise with the onset of ventricular contraction, the pressure differential between the atria and ventricles favors ventricular pressure, resulting in the abrupt closure of the AV valves, preventing the backflow of blood into the atria at the start of ventricular systole. **Isovolumetric contraction** occurs between the onset of ventricular contraction and prior to the opening of the aortic and pulmonary valves. Although isovolumetric contraction lasts less than 0.1 second, it is critically important in order to effectively build the driving pressure for the CV system. Notice that when the ventricle begins to contract, the QRS complex has occurred, the mitral valve is closed, and ventricular pressure begins a sharp rise (Fig. 1.9). Prior to opening of the aortic and pulmonary valves, and while the mitral and tricuspid valves are still closed, the ventricles have all the blood they will receive for that cardiac cycle. In this example, the ventricle has about 130 mL (ventricular volume curve). During this time period, the **end-diastolic volume** (EDV) of the ventricles can be measured.

When ventricular pressures exceed arterial pressures, the aortic and pulmonary semilunar valves open, expelling blood into the aorta and pulmonary artery very quickly and with high pressure. This period is called rapid ventricular ejection. After the blood is expelled into the aorta and pulmonary artery, the pressure in the ventricles begins to fall and eventually falls below the pressure of the arterial system. At this point, the aortic and pulmonary valves close, and the ventricles are in the isovolumetric relaxation phase of the cardiac cycle. This is the beginning of diastole. At this time, the blood remaining in the ventricle after ejection can be determined as the **end-systolic volume** (ESV), as shown (approximately 50 mL). *Try identifying EDV and ESV on the ventricular volume curve in Figure 1.9 and produce an equation that demonstrates the amount of blood ejected with each beat.*

The pressure in the ventricles continues to fall until ventricular pressure is below atrial pressure. At this point, the mitral and triscuspid valves open, and filling of the ventricles occurs. It is also during diastole that the myocardium receives its own blood supply, as the coronary arteries, unlike other arteries, do not fill during the systolic phase because the openings of the coronary main arteries are covered by the cusps of the aortic semilunar valve. Rather, the left and right main coronary arteries fill during diastole as blood backflows in the proximal aorta, which also allows for better perfusion of the heart to occur while the myocardium is relaxing.

Be aware that during the preceding discussion, reference was made to both right and left hearts. While only the left heart is represented in Figure 1.9, the same pressure curves would apply to the right heart, the only difference being that the right heart curves are of much smaller magnitude. *Why do you suppose this is so?*

As mentioned earlier, systole produces the systolic blood pressure, which is the peak force (pressure) exerted on the wall of the vessel by the blood during systole. This force is caused by the contracting ventricle. However, as the ventricle relaxes, some pressure (force) is still maintained in the vascular system. This pressure, the DBP, is caused by the same elastic recoil of the arterial tree that was responsible for maintaining the forward kinetic motion of blood during cardiac relaxation.

Veins are low-pressure tubes with the ability to constrict and dilate. At the end of the capillary bed, a driving force of about 7 mmHg is available to move blood back to the right heart. Low pressure in the veins occurs because the pressure drops across the systemic circulation as resistance to blood flow occurs. As blood leaves the aorta and flows into the arteries, the resting pressure is between 80 and 120 mmHg. As blood flows through the smaller arterioles, capillaries and veins, the pressure continues to drop until it is very low by the time the blood reaches the veins. Furthermore, during the resting state, the venous system contains about 70% of the total blood volume. Veins, therefore, function as **capacitance vessels** because of the large volume of blood they contain. The ability of veins to serve as storage vessels relates to the high degree of **compliance** inherent in them. Venous compliance is about 20 times greater than arterial compliance. The volume of the venous reservoir changes with postural shifts. For instance, in the supine position more blood is put in the heart, and **stroke volume** increases accordingly. Therefore, blood in the capacitance vessels dictates the size of the ventricular EDV, which in turn dictates SV (mechanism explained further on). When upright, the opposite occurs. Constriction of veins increases the driving force for returning blood to the heart.

During exercise, blood is diverted from the venous storage reservoir and transferred to the arterial system to sustain exercise metabolism. Several mechanisms explain how blood returns to the right atrium against gravity. The veins contain small flaps or valves that keep the blood moving forward, barring pooling of blood in the veins of the lower extremities (Fig. 1.10). The other mechanism that assists the flow of blood back to the heart is the skeletal muscle pump. Skeletal muscle contraction compresses the veins, propelling blood toward the heart. Without these two mechanisms, blood would pool more readily in the lower extremities.

When a person exercises, the flow of blood must be redistributed away from less active tissues to the working muscles. Figure 1.11 demonstrates flow redistribution as a percentage of the **cardiac output** ($\dot{Q}$) under the resting condition and three levels of exercise. This redistribution allows for transport of O_2 and other nutrients to and

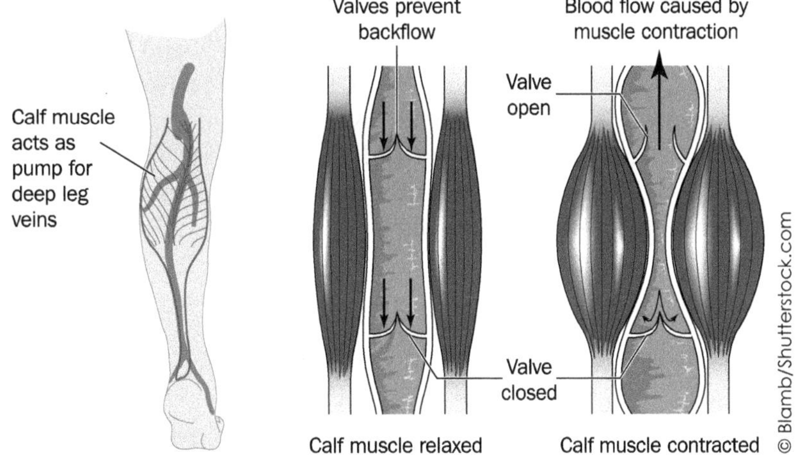

FIGURE 1.10 Action of the muscle pump in venous return from the legs. At rest, the venous valves are open, and blood flows upward toward the heart by virtue of the pressure generated by the heart and transmitted through the capillaries to the veins from the arterial side of the circulation. In exercise, muscle contraction compresses the vein, thus increasing local pressure and driving the blood toward the heart through the upper valve and closing the lower valve in the uncompressed segment of the vein. When the muscle relaxes again, pressure in the previously compressed segment of the vein falls, which causes the upper valve to close and the lower valve to open.

removal of waste products from the muscles as muscle metabolism increases. Notice that as $\dot{Q}$ increases from light to maximal exercise, blood flow to muscle progressively increases, whereas blood flow to most other tissues progressively decreases. Skin is the exception during light and heavy exercise because skin blood flow is greater at these times than at rest in order to facilitate dissipation of heat. However, as exercise intensity increases to the maximum, skin blood flow is greatly reduced to direct the necessary blood to the muscles. The heart is also an exception. As a percentage of the available $\dot{Q}$, cardiac blood flow is maintained, but an equal percentage of a larger pie means that absolute flow has increased. This is the case in cardiac blood flow during exercise as myocardial workload increases.

PHYSIOLOGIC STATE ($\dot{Q}$ L·min^{-1})	DIGESTIVE TRACT (%)	HEART (%)	KIDNEYS (%)	BRAIN (%)	SKIN (%)	MUSCLE (%)
Rest: $\dot{Q}$ = 5 L·min^{-1}	24	4	19	13 (.65 L/min)	9	21
Light Exercise: $\dot{Q}$ = 9 L·min^{-1}	12	4	9	8	16	47
Heavy Exercise: $\dot{Q}$ = 17 L·min^{-1}	3	4	3	4	12	71
Maximal Exercise: $\dot{Q}$ = 25 L·min^{-1}	1	4	1	3 (.75 L/min)	2	88

FIGURE 1.11 Distribution of cardiac output. During maximal exercise, the cardiac output increases fivefold. Note the large increases in blood flow to the skeletal muscle and the reduction in flow to the gastrointestinal tract. For the brain, blood flow, as a percentage of maximum, is reduced in maximal exercise, but total flow is increased from rest to maximal exercise.

Cardiac Output

Cardiac output ($\dot{Q}$) can be determined by systemic variables, not just those intrinsic to the heart (HR x SV). The average rate of blood flowing through the circulation is attributable to a combination of mean arterial pressure (MAP) and **total peripheral resistance** (TPR) because $\dot{Q}$ = MAP ÷ TPR. Based on this equation, a reduction in TPR, as occurs during endurance exercise primarily owing to **vasodilation** of the arteries in the active muscles, increases $\dot{Q}$. If TPR remained unchanged, it would necessitate large rises in MAP for $\dot{Q}$ to increase. For instance, $\dot{Q}$ can increase sevenfold or more in well-conditioned endurance athletes. If this magnitude of increase in $\dot{Q}$ were accomplished only via increases in MAP, there would also have to be a sevenfold increase in MAP, a pressure increase that would damage the heart.

However, as mentioned earlier in this chapter, $\dot{Q}$ is the product of SV and HR; therefore, these variables are more direct determinants of $\dot{Q}$. At rest, the average HR is 70 beats·min^{-1}, whereas the average SV is 70–80 mL of blood ejected per beat. Multiplying these two variables gives an average $\dot{Q}$ of about 5,000 mL of blood·min^{-1}or 5 L·min^{-1}. To meet metabolic needs of tissues at rest and during exercise, $\dot{Q}$ is adjusted by changes in SV and HR. The ability of the CV system to increase $\dot{Q}$ to meet the demands of exercise is very important to strike a steady-state match between metabolism and blood flow.

Heart Rate

Earlier in this chapter, the concept of autorhythmicity of the SA node was discussed. On its own, the SA node will depolarize approximately 60 to 100 times per minute. However, the SA node can be influenced to alter its discharge rate. Autonomic control, through both its sympathetic and parasympathetic divisions, provides a major mechanism for controlling the rate of SA node firing (Fig. 1.12).

The anotomic Neuros System

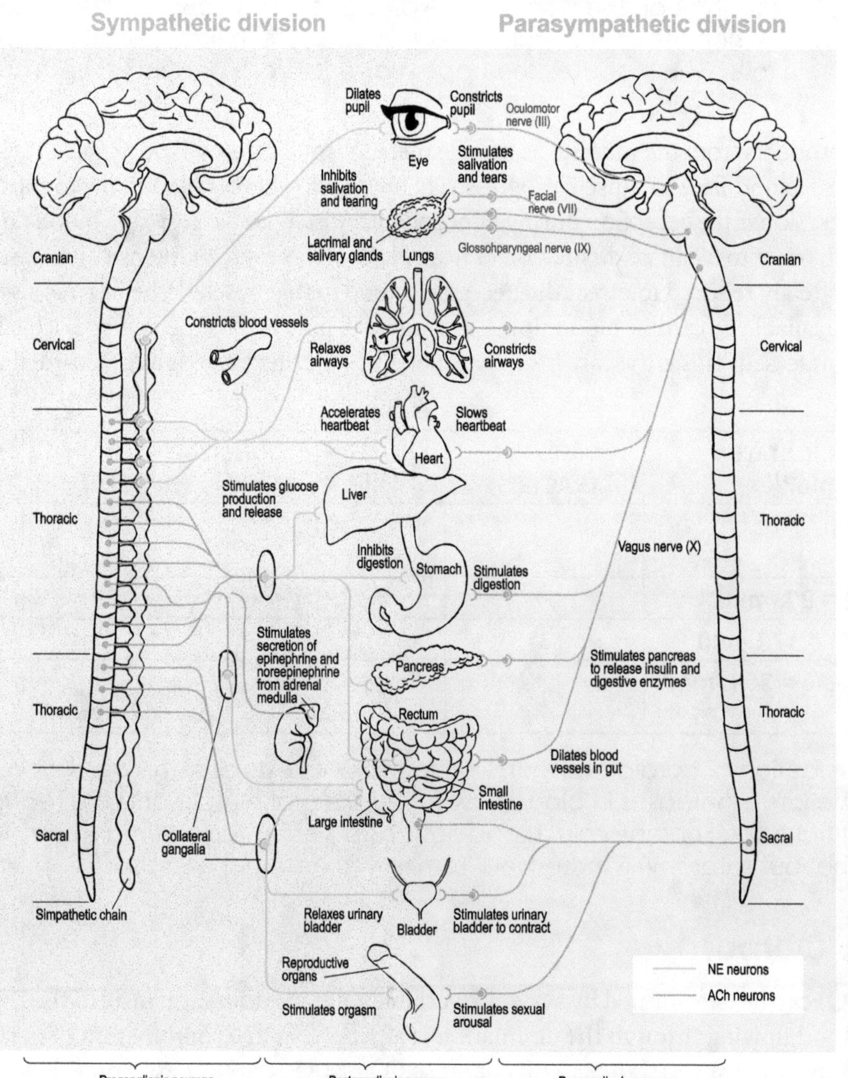

FIGURE 1.12 The activities of the SA and AV nodes can be altered by both the sympathetic and parasympathetic divisions of the autonomic nervous system.

The sympathetic branch of the autonomic nervous system supplying the heart originates in the cardiac accelerator nucleus of the medulla oblongata. These fibers innervate the SA node, the AV node, and to some degree the ventricles. When stimulated, norepinephrine is released, causing an increase in membrane permeability to Na^+ and Ca^{++}, enhancing both **chronotropic** (HR) and **inotropic** (force of contraction or contractility) capabilities of the heart. Parasympathetic innervation of the heart occurs via the vagus nerve and is controlled by the vasomotor center. When these fibers are stimulated, acetylcholine (ACh) is released from the nerve endings. ACh increases membrane permeability to K^+, hyperpolarizing the SA node, resulting in a negative chronotropic effect. To a more minor extent, ACh decreases membrane permeability to Ca^{++}, producing negative inotropic effects.

At rest, there is a balance between sympathetic and parasympathetic nervous tone, with parasympathetic dominating. With the onset of exercise, HR increases owing to decreased parasympathetic and increased sympathetic stimulation to the heart. The release of epinephrine from the adrenal medulla also augments HR and contractive force as exercise intensity approaches a moderate level (Fig. 1.13).

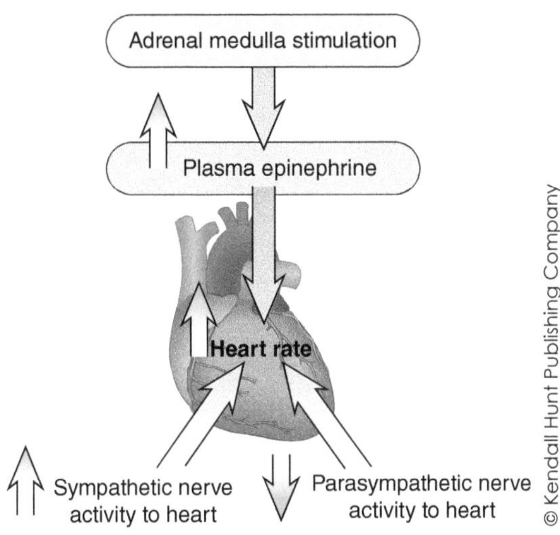

FIGURE 1.13 Factors affecting heart rate with onset of exercise.

Stroke Volume

Along with HR, SV is the other main determinant of $\dot{Q}$. SV is a function of ventricular filling and emptying, as reflected in the equation SV = EDV – ESV. As a factor controlling the level of $\dot{Q}$, SV is itself regulated by the two variables presented in this equation and by changes in TPR.

The amount of blood in the ventricle at the beginning of systole (the EDV) reflects the blood volume that was returned to the heart from the venous circulation (venous return). This regulatory factor is referred to as **preload**. Cardiac SV is regulated by preloading the ventricles with a certain volume of blood from one cardiac cycle to the next.

EDV serves as an index of ventricular preload affecting both SV and $\dot{Q}$ (Fig. 1.14). In the supine position (line A position 2), the ventricles are preloaded with an extra volume of blood owing to the removal of the pooling effect of upright posture. Postural shift from standing to supine results in the working point on the cardiac function curve moving from position 1 to position 2, as depicted by curve A.

SV is altered as the changing ventricular volume either increases (more EDV) or decreases (less EDV) the stretch to the myocardium, causing more forceful or less forceful myocardial contractions and producing a higher or lower SV, respectively. As illustrated, however, the ability of the ventricles to respond with a greater SV is limited, and, eventually, there are diminishing returns (curve A, position 3) with cardiac

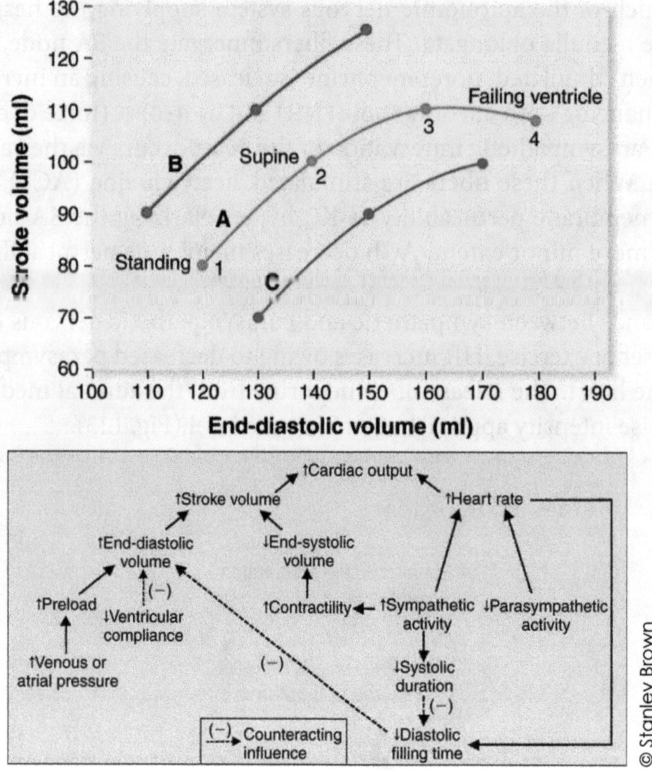

FIGURE 1.14 Cardiac function curves A–C (top figure). Curve A shows that SV is affected by postural positions through an increase in the EDV (preload) of the ventricle. Numbers 1–4 on curve A may also refer to a progressively higher EDV as endurance exercise intensity increases, thereby causing SV to increase. Notice that this increase in SV with increasing EDV does not continue indefinitely—there are diminishing returns in the SV response. Curve B represents a hyperdynamic heart (at any level of EDV, SV is higher) as caused by greater contractility (e.g., epinephrine infusion). Curve C represents a hypodynamic heart (at any level of EDV, SV is lower) as is the case in heart failure. The complex influence of stroke volume and heart rate on cardiac output is shown in the bottom figure.

pumping capacity lessening as even more blood is placed in the ventricle (curve A, position 4). SV can be enhanced or diminished by changes in EDV alone. The Frank-Starling "law of the heart" indicates that cardiac pump performance (i.e., SV) changes as a function of preload, or the degree of cardiac filling, measured as EDV. Another index of preload is the **central venous pressure** (CVP), which is the pressure in the right atrium and thoracic vena cava. However, SV can also be increased by contractility working through ESV.

A reduction in ESV during exercise increases SV even when EDV is unchanged; this is possible because of direct sympathetic stimulation to the ventricles and the stimulatory effect of circulating catecholamines. This was demonstrated experimentally by showing that the heart can increase SV by changing its contraction vigor without altering myocardial fiber length (preload). This phenomenon is usually demonstrated by plotting a "family" of ventricular function curves (curves B and C in Fig. 1.14), showing that the Frank-Starling relationship for the heart is not fixed but may be shifted to the right or left, and up or down, depending on various loading conditions. At a given EDV, ESV may, therefore, be elevated or depressed by altering the inotropic state of the myocardium, resulting in changes in SV. Contractility, like preload, is directly related to SV and is demonstrated clinically as a reduction in ESV when preload is constant. ESV, therefore, is considered a clinical index of contractility. Another clinical index of contractility is the cardiac **ejection fraction**, the ratio of SV to EDV (SV ÷ EDV).

Contractility can be augmented by positive inotropic drugs (i.e., norepinephrine) or by negative inotropic drugs (i.e., β blockers). A patient with heart failure, for instance, is often treated with digitalis (positive inotropic agent) to increase intracellular calcium, which enhances contractile force to increase SV.

Cardiac afterload is the resistance to ventricular emptying and can be quantified as either TPR or, more clinically relevant, MAP. Afterload is inversely related to SV. That is, SV decreases as afterload increases. The decrease in SV results primarily from the effect of aortic pressure on aortic valve function. Higher pressures lead to a shorter ejection time and decreased SV owing to the aortic valve not being open as long.

Vascular Function

In the regulation of $\dot{Q}$, afterload and preload are referred to as coupling factors because they couple cardiac with vascular function. The cardiac function curve defines how the heart responds to changes in preload; that is, $\dot{Q}$ (or SV) is dependent on EDV (an index of preload) (Fig. 1.14). We have already seen that $\dot{Q}$ (Y-axis) varies directly with preload (X-axis) over a wide range of preloads. Similarly, a second functional relationship describes the dependence of CVP on $\dot{Q}$. CVP is the blood pressure measured in the superior vena cava or right atrium and provides information about the function of the right heart, the circulating blood volume, vascular tone, and venous return. With respect to the vascular system, preload (as CVP; Y-axis) varies inversely with $\dot{Q}$ (X-axis), as illustrated in the vascular function curve (Fig. 1.15).

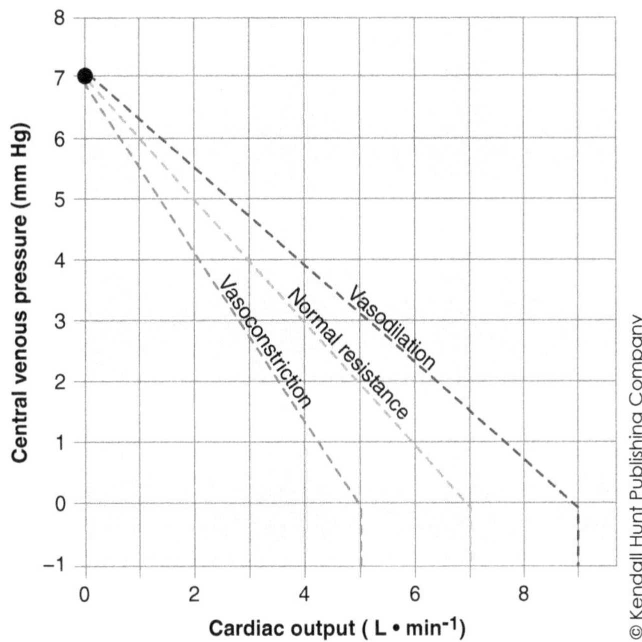

FIGURE 1.15 Vascular function curves showing the effects of increases or decreases in afterload on CVP and $\dot{Q}$. With respect to the vascular system, preload (i.e., CVP) varies inversely with $\dot{Q}$. The principal factors that govern the vascular function curve are the arterial and venous compliances and total blood volume.

The principal factors governing the vascular function curve are the arterial and venous compliances, the TPR, and the total blood volume. Figure 1.15 shows three vascular function curves and demonstrates the effect of an increase or decrease in afterload on $\dot{Q}$ and CVP (at any level of $\dot{Q}$). For instance, as afterload increases (i.e., **vasoconstriction** = increased arteriolar tone), $\dot{Q}$ is reduced at any level of CVP. The reverse is also true: at any level of $\dot{Q}$, an increased afterload decreases CVP.

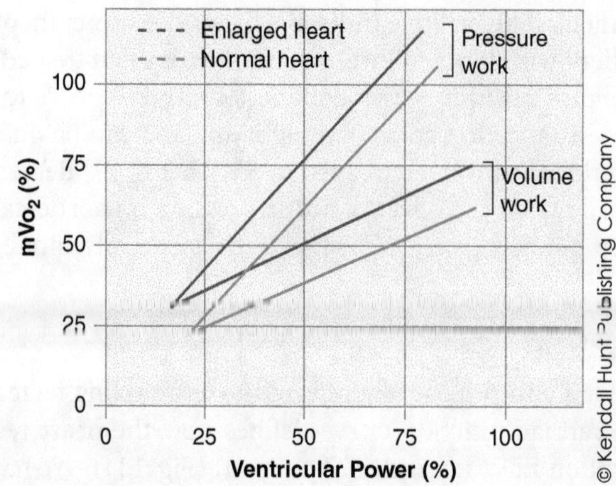

FIGURE 1.16 The effect of the type of ventricular work on myocardial O_2 cost (M$\dot{V}O_2$). If the predominant work is pressure load, M$\dot{V}O_2$ is greater at any level of ventricular power. M$\dot{V}O_2$ is greater still in an enlarged heart.

TPR is greatly reduced in exercise, which permits $\dot{Q}$ to increase as more blood is pumped at a lesser load and more efficiently than if TPR were unchanged from resting levels. The vascular function curve is also influenced by blood volume. For a given vascular compliance, CVP is increased when blood volume is expanded and decreased when blood volume is diminished. *Can you demonstrate how the decrease in TPR seen with exercise might alter the cardiac and vascular function curves?*

Myocardial Oxygen Consumption

Rate Pressure Product (RPP) is highly related to the work of the heart (measured as M$\dot{V}O_2$). The volume of O_2 consumed by the heart (M$\dot{V}O_2$, usually about 8 to 10 mL·min^{-1}·100 g^{-1} of myocardium at rest) is determined by the loading parameters the heart pumps against. RPP (SBP x HR ÷ 100) during resistance (**pressure-loaded**) exercise is typically greater than during endurance exercise (**volume-loaded exercise**). This leads to different myocardial metabolic requirements.

The O_2 requirements of the heart are greater for any given amount of left ventricular work (stroke work – the product of SV and the mean aortic pressure) when a major fraction of the total cardiac work is pressure work as opposed to volume work (Fig. 1.16). For example, an increase in $\dot{Q}$ at a constant aortic pressure (volume work) is accomplished with a small increase in left ventricular O_2 consumption. Conversely, pumping against an increased arterial pressure at a constant $\dot{Q}$ (pressure work) is accomplished by a large increment in M$\dot{V}O_2$. The reason pressure work is more costly in terms of M$\dot{V}O_2$ than the same amount of volume work is that in pumping against elevated arterial pressures (pressure-load work), the heart must generate a large amount of energy-consuming static force just to open the aortic valve.

The greater energy demand of pressure work compared to volume work is clinically significant. For example, in patients with aortic stenosis (narrowed opening of the aortic valve), there is an increase in left ventricular M$\dot{V}O_2$ which is caused by the extra energy needed to overcome the resistance to ventricular emptying offered by the stenotic aortic valve. This condition is usually also associated with a decreased coronary perfusion pressure, which can often lead to myocardial ischemia if the coronary arteries are not properly perfused. Figure 1.16 also shows that when the heart is enlarged, either form of work requires greater levels of energy output by the heart.

Chapter Questions

1. Why is the circulation separated into two circuits?
2. Why can't the cell respond to the next electrical stimulus too soon?
3. Explain the difference between preload and afterload.
4. Why must the heart's electrical function precede mechanical function?

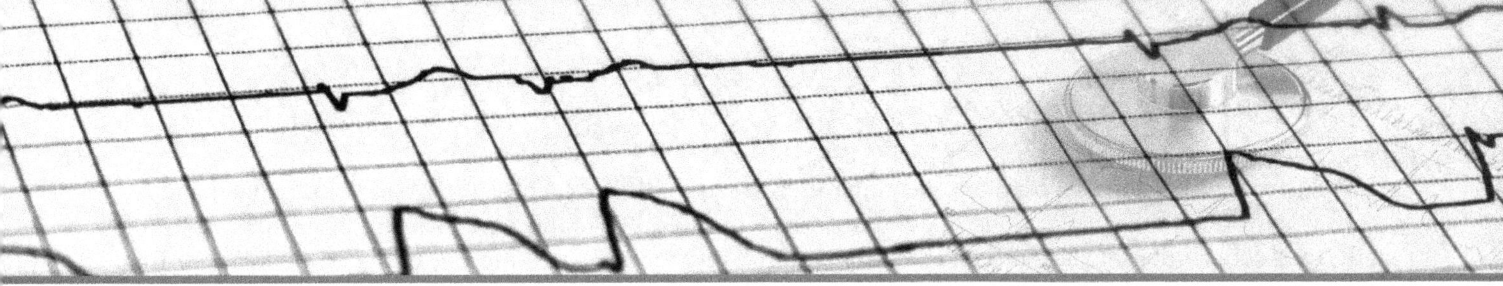

CHAPTER 2

Concepts of Pharmacology

Individuals in clinical exercise programs are usually on a course of prescriptive drug therapy appropriate to their pathophysiological involvement. Understanding the nature of the physiological limitations these patients experience is vital when using prescriptive exercise training as a therapeutic modality.

CONTENT OUTLINE

- Definition of Pharmacology
- Pharmacokinetics and Pharmacodynamics
- Pharmacokinetics and Age-Related Physiological Changes
- Pharmacodynamic Processes
- Cardiovascular Medications
- Organic Nitrates
- Beta-Blockers
- Calcium Channel Blockers
- Positive Inotropes
- Diuretics
- ACE Inhibitors
- Chapter Questions

Health care professionals most often encounter individuals in clinical exercise programs who are older and on a course of multiple medications. Older individuals consume 30% of the prescribed and from 40% to 50% of the over-the-counter medications taken in this country, yet they make up only 13% of the US population. This **polypharmacy** has several features:

- Medications are given that are not always necessary.
- Duplicate medications are often given.
- Persons are often on a course of concurrently interacting medications.
- Individuals are taking inappropriate dosages.
- When adverse **drug** reactions ensue, drug treatment often follows.
- Once the course of polypharmacy is discontinued, improvement follows.

The combination of physiological changes accompanying aging, the negative effects of polypharmacy, and the physiological responses to acute exercise place older patients at risk of adverse effects during therapeutic exercise training. For therapy to be effective, patients must adhere appropriately to both their medical and therapeutic exercise regimens. Because exercise and medications, often working in opposition, alter the magnitude and direction of physiological variables, **pharmacology** is an important topic for an exercise electrocardiography text. Health care professionals need to understand the effects and potential side effects of the drug regimen of their patients and how exercise training interacts with this medication regimen. *How might regular exercise training help older individuals overcome the problems inherent in chronic polypharmacy?*

Definition of Pharmacology

Pharmacology is defined as the study of the interactions between physiological processes and drugs. Drugs, by definition, alter bodily function by interactions, starting at the molecular and cellular levels, and then progressing to the organ and, finally, the systemic level. A complicating factor in the prescription of medication is that of interindividual variability. Not all individuals react the same way to a given drug dosage because drug metabolism is variable among individuals. The goal of the physician is to prescribe appropriate therapeutic dosages to better the medical status of their patients. Therefore, the goal of drug therapy is to fit the right kind of medication and an appropriate dose to the individual needs of the patient at a given moment in time (Case Study 2.1).

CASE STUDY 2.1: ANTIARRHYTHMIA PRESCRIPTION

Bill is a 65-year-old manager who complained to his physician about "flutters" accompanied by light-headedness. Three years earlier, he had suffered a lateral wall myocardial infarction and has since been on a course of isordil, atenolol, and diltiazem. The symptoms occurred while in the doctor's office. The nurse could not feel a pulse every other beat. The physician promptly ordered Bill to be placed on a 24-hour Holter monitor to "capture" such episodes on tape. Subsequent analysis showed that Bill experienced an irregular heart rhythm known as ventricular bigeminy (premature ventricular complexes every other beat) with occasional couplets.

Description

Cardiac **arrhythmia** is an alteration in rhythm or rate of the heartbeat and may be serious enough to warrant medical intervention. An arrhythmia is a change from the normal rhythm of the heart. Where the changes are under the influence of the sinoatrial (SA) node, the term sinus arrhythmia is used. Sometimes, rhythms are generated outside of the SA node. These are separated into supraventricular and ventricular, depending on their origin. In Bill's case the locus was in the ventricle. In ventricular rhythms, the depolarization wave spreads through the ventricles by an irregular and therefore slower pathway. Thus, the QRS complex is wide and abnormal. Repolarization pathways are also different, causing the T wave to have an unusual morphology. Above 100 beats per minutes, this rhythm is termed ventricular tachycardia and may pose a serious threat.

Intervention

Bill's physician prescribed quinidine to control the ventricular ectopy. Bill subsequently could not tolerate the quinidine well and experienced gastrointestinal (GI) symptoms. He was taken off the quinidine and placed on procainamide, which alleviated the GI problems. After months on this regimen, Bill again began to have symptoms of flutter and dizziness. His physician again ordered Holter monitoring, which showed that his original ventricular ectopy had returned. Bill also noticed joint pain, which caused him to cease the exercise prescription he had been placed on. The physician stopped the procainamide treatment, and Bill was admitted to the hospital, where he underwent exercise thallium testing to determine the extent of myocardial perfusion during exercise and to determine whether the ectopy was ischemia induced. The test was negative for ischemia but positive for anterior wall **dyskinesis**, consistent with a ventricular aneurysm. Bill also underwent electrophysiological testing to induce ventricular tachycardia. Bill was put on a course of mexiletine. Subsequently, Bill was retested to reinduce the ventricular tachycardia, which was unsuccessful. Bill was discharged on mexiletine and to resume his monitored cardiac rehabilitation program.

Pharmacokinetics and Pharmacodynamics

The foundation of medical prescription rests on two important concepts within pharmacology: **pharmacokinetics** and **pharmacodynamics**. Pharmacokinetics, how the body handles drugs, has five aspects:

1. Absorption: how and where the drug is introduced to the body
2. **Bioavailability**: the availability of an amount of a drug at the site of drug action
3. Distribution: how the drug moves to different locations in the body
4. Metabolism: how the drug is transformed from its active to its inactive state
5. Excretion: how the drug passes out of the body

Pharmacodynamics is concerned with processes involved in the interaction between a drug and an effector organ that results in a clinical response, either a therapeutic (efficacious) or an adverse (toxic) effect. Pharmacodynamics measures the intensity, peak, and duration of action of a medication. Figure 2.1 shows the interaction of these two concepts in the patient. The pharmacokinetic effect precedes, and largely causes, the pharmacodynamic effect.

Absorption and bioavailability are affected by dosage and route of administration of a drug. Typically, dosage considers three variables:

1. Amount of the drug given at one time
2. Method and route of administration
3. Duration of drug prescription

Method of drug administration includes *continuous* (e.g., wearing a transcutaneous nitroglycerin patch) or *intermittent* (the time interval between doses taken by any route) input. Likewise, there are two basic access routes of administration: **enteral** or **parenteral**. Enteral means that the drug enters the gastrointestinal (GI) system before it enters the circulation. It can enter the GI system by mouth or through the rectum. Parenteral means that the drug enters via a route other than the intestinal route. In this access route, the drug can enter through any of the following means: intravenous injection (IV), subcutaneous injection (SubQ), intramuscular injection (IM), intrathecal injection (Spinal), intraperitoneal injection, sublingual, or inhalational.

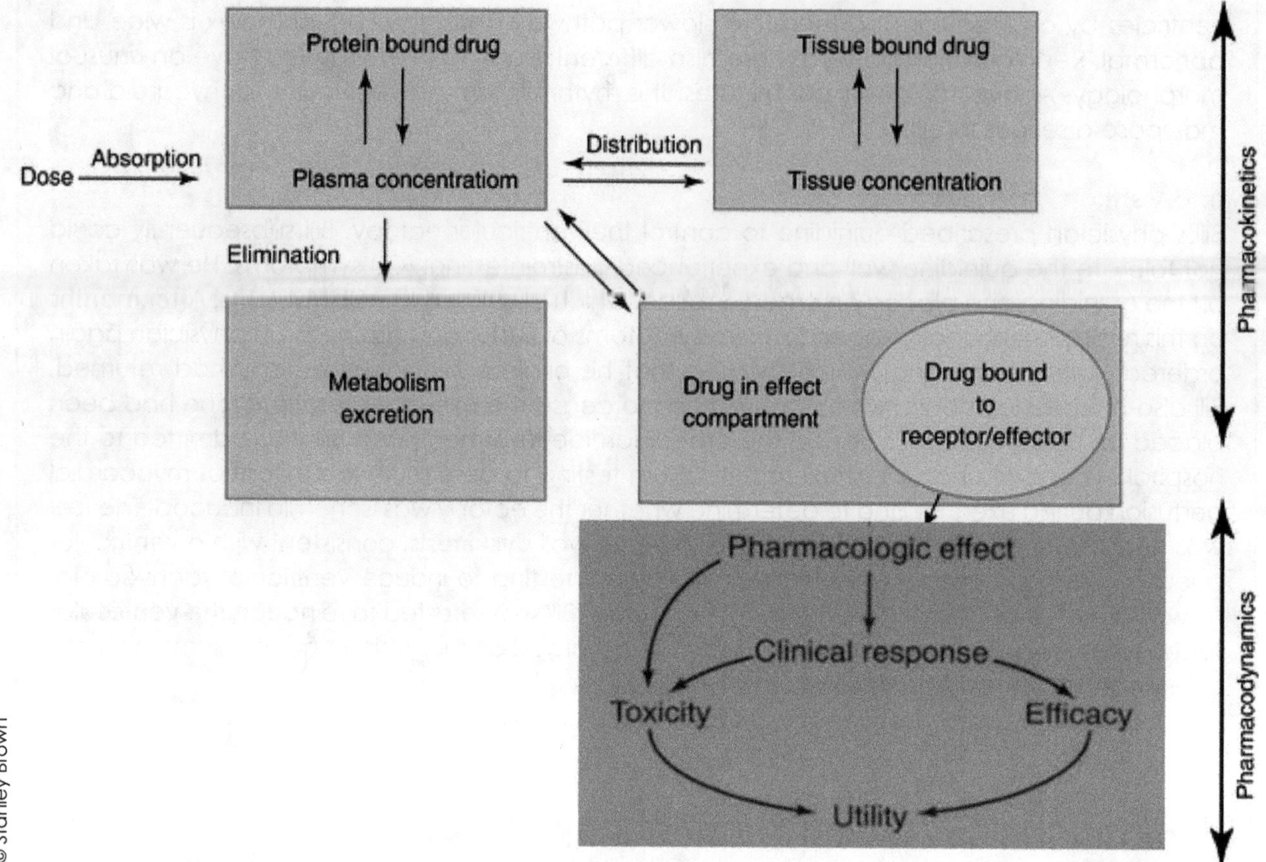

FIGURE 2.1 Interplay between pharmacokinetics and pharmacodynamics.

Pharmacokinetics and Age-Related Physiological Changes

Because clinical exercise programs are most often populated with older individuals, it is necessary to review the interactions between age-related physiological changes and the concept of pharmacokinetics. A brief review is presented in Table 2.1.

GI motility is decreased in older adults, which may prolong the absorption phase of the drug as it stays in one locale within the intestinal tract for a longer time period. The likelihood of a decreased mucosal cell count in elderly individuals coupled with reduced intestinal blood flow may also affect absorption in elderly individuals. This increases the bioavailability of the drug by reducing its availability to the hepatic portal circulation, where it first passes before entering the systemic circulation. Box 2.1 provides additional information about the hepatic portal circulation.

Bioavailability refers to that proportion of a drug that reaches the systemic circulation unchanged after a route of administration. When drugs are taken orally, their bioavailability is determined by factors in the drug, including the nature of the molecule, its stability, and the formulation administered. Bioavailability is also determined by factors in the patient such as a reduced intestinal surface area as a result of coeliac disease or intestinal resection. Whether or not the drug is taken with a meal also affects bioavailability. If less of the drug is sent to the liver because of poor portal circulatory uptake, there is the potential for reduced inactivation of the drug by the liver and for greater bioavailability resulting from a reduced **first pass effect** of the drug. The liver primarily dictates the magnitude of the first pass effect. In addition, this effect may also be enhanced by the reduced renal function seen with aging. As kidney competency declines with age attributable to reduced renal blood flow, drug accumulation and the potential for **toxicity** ensues. Bioavailability is also increased by the parenteral route of administration. Typical among these are injection and sublingual administration, which are particularly fast acting.

TABLE 2.1 Pharmacokinetics Altered by Age-Related Physiological Changes

System	*Change*
Gastrointestinal	• drug–drug interaction alters absorption • splanchnic blood flow decreases with no effect on drug absorption
Liver	• decrease in hepatic blood flow often associated with decreased first-pass metabolism • phase I drug metabolism decreased • phase II drug metabolism unaffected

Fluid and Tissue Compartments	• decrease in total body water
	  • decrease in plasma volume
	  • decrease in extracellular fluid
	• increase in fat compartment
	• decrease in muscle mass

Plasma drug-binding proteins	• decrease in serum albumin • decrease in plasma globulin
Kidneys	• decrease in renal blood flow • decline in creatine clearance • decline in tubular secretion • decrease in glomerular filtration rate
Cardiorespiratory	• decrease in cardiac index • decrease in vital capacity • decrease in cardiac output • decrease in splanchnic and renal blood flow

BOX 2.1: HEPATIC PORTAL CIRCULATION

There are three types of circulatory systems, two of which (systemic circulation and pulmonary circulation) depend on the heart to pump blood. The third type of circulation is known as a portal system, comprising specialized channels connecting one capillary bed site to another, but they do not depend directly on a central pump. The largest of these in the human is the hepatic portal system, connecting the intestines to the liver. Normally, there is only one capillary bed for each branch of a circuit; however, there are a few instances where there are two capillary beds, one after each other, in series. These are known as portal systems or portal circulations. Part of the blood supply to the liver is venous blood coming directly from the gastrointestinal (GI) tract and spleen via the hepatic portal vein. This arrangement enables the digested and absorbed substances from the gut to be transported directly to the liver, where many of the body's metabolic requirements are synthesized. Thus, there are two microcirculations in series, one in the gut and the other in the liver. The hepatic portal circulation serves the intestines, spleen, pancreas, and gall bladder. The liver receives its blood from two main sources—the hepatic artery, which is a branch of the aorta that supplies oxygenated blood to the liver, and the hepatic portal vein, which is formed by the union of veins from the spleen, the stomach, pancreas, duodenum, and colon. The hepatic portal vein transports the following to the liver.

- Absorbed nutrients from the duodenum
- White blood cells (added to the circulation) from the spleen
- Poisonous substances, such as alcohol, which are absorbed in the intestines
- Waste products, such as carbon dioxide, from the spleen, pancreas, stomach, and duodenum.

The hepatic artery and hepatic portal vein open into the liver sinuses, where the blood is in direct contact with liver cells. The deoxygenated blood, which still retains some dissolved nutrients, eventually flows into the inferior vena cava via the hepatic veins.

After absorption, drugs enter the general circulation and are distributed. Solubility in lipid and the extent of protein binding dictate distribution. Distribution refers to the amount of drug free to bind to its specific receptor site at the plasma membrane of the target tissue. Thus, if too much protein binding occurs, less of the drug is available for action at target tissues. To be pharmacologically active, higher free drug levels must exist. Given these facts, many elderly people are susceptible to increased pharmacological activity. For example, the dietary protein intake of many elderly individuals is often less than adequate. In this situation, these people may become **hypoproteinemic** and have lower levels of albumin (plasma protein), resulting in higher plasma-free drug concentration and an increased pharmacological effect. This effect, however, may be countered by the reduced resting cardiac output seen in elderly individuals. Lower cardiac output leads to a decreased peripheral blood flow, less distribution of the drug, and lower pharmacological effect.

Drug metabolism takes place in the liver. In older individuals, drug metabolism is slow owing to a smaller liver mass and less hepatic blood flow. This increases drug bioavailability. Drug metabolism by the liver is classified into phase I and phase II metabolism, during which the drug is first converted to a more easily excreted metabolite (phase I), and then the drug or its metabolite is coupled with an endogenous substrate (phase II). As shown in Table 2.1, phase I metabolism is decreased with age, which allows more of the biologically active drug remaining to have a pharmacological effect. Phase II metabolism is unaltered by age. The changes in phase I metabolism with age allow drug **half-life** to increase in older individuals. Half-life is the time it takes for a drug to be reduced to 50% of its initial plasma concentration. If half-life increases, the effects of the drug will be longer lasting, increasing bioavailability. Drug half-life dictates the frequency of its administration. Typically, the following frequencies are commonly prescribed:

qid (4x/day), tid (3x/day), bid (2x/day), qd (1x/day).

Because these frequencies are linked to the half-life of the drug, medications should always be taken at consistently regular intervals. If these intervals are not adhered to consistently, drug plasma concentrations will be altered, and the proper therapeutic dose will be lost.

The renal system is chiefly responsible for clearing or eliminating a drug from the body. Unfortunately, this system is affected by age because of decreases in kidney mass by about 20% by the eighth decade of life and a 10 $mL \cdot min^{-1}$ per decade reduction in renal blood flow after age 30. Reduced elimination because of decreased kidney function means that bioavailability is increased in elderly individuals.

Pharmacodynamic Processes

Pharmacodynamics is concerned with the intensity, peak, and duration of action of a drug. At the effector organ, a drug's effect is dictated by receptors, which are membrane-bound macromolecules. Receptors are of four general types: regulatory proteins, enzymes, transport proteins, or structural proteins. Receptors function in a nonspecific manner common to many cells; therefore, drugs produce multiple effects at many sites of action. These effects are classified as *primary, secondary, and side effects*. An individual's tolerance for the drug is determined by considering all possible effects so that toxicity is avoided.

Although a drug's activity is nonspecific, if the concentration is great enough, a drug does prefer one group or subgroup of receptors. This selectivity is based on the traditional "lock and key" complementary relationship formed between drug and receptor, much like the enzyme–receptor complementary relationship. Receptor sites are found all over the body. For example, common receptor sites for cardiac medications are found in the autonomic nervous system, kidneys, and vascular smooth muscle. Receptors of the autonomic nervous system are specific to one of its two branches: sympathetic and parasympathetic. Sympathetic branch activity secretes norepinephrine (adrenaline), and parasympathetic branch activity secretes acetylcholine from their respective postganglionic fibers. Therefore, the receptors for each of these branches are referred to as adrenergic and cholinergic, respectively. Subdivisions of these receptor types are classified as follows:

- Adrenergic receptors—alpha (α_1 & α_2), beta (β_1 & β_2), and dopamine
- Cholinergic receptors—muscarinic (M_1 & M_2) and nicotinic.

TABLE 2.2 Autonomic Receptor Types and Function

Receptor types	*Location*	*Function*
Cholinergic muscarinic	CNS neurons, atrial myocardium, SA and AV node smooth muscle, smooth muscle of secretory glands, bronchi	decrease contractility, decrease heart rate, decrease peripheral vascular resistance, broncho-constriction
Cholinergic nicotinic	skeletal muscle end-plates, autonomic ganglion cells	stimulation of neuromuscular junction
Adrenergic alpha	vascular smooth muscle, papillary dilator muscle, pilomotor smooth muscle, and smooth muscle of bronchi, GI tract, uterus & bladder	vasoconstriction, iris dilatation, intestinal relaxation, intestinal sphincter contraction, pilomotor contraction, bladder sphincter contraction
Adrenergic beta	heart, fat cells, respiratory, uterine, and vascular smooth muscle, skeletal muscle, liver	vasodilation (β_2), cardioacceleration (β_1), increased myocardial strength (β_1), intestinal relaxation (β_2), uterus relaxation (β_2), calorigenesis (β_2), glycogenolysis (β_2), lipolysis (β_1), bladder wall relaxation (β_2)

There is less distinct division of the alpha-adrenergic receptors than there is of the beta-adrenergic receptors. Alpha receptors are activated more strongly by norepinephrine than by **isoproterenol**, and the opposite is true of beta receptors. **Phenoxybenzamine** can be used to block alpha-adrenergic receptors, and **propranolol** can be used to block beta-adrenergic receptors. Other selective antagonists are also available for adrenergic receptors.

Cholinergic receptors are so named because of the chemicals that can activate them to the exclusion of the other. Muscarine is a poison from toadstools that activates only muscarinic cholinergic receptors (these receptors are blocked by **atropine**), while nicotine activates only nicotinic cholinergic receptors (these receptors are blocked by **curare**). Obviously, acetylcholine activates both types of cholinergic receptors.

These major receptors are classified by their sensitivity to **agonist** and **antagonist** drugs. An agonist drug is one that produces biochemical and physiological changes within the cell. Antagonist drugs interact with receptors to block a response. Drugs that mimic the activity of sympathetic neurotransmitters (i.e., epinephrine, norepinephrine, and dopamine) are called **sympathomimetics** (adrenergic agonists). Drugs that block sympathetic nervous system action are called **sympatholytics** (adrenergic antagonists). Likewise, drugs that simulate parasympathetic activity are known as **parasympathomimetics** (cholinergic agonists), and drugs that block cholinergic activity are called **parasympatholytics** (cholinergic antagonists). Table 2.2 lists the autonomic receptor types by name, location, and action.

The following sections highlight several major classes of drugs encountered most often in therapeutic exercise programs. Cardiovascular physiology is altered by disease in such a way as to disrupt the attempt of homeostatic mechanisms to return function to normal. Because of this, drugs are used to help restore proper function. The available pharmaceuticals used in the treatment of the conditions presented in this section are extensive, and, therefore, only a basic overview will be given of a few of the most important classes of drugs.

Cardiovascular Medications

Modern pharmacotherapy for patients with chronic illnesses has been very successful and has contributed to the longevity of elderly persons. For example, the management of cardiac dysfunction involves the prescription of a multifaceted drug regimen to produce an efficacious clinical response in patients with disease and disability. Clearly, the use of prescriptive medications has allowed many people to live much longer with chronic diseases.

Physiological side effects may occur in patients as exercise responses and drugs interact in a synergistic fashion. For example, patients may develop symptoms when medications that cause peripheral vasodilation are taken with aerobic exercise interventions that also produce peripheral vasodilation. The symptoms, for example, hypotension, dizziness, and **syncope,** may be present only when both exercise and drug intervention occur simultaneously. In a similar manner, drugs may blunt the physiological effects of exercise, as is the case when taking beta-blocking medications. Beta-blockers limit the normal increase in heart rate that occurs with an imposed exercise load. In addition, health care professionals who provide exercise therapy need to be alert to the potential side effects of cardiovascular medications, some of which can be exacerbated by exercise. These are presented in Table 2.3.

The goal of pharmacological treatment of coronary artery disease (CAD) is to prevent myocardial ischemia and infarction and to maximize and improve cardiovascular function. Table 2.4 presents the major medical conditions with the predominant cardiovascular medications used in treatment. The following brief descriptions highlight many of these drugs.

TABLE 2.3 Common Side Effects of Cardiopulmonary Drugs and the Proper Patient Response

Side Effects	*Action*
Abdominal pain	Visit physician
Asthmatic attacks	Visit physician
Bradycardia	Visit physician
Cough	None
Dehydration	None
Difficulty breathing or swallowing	Visit physician
Dizziness or fainting	Visit physician
Drowsiness	None
Easy bruising	None
Fatigue	None
Headache	None
Insomnia	Call physician
Joint pain	Visit physician
Loss of taste	None
Muscle cramps	Call physician
Nausea	None
Nightmares	Call physician
Orthostatic hypotension	Call physician
Palpitations	Call physician
Paralysis	Visit physician
Sexual dysfunction	Call physician
Skin rash	Call physician
Stomach irritation	Call physician
Swelling of feet or abdomen	Call physician
Symptoms of congestive heart failure (shortness of breath, swollen ankles, coughing up blood)	Visit physician
Tachycardia	Call physician
Unexplained swelling, unusual or uncontrolled bleeding	Call physician
Vomiting	Call Physician
Weakness	None

TABLE 2.4 Commonly Prescribed Cardiovascular Medications

Conditions	*Drug Class*
Angina pectoris	Organic nitrates
	Beta-blockers
	Calcium channel (Ca^{2+}) blockers
Arrhythmias	Beta-blockers
	Calcium channel (Ca^{2+}) blockers
	Agents prolonging depolarization
Congestive heart failure	Positive inotropes (digitalis)
	Diuretics
	ACE inhibitors
	Vasodilators
Hypertension	Diuretics
	Beta-blockers
	ACE inhibitors
	Vasodilators
	Calcium channel (Ca^{2+}) blockers

Organic Nitrates

Common nitrates are those that are longer acting, such as isosorbide mononitrate and isosorbide dinitrate (Isordil), and those that are rapidly acting, such as nitroglycerin. The purpose of nitrate administration, as shown in Figure 2.2, is to: (1) redistribute blood flow along collateral channels and from epicardial to endocardial regions, (2) relieve coronary artery spasm, and (3) induce peripheral vasodilation to unload the heart by reducing afterload (reduced blood pressure) and preload. The vasodilatory effect of nitrates on the peripheral

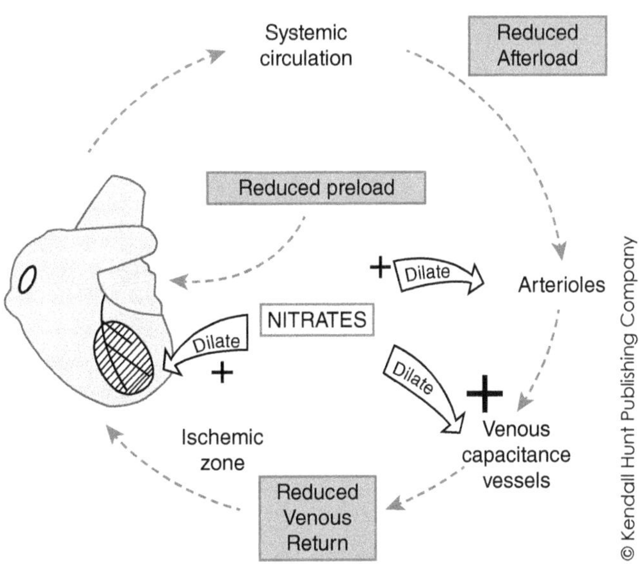

FIGURE 2.2 The effects of nitrates on the circulation. The major effect of nitrates is on venous capacitance vessels, but there are also coronary and peripheral arteriolar dilation effects.

vasculature causes pooling of blood. This lowers the venous return and ventricular volume, which reduces preload. Because the ventricle is now on a reduced stretch, mechanical stress on the myocardial walls is also lower, thereby reducing myocardial O_2 demand.

Organic nitrates act directly on arterial and vascular smooth muscle to produce arterial and venous vasodilation. By reducing preload and afterload, nitrates reduce myocardial O_2 consumption and restore the balance between O_2 supply and demand. However, coronary blood flow is unaltered. Concomitant with a decrease in mean blood pressure is the activation of the sympathetic nervous system. Increases in heart rate and **contractility** partially reverse the decrease in myocardial O_2 consumption produced by arterial and venous vasodilation. In patients with variant angina, organic nitrates can prevent or reverse coronary artery spasm. Nitrates increase the exercise capacity of patients with angina because they reduce cardiac workload during exercise.

Individuals with CAD should be administered sublingual nitrate at the onset of chest pain. Blood pressure should be monitored, and the patient should be recumbent to prevent hypotension. The patient should return to the upright position slowly after administration. If pain is not relieved, emergency medical care should be implemented immediately.

Beta-Blockers

Beta-blockade therapy attempts to strike a balance between O_2 supply and demand in the ischemic heart. To do this, beta-blockade produces negative chronotropic, **dromotropic**, and inotropic effects on the sinoatrial (SA) node, atrioventricular (AV) node, and on myocardial contraction, respectively (Fig. 2.3). The consequent

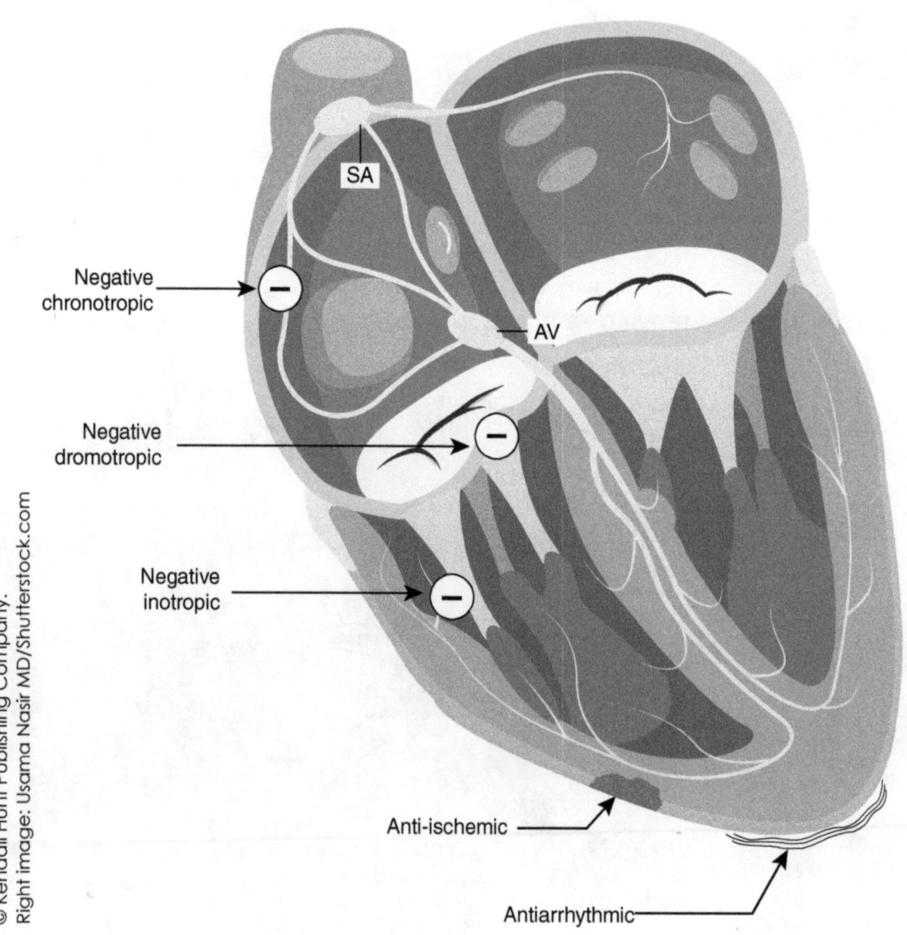

FIGURE 2.3 Effects of beta-adrenergic blocking drugs on SA node, AV node, myocardial oxygenation, and rhythmicity.

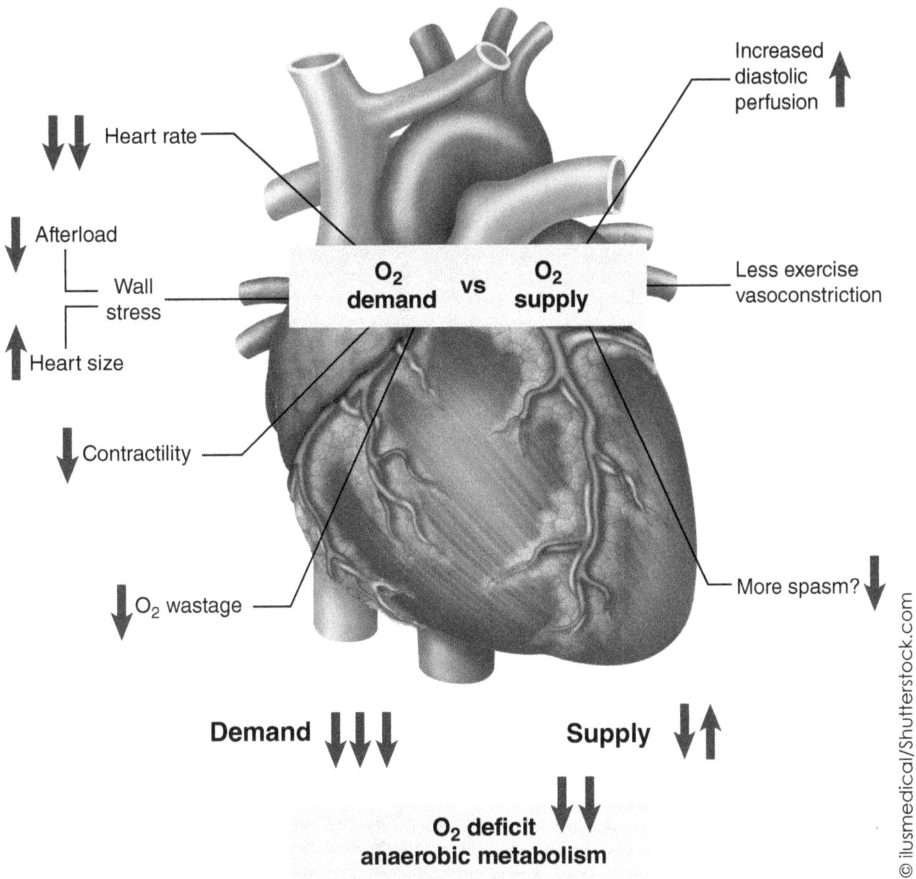

FIGURE 2.4 Effects of beta-blockade on the ischemic heart. Beta-blockers reduce angina by decreasing demand for O_2, not supply of O_2.

reduction in myocardial O_2 demand is therapeutic for angina pectoris. As shown in Figure 2.4, beta-blockade decreases the heart's demand for O_2 by reducing wall stress. There is a large reduction in O_2 demand and a negligible increase in O_2 supply. Wall stress is reduced through qualitative changes in the factors shown in Figure 2.4. As a result, there is less O_2 deficit and decreased reliance on anaerobic metabolism. Beta-blockade therapy to control atrial and ventricular **tachyarrhythmias** is also effective, with three proposed mechanisms (Fig. 2.5). These include inhibiting phase 0 depolarization (class I), inhibiting spontaneous depolarizations (class II), and increasing the duration of the cardiac action potential (class III).

Beta-blockers are not prescribed for patients with hypotension, congestive heart failure (CHF), bradycardia, AV blocks, and chronic obstructive pulmonary disease (COPD). These agents increase the exercise capacity of patients with angina. Higher levels of activity can be attained before the ischemic threshold is reached. Patients on beta-blocker drugs will have a lower heart rate than usual at the same level of exercise. If exercise testing and prescription are given, any change in the drug dosage may necessitate a repeat test and prescription.

Calcium Channel Blockers

Calcium channel blockers (CCB) work by blocking the entry of Ca^{++} through the Ca^{++} channels in smooth and cardiac muscle. Muscle contraction is thus attenuated, producing vasodilation in smooth muscle and a negative inotropic effect in cardiac muscle. The vasodilatory effect reduces total peripheral resistance (TPR) (decreased afterload), which helps in the medical management of angina pectoris, hypertension, and coronary spasm. These effects increase O_2 supply more than they decrease O_2 demand, and, like beta-blockers, the heart relies less on anaerobic metabolism (decreased O_2 deficit). Mechanisms of the anti-ischemic effect of calcium channel blockade are shown in Figure 2.6.

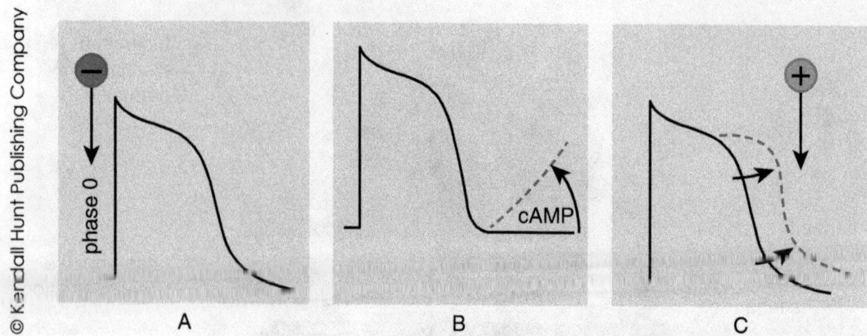

FIGURE 2.5 Antiarrhythmia properties of different types of beta-blockade drugs showing types of restraint during depolarization: (A) Class I has membrane stabilizing effects working to inhibit Phase 0, (B) Class II inhibiting spontaneous depolarizations (all β blockers do this), and (C) Class III increasing the duration of the action potential (Phase 2), which is specific to Sotalol.

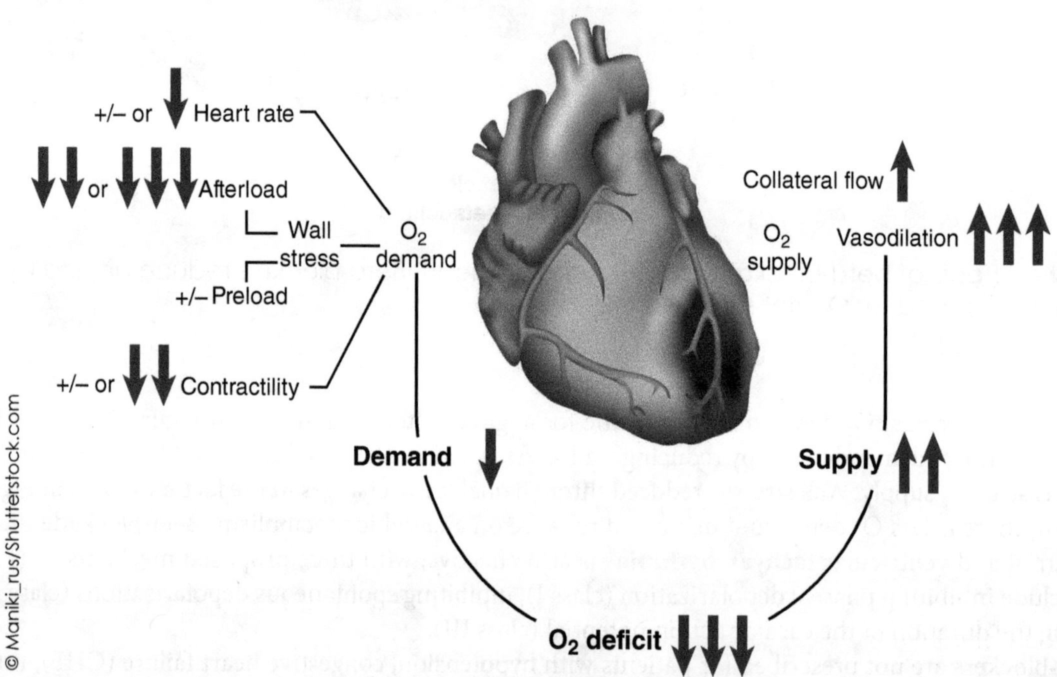

FIGURE 2.6 Effects of calcium channel blockade on the ischemic heart. The drug affects O_2 demand and supply in the ways shown in the figure.

CCB are of two general classifications: dihydropyridine (DHP) and non-DHP. DHP CCB tend to affect primarily smooth muscle, causing vasodilation of both peripheral and coronary arteries, whereas non-DHP CCB exert their effects primarily on cardiac muscle, producing negative chronotropic and inotropic effects. Although working through different mechanisms, both subclasses have a similar capacity to lower BP. Non-DHP CCB are verapamil and diltiazem, whereas DHP CCB end in the suffix "dipine" (i.e., amlodipine, felodipine).

CCB increase the exercise capacity of patients with angina because the drug decreases myocardial O_2 demand and increases myocardial blood supply. As with other medications that lower blood pressure, patients should be observed for postural hypotension.

Positive Inotropes

Positive inotropes improve the pumping capacity of the heart in chronic or **acute heart failure.** In **chronic heart failure,** positive inotropes are not used until pump failure is severe. However, in acute heart failure, positive inotropic therapy is commenced immediately. Digitalis is an important drug to improve pump function during CHF. Digitalis has both neural and myocardial cellular effects (Fig. 2.7). Digitalis activates the parasympathetic nervous system and inhibits the sympathetic nervous system. This results in a slower heart rate and conduction through the AV node. The positive inotropic effect of digitalis comes about through sodium–calcium exchange (Fig. 2.7, insert), whereby cytosolic Ca^{++} concentration is increased, which enhances myocardial contractility (more forceful muscle contraction) and pump performance. Digitalis increases the exercise capacity of patients with CAD because of improved ventricular performance. Exercise personnel should be aware of the effects of digitalis on the electrocardiogram (ECG), such as a sagging ST segment, which mimics the ST depression seen in ischemia.

Diuretics

Diuretics are not only used to treat symptomatic heart failure, primarily to control pulmonary and peripheral symptoms of congestion, but are also important in the treatment of hypertension. The three major groups of diuretics are the loop diuretics, the thiazides, and the potassium-sparing diuretics, each acting at different sites of the nephron of the kidneys (Fig. 2.8).

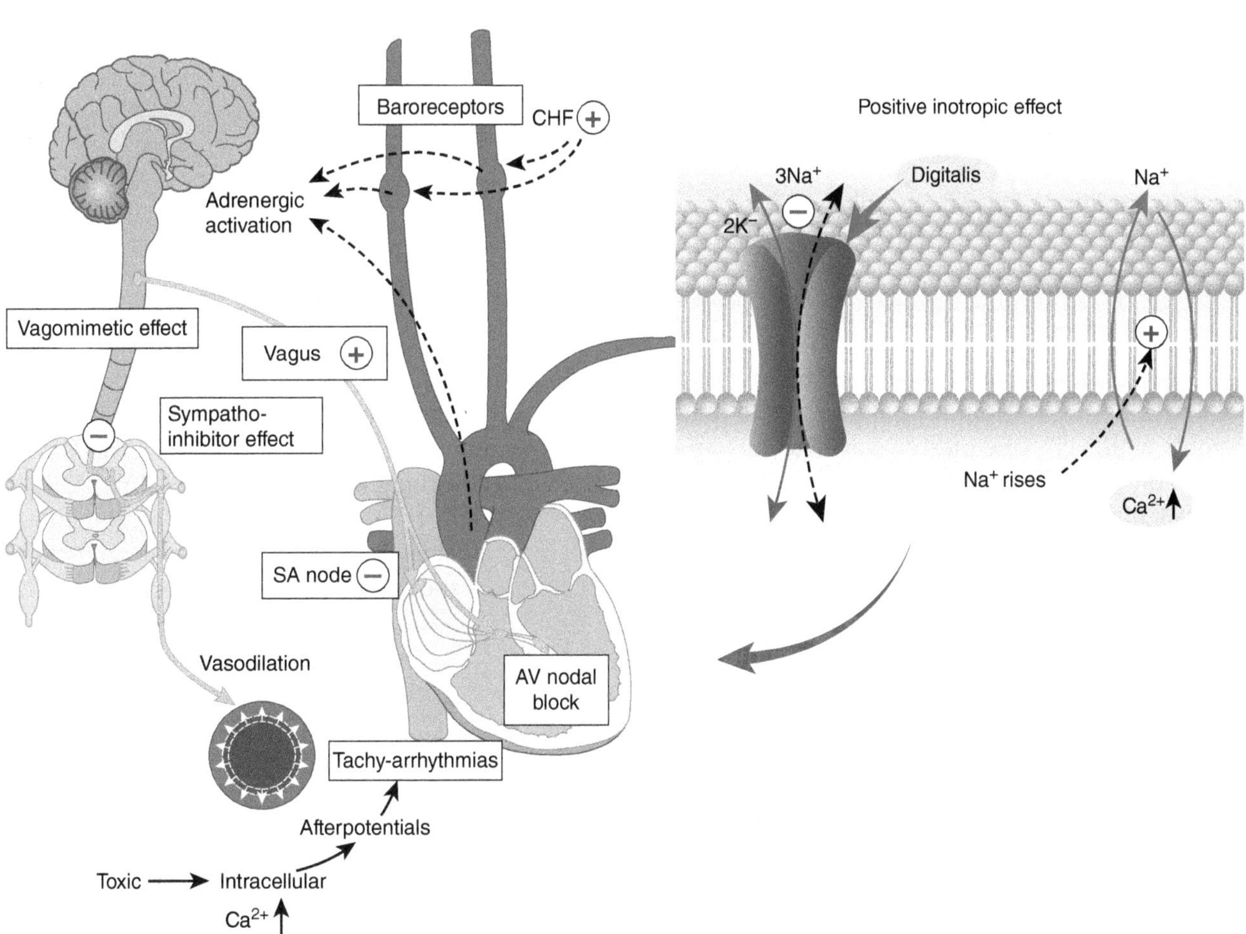

FIGURE 2.7 The inotropic effect of digitalis is due to inhibition of the sodium pump in myocardial cells, whereby Ca^{++} influx to the cytosol via exchange with sodium is promoted. Digitalis also slows the heart rate, inhibits the AV node, and decreases sympathetic drive.

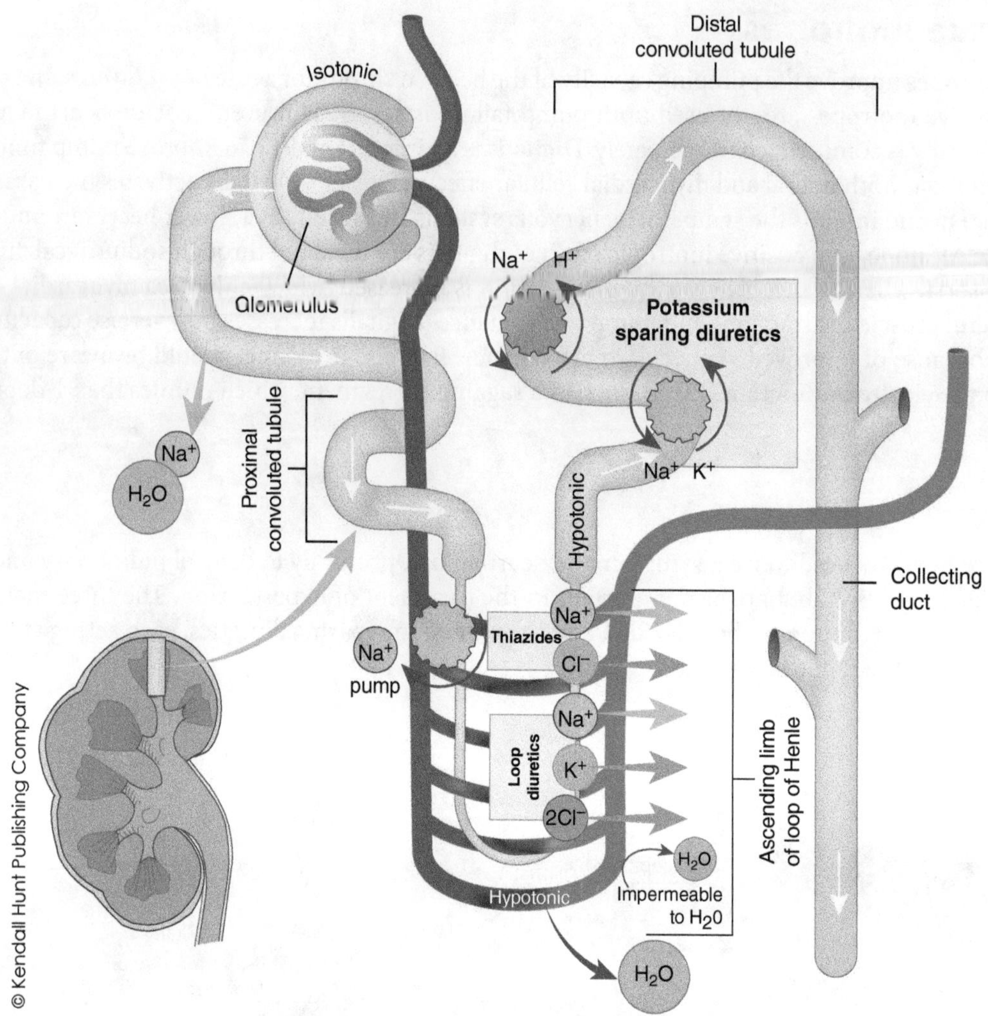

FIGURE 2.8 The kidney nephron showing sites of action of diuretics.

Loop diuretics constitute a family of drugs that remove water from the body. They are used to lower blood pressure in people with hypertension and to reduce the workload of the heart, allowing it to pump better in people with CHF. The most widely used loop diuretic is furosemide (Lasix). The "loop" refers to the drug's action on the loop of Henlé, a structure of the kidney involved in reabsorbing water. Kidneys control the extracellular fluid (ECF) volume by adjusting sodium chloride (NaCl) and H_2O excretion. Each day, the kidney filters more than 22 moles of Na. To maintain NaCl balance, approximately 1.4 kg of NaCl must be reabsorbed by the renal tubules daily. Thus, the body maintains blood pressure at the expense of ECF volume. When NaCl intake is greater than output (as in CHF or renal failure), edema develops. Loop diuretics act primarily by blocking the $Na^+/K^+/Cl^-$ co-transporter in the membrane of the thick ascending limb of Henle's loop. Because this is the same site responsible for concentrating and diluting urine, loop diuretics decrease maximal urinary concentrating and diluting. The thick ascending limb is a major site of Ca^{++} and Mg^{++} reabsorption, processes that are dependent on normal Na^+ and Cl^- reabsorption. Therefore, loop diuretics increase urinary water, Na^+, K^+, Ca^{++}, and Mg^{++} excretion.

Loop diuretics are more potent than thiazide diuretics, but thiazides are the most commonly prescribed class of diuretics. They inhibit Na^+ and Cl^- transport in the cortical thick ascending limb and early distal tubule. They have a milder diuretic action than do the loop diuretics, because this nephron site reabsorbs less Na^+ than the thick ascending limb. Potassium-sparing diuretics act in the distal tubules of the nephron and are often given to avoid the hypokalemia (decrease K^+ concentration) that accompanies the agents previously described. They should never be given in the setting of hyperkalemia (increase K^+ concentration) or in patients on drugs or with disease states likely to cause hyperkalemia. Diuretics increase the exercise capacity of patients with CHF.

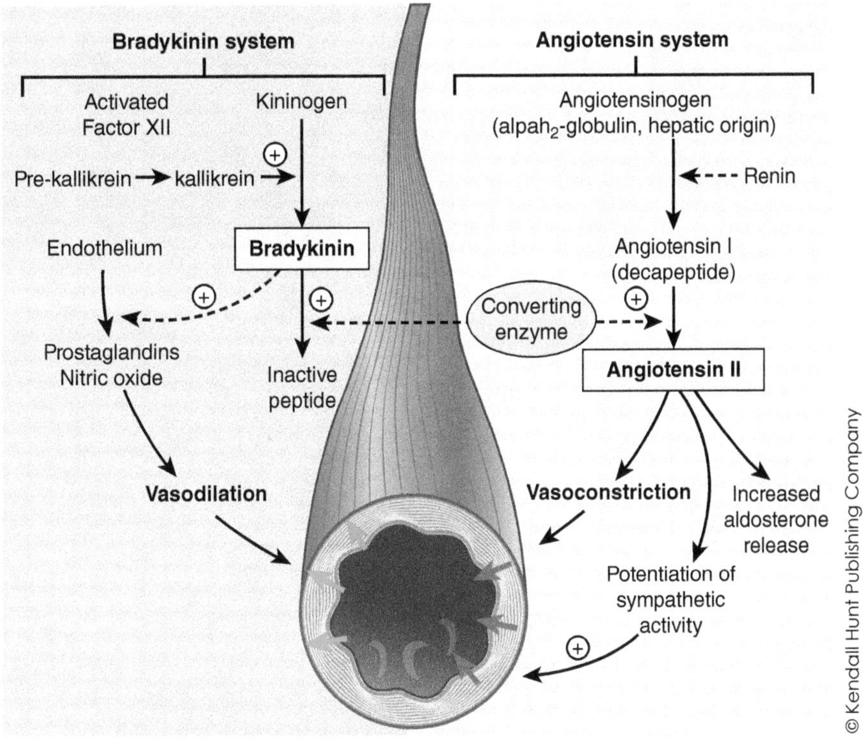

FIGURE 2.9 The dual vasodilatory actions of ACE inhibitors.

ACE Inhibitors

Angiotensin-converting enzyme (ACE) inhibitors interrupt the molecular messengers that constrict blood vessels. These drugs have dual vasodilatory actions, working principally through the renin–angiotensin aldosterone system but also influencing the bradykinin system (Fig. 2.9).

Working through the renin–angiotensin–aldosterone system, ACE inhibitors inhibit the normal vasoconstriction that follows angiotensin II release. Working through bradykinin, ACE inhibitors lead to the formation of vasodilatory nitric oxide and prostaglandins. ACE inhibitors improve heart function in individuals with heart failure and are also used to treat hypertension. The most common ACE inhibitors are captopril (Capoten), enalapril (Vasotec), lisinopril (Zestril, Prinivil), ramipril (Altace), and moexipril (Univasc). Common side effects are cough, hypotension, rash, swelling of face, lips, and tongue, GI disturbances, headache, dizziness, lightheadedness, and fatigue. Patients on diuretic therapy may be more prone to hypotension with ACE inhibitor therapy, so patients need to be cautioned to change body position slowly. ACE inhibitors increase the exercise capacity of patients with CHF.

Chapter Questions

1. Compare and contrast pharmacodynamics with pharmacokinetics.
2. Why must drug prescription be considered when writing an exercise prescription?
3. Why would a heart patient require a nitrate versus an inotropic agent?

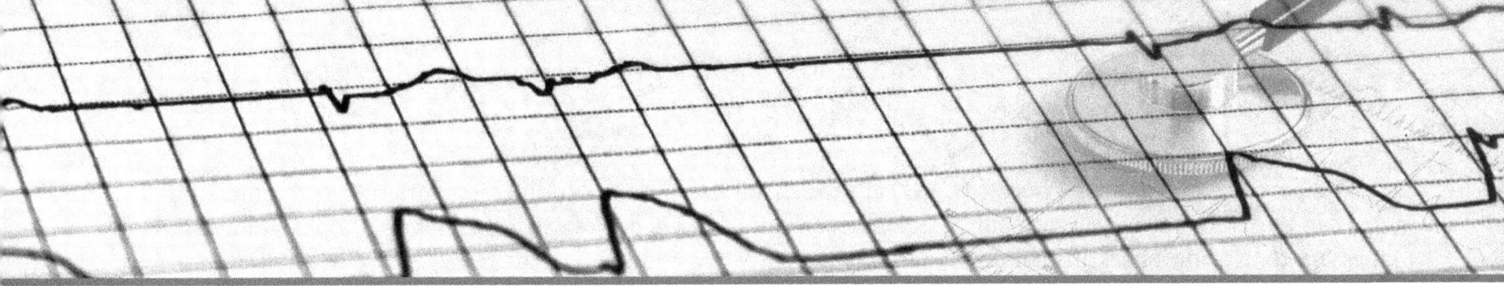

CHAPTER 3

Concepts of Pathophysiology

The list of cardiovascular diseases, conditions that affect the structures and function of the heart, includes arrhythmias, aorta disease and Marfan syndrome, congenital heart disease, coronary artery disease, deep vein thrombosis and pulmonary embolism, heart attack, heart failure, cardiomyopathy, heart valve disease, pericardial disease, peripheral vascular disease, rheumatic heart disease, stroke, and vascular disorders.

CONTENT OUTLINE

The list of cardiovascular diseases (CVD) at the start of the chapter is quite long, and therefore none of them can be given extensive treatment here. However, some knowledge of cardiovascular pathophysiology is necessary to provide a backdrop of understanding for parts two and three of the text.

CVD is the leading cause of death in industrialized nations, with an estimate of one person dying every 36 seconds in the United States, or about 655,000 American deaths from heart disease each year (one in every four deaths). Coronary artery disease (CAD) is the most common type of CVD. About 18.2 million adults aged 20 and older have CAD, and about 2 in 10 deaths occur in adults less than 65 years old. Each year approximately 805,000 Americans have heart attacks: 605,000 are a first heart attack and 200,000 have had a previous heart attack. One in five heart attacks are silent. CVD costs the United States about $219 billion each year. This includes the cost of health care services, medicines, and lost productivity. Additionally, about two million Americans suffer from congestive heart failure (CHF), with 400,000 new cases annually, requiring 900,000 hospitalizations per year. Despite these grim statistics, over the last few decades there has been a steady decline in mortality from CVD. During the last 50 years, it is estimated that the 73% decline in total death rate was mostly attributable to the 56% decrease in CVD death rate and the 70% decrease in stroke death rate. The percentages of all deaths caused by CVD in 2015 is listed by ethnicity, race, and sex in Table 3.1.

The following signs and symptoms associated with CVD are considered common:

- Chest pain: pain radiating to the neck, jaw, upper trapezius muscle, upper back, shoulder, or arms. Cardiac origin secondary to angina, myocardial infarction (MI), pericarditis, mitral valve **prolapse** or dissecting aortic **aneurysm**. Case study 3.1 distinguishes noncardiac from cardiac chest pain. Pain pattern usually specific to the condition (Fig. 3.1–3.3). Box 3.1 is a laboratory exercise helpful to students learning to distinguish chest pain patterns.

TABLE 3.1 CVD Prevalence by Ethnic Group

Race of Ethnic Group	*% of Deaths*	*%Men*	*%Women*
American Indian or Alaska Native	18.3	19.4	17.0
Asian American or Pacific Islander	21.4	22.9	19.9
Black (Non-Hispanic)	23.5	23.9	23.1
White (Non-Hispanic)	23.7	24.9	22.5
Hispanic	20.3	20.6	19.9
All	23.4	24.4	22.3

CASE STUDY 3.1: DIFFERENTIATING CHEST PAIN

Sally is a 60-year-old woman employed at a sawmill with work requiring repetitive shoulder flexion and extension and lifting tasks. She was diagnosed with left anterior chest pain after a history of hysterectomy and is a 4-pack-per-day smoker for 30 years. Her chest pain was sudden and crushing. Tests after treatment in the emergency room were negative for cardiac involvement. Blood pressure was 195/115 mmHg on admittance. Diagnosis: stress-induced chest pain. She described the pain as radiating around the chest, under the armpit, and to the upper back. No numbness and tingling were noticed. The pain did not radiate down the arm.

Most causes of chest pain are not related to cardiac problems. The following are broad causative categories, followed by examples and specific clues to distinguish each:

- Cancer—mediastinal tumors: weight loss though chronically inactive, pain that does not respond to treatment, nocturnal pain
- Pleuropulmonary—pulmonary hypertension: pain not palpable, pain worsens in the lying position, presence of associated signs and symptoms such as persistent cough or dyspnea

- Epigastric—esophageal spasm: symptoms relieved by antacids, symptoms are not reproduced or aggravated by effort or exertion, presence of nausea, vomiting, dark urine, jaundice, indigestion, abdominal fullness or bloating
- Breast—mastitis: lump, nodule, skin puckering, recent childbirth and/or breast feeding, association between painful symptoms and menstrual cycle
- Neuromusculoskeletal—Tietze's syndrome: aching, burning and hot, pain is unrelated to effort and lasts for hours or weeks to months, symptoms are relieved by heat and stretching
- Cardiac—myocardial infarction: pain associated with physical activity, pain related to temperature changes, emotional reactions, or large meal. Dyspnea, arrhythmias, syncope

Intervention

A neurological screen was negative. Tests included deep tendon reflexes (within normal limits), strength testing (limited by pain), and no changes in sensation, two-point discrimination, or proprioception were observed. Left pectoral palpation revealed pain with tenderness and swelling at the second, third, and fourth costochondral joints. Resisted shoulder horizontal adduction produced pain and radiating symptoms. Active shoulder range of motion was normal but painful on the left. Pain in the chest, arm, and upper back region was not altered by respiratory movements (deep breathing or coughing). The supine position did not produce pain. The diagnosis was Tietze's syndrome secondary to repetitive motion and exacerbated by emotional stress. The patient also had shoulder impingement syndrome. The pain and movement dysfunction were relieved after 6 weeks of physical therapy.

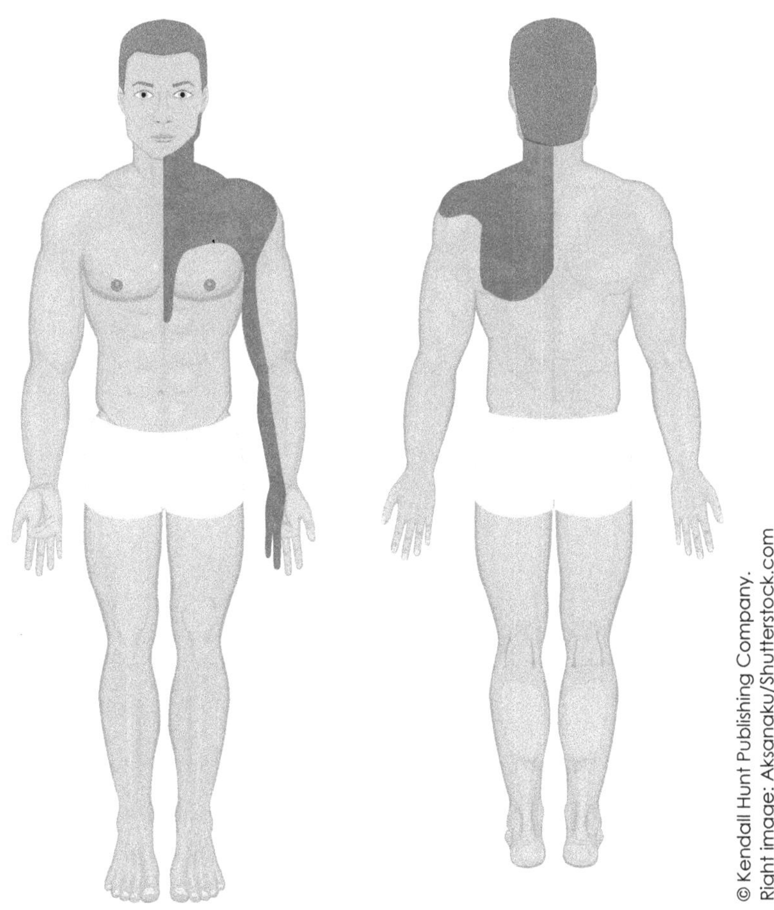

FIGURE 3.1 Angina chest pain pattern. Left figure illustrates area of substernal discomfort projected to the left shoulder and arm over the distribution of the ulnar nerve. Right figure illustrates that anginal pain may be referred to the back (left scapula).

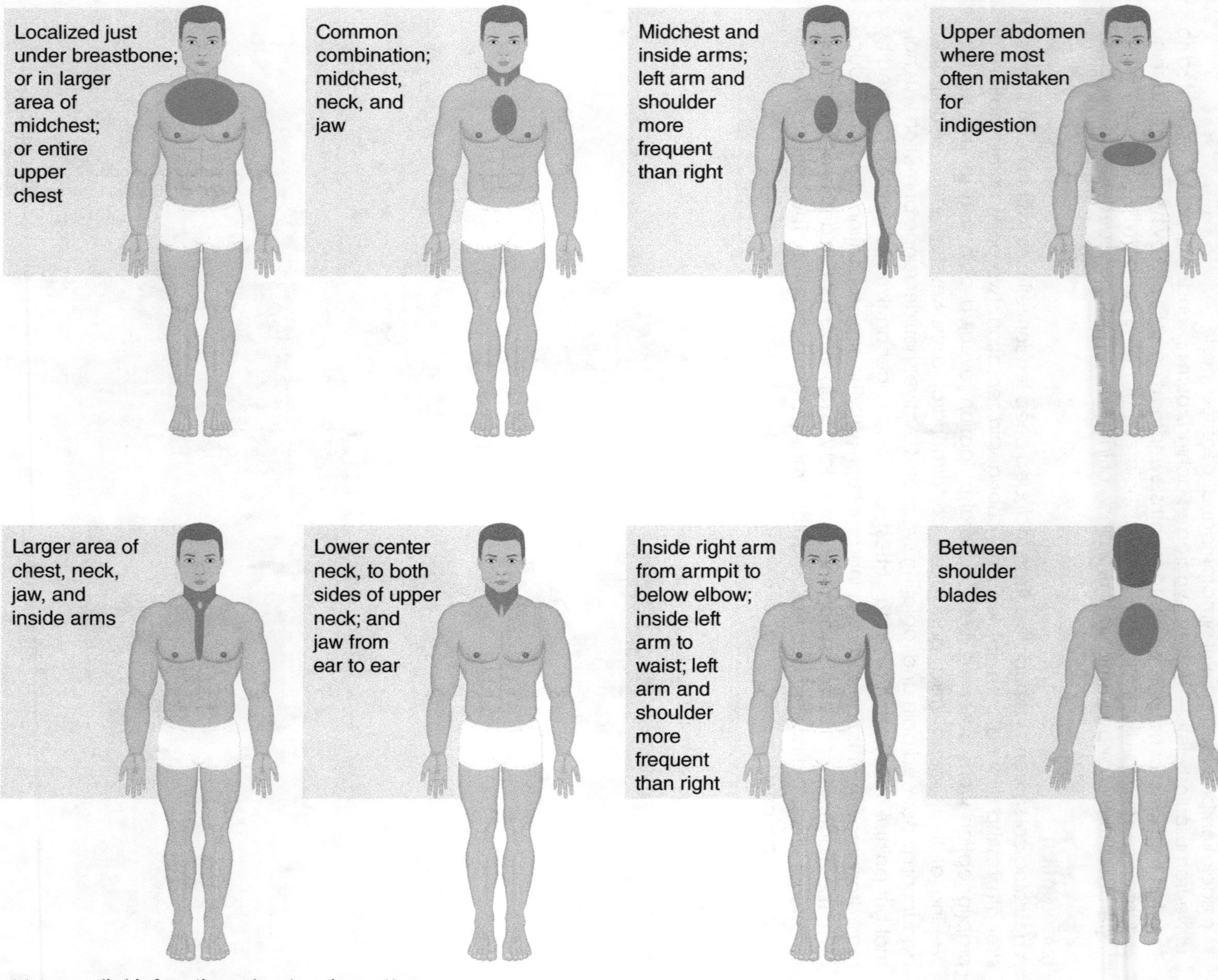
Localized just under breastbone; or in larger area of midchest; or entire upper chest
Common combination; midchest, neck, and jaw
Midchest and inside arms; left arm and shoulder more frequent than right
Upper abdomen where most often mistaken for indigestion
Larger area of chest, neck, jaw, and inside arms
Lower center neck, to both sides of upper neck; and jaw from ear to ear
Inside right arm from armpit to below elbow; inside left arm to waist; left arm and shoulder more frequent than right
Between shoulder blades

FIGURE 3.2 Myocardial infarction chest pain pattern.

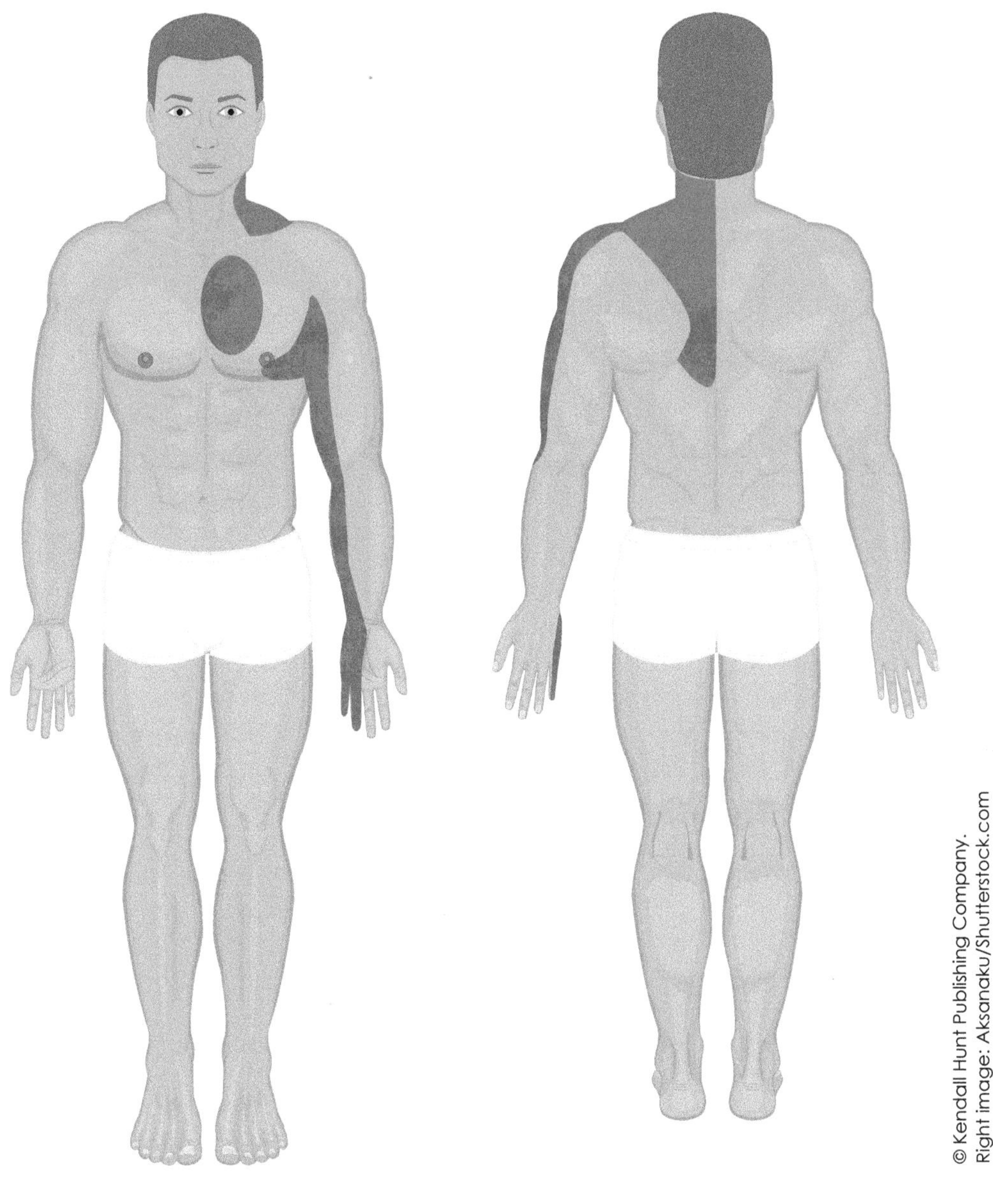

FIGURE 3.3 Pericarditis chest pain pattern. Left figure illustrates substernal pain associated with pericarditis may radiate anteriorly to the costal margins, neck, upper back, upper trapezius muscle, and left supraclavicular area or down the left arm.

BOX 3.1: DISCUSSING DIFFERENTIAL DIAGNOSIS OF CHEST PAIN

Therapists monitoring exercise sessions should understand the differential diagnosis of chest pain. This laboratory exercise focuses on chest pain originating as anginal pain, pain from a myocardial infarction (MI), and pain caused by pericarditis. Referring to Figures 3.1 to 3.3, the following descriptions should be thoroughly studied.

Anginal Chest Pain Pattern

Location: Substernal/Retrosternal; Referral: Neck, jaw, back, shoulder, or arms (more common in the left arm), occasionally radiates to the abdomen; Description: Viselike pressure, squeezing, heaviness, burning indigestion; Intensity: Mild to moderate (builds up gradually or may be sudden); Duration: Usually less than 10 minutes (never more than 30 minutes), Average 3 to 5 minutes; Associated Signs And Symptoms: Extreme fatigue, lethargy, weakness, shortness of breath, nausea, diaphoresis, anxiety, belching, heartburn; Relieving Factors: Rest or Nitroglycerin; Aggravating Factors: Exercise or physical exertion, cold weather, heavy meals, emotional stress

Myocardial Infarction Chest Pain Pattern

Location: Substernal, anterior chest; Referral: May radiate like angina, frequently down both arms; Description: Burning, stabbing, viselike pressure, squeezing, heaviness; Intensity: Severe Duration: Usually at least 30 minutes, may last 1 to 2 hours; Associated Signs And Symptoms: None with a silent MI, dizziness, feeling faint, nausea, vomiting, pallor, diaphoresis, severe anxiety, fatigue, sudden weakness, shortness of breath; Relieving Factors: None (unrelieved by rest or nitroglycerin taken every 5 minutes for 20 minutes); Aggravating Factors: Not necessarily anything, may occur at rest or may follow emotional stress or physical exertion

Pericarditis Chest Pain Pattern

Location: Substernal or over the sternum, sometimes to the left of midline toward cardiac apex; Referral: Neck, upper back, upper trapezius muscle, left supraclavicular area, down the left arm, costal margins; Description: More localized than pain of MI; Intensity: Moderate to severe; Duration: Continuous, may last hours or days with residual soreness following; Associated Signs And Symptoms: Usually medically determined associated symptoms (e.g., by chest auscultation using a stethoscope); Relieving Factors: Sitting upright or leaning forward; Aggravating Factors: Muscle movement associated with deep breathing (e.g., laughter, inspiration, coughing), left lateral (side) bending of the upper trunk, trunk rotation (either to the right or to the left), supine position

Laboratory Exercise

In groups perform mock cases of individuals presenting with any of the three foregoing patterns. One student serves as the patient, and the others practice any of the following scenarios using one of the pain patterns: (1) An outpatient during cardiopulmonary rehabilitation doing ergometer exercise complains of chest pain; (2) An inpatient doing bedside range of motion exercise complains of chest pain; (3) A patient performing a prescribed home exercise routine calls in to the center complaining of chest pain.

- **Palpitation**: an arrhythmic heartbeat, it can have several origins ranging from benign (mitral valve prolapse anxiety) to severe (CVD, cardiomyopathy, atrioventricular valve disease) conditions. Physical sensation is often referred to as a pounding in the chest and may produce light-headedness. The duration and frequency of occurrence are significant to observe, that is, lasting from less than six per minute (benign) to several hours (pathologic when occurring with pain, shortness of breath, fainting, or severe light-headedness).
- **Dyspnea**: shortness of breath; it can be of cardiovascular or pulmonary pathology, or it may occur in relatively benign conditions (fever, medications, allergies, poor physical conditioning, or obesity). When of cardiovascular origin, dyspnea is related to poor left ventricular pumping, resulting in fluid backup to the lungs and shortness of breath.
- Syncope: fainting caused by reduced O_2 delivery to the brain can be caused by various cardiovascular conditions, such as arrhythmias, **orthostatic hypotension** (sudden drop in blood pressure), poor ventricular function, CAD, and vertebral artery insufficiency. Noncardiac conditions may also cause syncope via a vasovagal maneuver from hyperventilatory responses initiated by anxiety or emotional stress.
- Fatigue: may be cardiac in origin when accompanied by symptoms such as dyspnea, chest pain, palpitations, or headache. Fatigue may also be secondary to neurologic, muscular, metabolic, or pulmonary conditions. Fatigue may also be due to deconditioning.

- Cough: associated with pulmonary conditions or cardiac conditions with associated pulmonary complications. In CHF, a cough is the result of fluid backup to the lungs.
- **Cyanosis**: discoloration of the lips and nail beds resulting from a lack of O_2 is usually of pulmonary or cardiac origin.
- **Edema**: may be of cardiac origin, where symptoms of right-sided CHF include swelling of the ankles, abdomen, hands, dyspnea, fatigue, and dizziness. Most often, the cause of right heart failure is left heart failure.
- **Claudication**: leg pain and occurs in peripheral vascular disease as arteries or veins become narrowed owing to the process of atherosclerosis. Skin discoloration also occurs.

Disorders Affecting the Heart Muscle

In most cases, a cardiac pathologic condition can be traced to one of three processes: (1) obstruction or restriction, (2) inflammation, or (3) dilation or distension. Combinations of these problems can cause pain in the chest, neck, back, and/or shoulder. Table 3.2 presents six specific pathologic processes with associated signs and symptoms.

TABLE 3.2 Diseases/Disorders Affecting the Heart Muscle

Disease/ Disorder	*Underlying Pathologic Process*	*Clinical Signs and Symptoms*
Coronary Artery Disease	Atherosclerotic process leading to narrowing of coronary artery lumen, which restricts blood flow to the muscle	Asymptomatic until a critical deficit of blood supply is reached; symptoms usually appear when the artery narrows by 75%.
Angina Pectoris	Imbalance between myocardial O_2 demand and supply caused by advanced atherosclerosis and leading to myocardial ischemia	Chest pain (radiating to left shoulder and arm, neck, jaw, teeth, upper back, and abdomen). Burning indigestion present with nausea, dyspnea, and exercise intolerance; relieved by rest and nitrates; Figure 3.1.
Myocardial Infarction	Sudden decrease in coronary perfusion, leading to myocardial tissue death	Same as angina, but that pain not relieved by rest or nitrates. Syncope; Figure 3.2
Pericarditis	Inflammation of the pericardium as caused by a number of different diseases (secondary pericarditis), or it may be primary pericarditis	Chest pain (similar to myocardial infarction [MI] but aggravated by deep breathing and trunk movements), dyspnea, increased pulse rate and core temperature; Figure 3.3
Congestive Heart Failure	Decreased pump function secondary to intrinsic myocardial disease or structural defects; left sided heart failure is the principle cause of right sided heart failure	Left-sided heart failure causes fatigue and dyspnea upon exercise and is associated with persistent cough, orthopnea, tachycardia, edema, and decreased renal function; right-sided heart failure causes fatigue and is associated with dependent edema (i.e., feet & ankles), cyanosis of the nail beds, and distended neck veins
Aneurysm	Weakened vessel wall created from a trauma, congenital vascular disease, infection, or atherosclerosis. Can occur in thoracic, abdominal, and peripheral arteries.	Chest pain, awareness of a pulsating mass in the abdomen (with abdominal and back pain), extreme pain along the base of the neck along the back between the scapular blades, groin and leg pain, tachycardia, systolic hypotension (<100 mmHg).

Disorders Affecting Heart Valves

Table 3.3 presents conditions that occur secondary to impairment of the valves caused by disease (rheumatic fever), infection (endocarditis), or congenital deformity (mitral valve prolapse). Three types of valvular deformity affect the aortic, mitral, tricuspid, or pulmonic valves: stenosis (narrowing that prevents the valve from opening fully), *regurgitation* (improper closure of the valve that allows blood to flow back into the heart chamber) or *prolapse* (specific only to the mitral valve and refers to the bulging backward of the valve leaflets into the upper chamber). These conditions cause the heart to pump harder to force blood through a stenosed valve or to maintain adequate flow if blood is reentering the atrium.

Disorders Affecting the Cardiac Nervous System

The heart's nervous system can fail to conduct normal electrical impulses, leading to a cardiac arrhythmia. Arrhythmias can induce tachycardia or bradycardia and may cause extra beats and fibrillations. Circulatory dynamics change, leading to mild or severe symptoms (Table 3.4).

TABLE 3.3 Diseases/Disorders Affecting the Heart Valves

Disease/ Disorder	*Underlying Pathologic Process*	*Clinical Signs and Symptoms*
Rheumatic Fever	Streptococcal bacterial infection resulting in scarring and deformity of the heart valves.	Fever and sore throat followed by migratory joint symptoms in the knees, shoulders, feet, ankles, elbows, fingers, or neck. Weakness, malaise, weight loss, and anorexia may accompany the fever.
Endocarditis	Bacterial infection inflaming the cardiac endothelium, damaging the tricuspid, aortic, or mitral valve	Musculoskeletal symptoms, including arthralgia, arthritis, low back pain, and myalgias; dyspnea, chest pain; and cold and painful extremities.
Mitral Valve Prolapse	Slight variation in the shape of the mitral valve, causing prolapse upon closer of the valve.	Common "triad" of symptoms include palpitations, fatigue, and dyspnea. Other symptoms include tachycardia, anxiety, depression, panic attacks, migraine headaches, and chest pain.

TABLE 3.4 Diseases/Disorders Affecting the Cardiac Nervous System

Disease/ Disorder	*Underlying Pathologic Process*	*Clinical Signs and Symptoms*
Arrhythmias	Disorders of the heart rate and rhythm caused by disturbances in the conduction system. This disorder may be due to underlying coronary artery disease.	Fibrillation may be felt as palpitations, sensations of fluttering, skipping, or pounding. Dyspnea, chest pain, anxiety, pallor, nervousness, and cyanosis are often the outcome.
Sinus Tachycardia	Normal physiologic response to conditions such as fever, exertion, hypotension, hypovolemia, congestive heart failure, shock, anemia, anxiety, and thyrotoxicosis. It is especially problematic in patients with organic myocardial disease.	Rapid rate (>100 bpm) may produce palpitation, restlessness, chest pain or discomfort, agitation, anxiety.
Sinus Bradycardia	Normal in fit individuals but could be a result of sinus node pathology.	Reduced rate (<60 bpm) may produce syncope.

Occlusive Heart Disease

Atherosclerotic occlusive disease refers to processes that result in arterial obstruction by the formation of lesions, leading to reduced perfusion of arteries that supply blood to the myocardium (CAD) or to the extremities (peripheral vascular disease). The result is tissue ischemia, which can affect the heart and skeletal muscle. Myocardial ischemia is one of the 10 most common primary pathologies leading to cardiac muscle dysfunction, and, ultimately, heart failure. The major disorders caused by insufficient blood supply to the myocardium are angina pectoris, CHF, and MI. Occlusive heart disease (CAD) results from a complex genetic makeup and interactions with the environment. Environmental interactions include nutrition, activity levels, and history of smoking. The underlying disease process is atherosclerosis, a progressive disorder beginning in childhood and occurring in any artery in the body, but most commonly in medium-sized arteries of the heart, brain, kidneys, and legs.

Congestive Heart Failure

Congestive heart failure (CHF) is a major health care problem today. CHF leads to the inability of the heart to maintain normal blood pressure and tissue perfusion via reduced cardiac output. Figure 3.4 shows the process of neurohumoral adaptation in CHF. The reduced organ perfusion is especially important for kidney function as renal ischemia sets in, which results in enhanced renin release. Enhanced renin release is also potentiated by the increase in sympathetic discharge that comes about because of the baroreceptor reflex activated by hypotension. Sympathetic discharge stimulates β_1 renal receptors involved in renin release. This reflexive neurohumoral activation leads to peripheral vasoconstriction via the increased formation of angiotensin II (Fig. 2.9), which increases peripheral vascular resistance and cardiac afterload. This scenario causes left ventricular function to fall further. With the increased afterload, the ventricle is not able to empty properly, and this leads to an increased preload (ventricular dilation). In the face of the high preloads and afterloads, ventricular wall stress is increased, according to the law of LaPlace:

$$\text{wall stress} = (\text{pressure} \times \text{radius}) \div (2 \times \text{wall thickness})$$

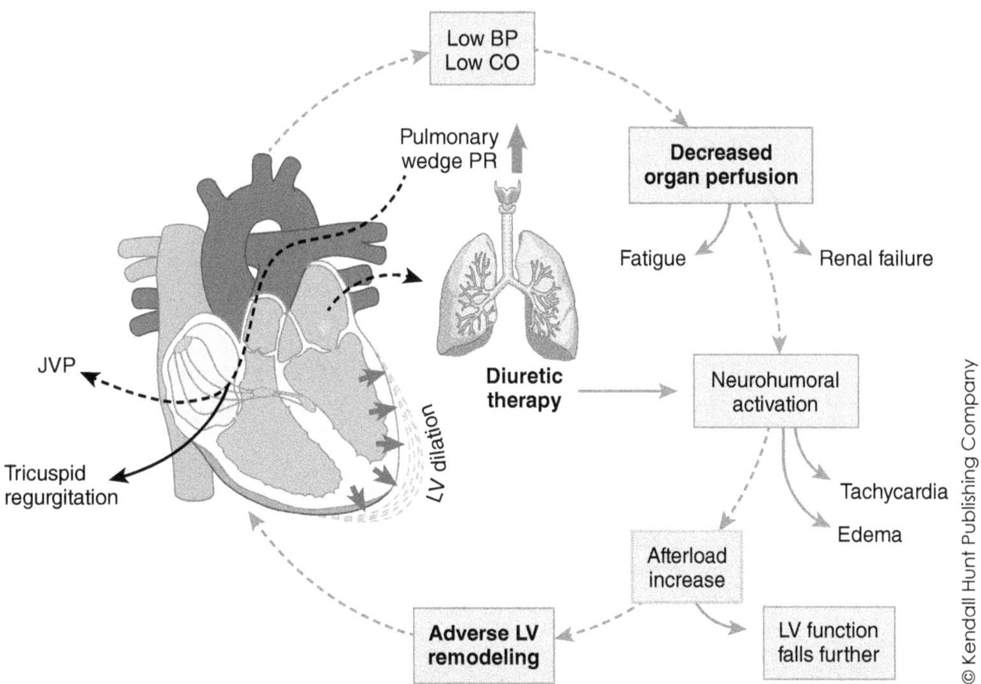

FIGURE 3.4 Neurohumoral adaptation in CHF. When the left ventricle (LV) fails, there is the inability to maintain normal blood pressure and normal organ perfusion. The failed LV leads to an increase in the pulmonary wedge pressure with consequences through the right heart. LV failure also eventually leads to neurohumoral activation to compensate. However, this scenario inevitably leads to abnormal left ventricular hypertrophy.

CHF leads to a progressive ventricular dilation, the ventricle undergoing wall remodeling leading to further loss of function. Wall stress is one of the major determinants of myocardial oxygen consumption. A key point of medical therapy for CHF is to improve myocardial O_2 balance by reducing the radius of the left ventricle, which decreases wall stress and O_2 demand. As pulmonary edema increases, pulmonary capillary wedge pressure increases, leading to backflow into the right heart and, eventually, right heart failure.

Peripheral Vascular Disorders

Peripheral vascular disease (PVD) can affect the arterial, venous, or lymphatic circulatory system. The underlying process is usually atherosclerosis, causing disturbances of circulation to the extremities, resulting in significant loss of function or either the upper or lower extremities. Other causes of PVD are embolism, thrombosis, trauma, vasospasm, inflammation, or autoimmunity (Table 3.5).

TABLE 3.5 Peripheral Vascular Disorders

Disease/Disorder	*Underlying Pathologic Process*	*Clinical Signs and Symptoms*
Occlusive Arterial Disease	Atherosclerotic process leading to disturbances in circulation to the extremities and peripheral ischemia	Loss of hair on the toes, intermittent claudication producing deep muscle pain or cramping due to ischemia which increases during exercise and is relieved by rest. Pain location is determined by site of major arterial occlusion. Other symptoms include decreased skin temperature; dry, scaly, or shiny skin, poor nail and hair growth; ulcerations and possible gangrene on weight bearing surfaces
Raynaud's Disease	Vasomotor disorder associated with hypersensitivity of the digital arteries to cold, release of serotonin, disposition to vasospasm	Digital pallor increasing to cyanosis with cold, numb, red, and painful digits
Thrombophlebitis	May be superficial (often iatrogenic, associated with insertion of intravenous catheters) or deep (one-third of individuals above 40 who have had major surgery or MI). Associated with venous stasis, hypercoagulability, or injury to the venous wall	Venous distension with a palpable, hard cord running with the vein. Other signs include redness, warmth, and swelling
Lymphedema	Excessive accumulation of fluid in tissue spaces secondary to an obstruction of the lymphatic system from trauma, infection, radiation, or surgery	Symptoms include edema of the dorsum of the foot or hand and decreased range of motion. Usually worsens after prolonged dependency
Hypertension	Essential hypertension is of unknown origin or no identifiable cause. Secondary hypertension may have a number of underlying causes, such as renal artery stenosis, oral contraceptive use, hyperthyroidism, adrenal tumors, and medication use	May be entirely asymptomatic in early stages, but may include the following symptoms: occipital headache, dizziness, flushed face, vision changes, spontaneous nosebleeds, and nocturnal urinary frequency

Disease/Disorder	*Underlying Pathologic Process*	*Clinical Signs and Symptoms*
Transient Ischemic Attack	Hypertension	Sudden difficulty with speech, temporary blindness, paralysis or extreme weakness affecting one side of the body
Orthostatic Hypotension	May occur as a normal consequence of aging or secondary to the effects of drugs such as antihypertensives, diuretics, and antidepressants	Light-headedness, syncope, visual blurring, sense of weakness

Chapter Question

1. Distinguish between angina and a heart attack. How would you approach each in a first aid emergency?

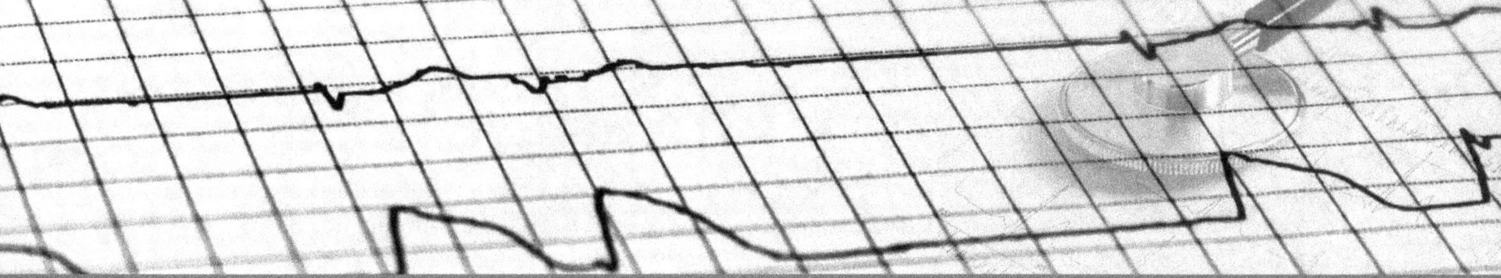

CHAPTER 4

Concepts of Clinical Exercise Testing

Determining functional capacity via clinical exercise testing is a necessary first step in the rehabilitation of heart patients. Once functional capacity is known, exercise prescriptions can be written that result in an increase in cardiovascular endurance, ultimately reducing functional limitations and disabilities.

CONTENT OUTLINE

Therapeutic exercise intervention is a key ingredient in improving cardiovascular health. Cardiovascular health is related to **functional aerobic capacity** (FAC), the decline of which is itself a consequence of the combined effects of aging and chronic disease. Regardless of the causative factor, a reduced FAC hampers patients' ability to adequately perform activities of daily living. There is a growing expectation of long-term benefits from enhanced fitness, including a reduction of morbidity, disability, and mortality from chronic disease, especially cardiovascular disease (CVD). When improved function occurs, patients experience reduced functional limitations and, potentially, can regress their disability leftward (Fig. 4.1), an achievement with important ramifications for the personal lives of these individuals and for society at large. Exercise intervention, therefore, ultimately allows individuals to maintain productive lives. Accordingly, therapeutic programs for people with multiple chronicities requires proper assessment procedures on which to base activity prescriptions.

Active Pathology ⟷ Impairment ⟷ Functional Limitation ⟷ Disability

FIGURE 4.1 Nagi's disablement model. The model shows the progression (rightward movement) to disability, but regression (leftward movement) can occur with proper treatment.

Source: "Nagi S. Disability consepts revisited: implications for prevention. In: Pope A, Tarlov A, eds. Disability in America: toward a national agenda for prevention. Washington, DC: Institute of Medicine, National Academy Press, 1991.

Measuring Functional Aerobic Capacity

When exercise is performed in a continuous and rhythmic manner for a prolonged period of time, cardiovascular endurance involves the capacity of the cardiopulmonary system to sustain elevated levels of O_2 metabolism. Therefore, cardiovascular endurance is the degree to which an individual can marshal cardiovascular, pulmonary, and muscular (metabolic) reserves to deliver and utilize O_2 during exercise.

FAC or maximal oxygen consumption ($\dot{V}O_{2max}$) defines the functional limits of the cardiovascular system. Cardiovascular endurance is usually quantified as $\dot{V}O_{2max}$ (also referred to as aerobic power or aerobic capacity), the maximal volume of O_2 consumed in mitochondrial respiration during maximal effort rhythmic exercise involving large muscle groups. The level of fitness (i.e., the amount of endurance) largely determines such things as biological age, disease risk, general health, and the ability to perform daily physical tasks. The ability to walk vigorously, perform household or employment tasks, or recreate without becoming "winded" requires an adequate level of cardiovascular endurance. Being able to accurately determine cardiovascular endurance is extremely important in adequately assessing heart patients. Therefore, knowledge of a patient's FAC helps determine therapeutic parameters.

When considering the FAC of individuals, $\dot{V}O_{2max}$ is the variable that most directly defines the concept and is accepted as the criterion measure of cardiovascular endurance, providing the clinician with knowledge of the individual's functional ability.

Regardless of the objectives of the therapeutic exercise program, $\dot{V}O_{2max}$ is accepted as the most important measure of cardiovascular endurance impairment. For this reason, direct measurement of, or at least a valid estimation of, $\dot{V}O_{2max}$ is essential to the successful administration of preventive and rehabilitative exercise programs. Therefore, the purpose of determining $\dot{V}O_{2max}$ includes the following:

- Provides data helpful in the development of exercise training prescriptions
- Collection of baseline and follow-up data allows for evaluation of progress
- Increases motivation for entering and adhering to exercise programs
- Assists in diagnosis and treatment of hypokinetic diseases
- Educates participants as to the benefits of cardiovascular fitness and endurance exercise

Knowing a patient's $\dot{V}O_{2max}$ allows the clinician to identify vocational and leisure activities that may be included or excluded on the basis of the individual's FAC. Decisions to allow return to work or to classify as disabled may also be justified using the $\dot{V}O_{2max}$ score. For example, a $\dot{V}O_{2max}$ below 15 $mL{\cdot}kg^{-1}{\cdot}min^{-1}$ defines a moderately impaired respiratory system in pulmonary patients. For purposes of employment, scores less than 15 $mL{\cdot}kg^{-1}{\cdot}min^{-1}$ are indicative of physical impairment.

$\dot{V}O_{2max}$ can also be accurately estimated without having to rely on expensive laboratory equipment required for directly measuring the variable. Procedures used for predicting $\dot{V}O_{2max}$ have proven to be valid and reliable. When valid and reliable methods to estimate $\dot{V}O_{2max}$ are chosen, there is a close relationship between the estimated and actual $\dot{V}O_{2max}$ values. This saves the time and expense of performing direct measurements. The absence or presence of the following factors affects the association between estimated and actual $\dot{V}O_{2max}$:

- **Habituation**—familiarization with the testing ergometer improves the association between predicted and actual values, and the variability between these scores decreases
- **Fitness**—increased fitness levels decrease the variability between actual and predicted scores —$\dot{V}O_{2max}$ is overpredicted in well-trained individuals, whereas $\dot{V}O_{2max}$ is underpredicted in untrained individuals
- **Heart disease**—predicted values are higher than actual values in these patients
- **Handrail holding**—overpredicts $\dot{V}O_{2max}$ as predicted values are greater than actual values
- **Exercise protocol**—as the exercise testing protocol becomes more demanding (i.e., the incremental stages of the test progress more vigorously in intensity from stage to stage), $\dot{V}O_{2max}$ is overpredicted and variability increases.

Choosing when to measure $\dot{V}O_{2max}$ versus when to estimate it can be difficult. For research purposes, the measurement of $\dot{V}O_{2max}$ is required. For clinical purposes, a determination should be made as to the degree of accuracy required of the values. Clearly, if prediction techniques significantly over- or underestimate the actual value of a patient's FAC, subsequent exercise prescriptions will not be as precise as they could be. $\dot{V}O_{2max}$ can be predicted using submaximal or maximal laboratory exercise tests (or field exercise tests) and associated prediction equations. An example is the use of the Bruce Protocol in stress testing patients. Once the endpoint is reached, the following equations can be applied to predict the FAC of the individual:

- Men: $\dot{V}O_{2max} = 14.8 - (1.379 \times T) + (0.451 \times T^2) - (0.012 \times T^3)$
- Women: $\dot{V}O_{2max} = (4.38 \times T) - 3.9$

In using these equations, T stands for total time on the treadmill, measured as a fraction of a minute. For example, a test time of 9 minutes and 30 seconds would be written as $T = 9.5$.

Types of Exercise Tests

Choosing an appropriate exercise test for the purpose of documenting a patient's FAC is an important decision. The decision involves matching the proper exercise mode and exercise protocol to the patient. Consideration should be given to test **specificity** and **sensitivity**, the physical limitations of the patient, and the reason for testing. Individuals must be able to perform the exercise mode chosen so that the cardiopulmonary system can be adequately stressed. In some instances, it may be appropriate to match exercise mode to the job task of the individual, which is especially important when testing for job-related fitness. Typically, most individuals are more accustomed to walking than to other exercise modes, making treadmill tests extremely popular. However, patients may have orthopedic limitations that preclude one test versus another. The key is to determine which exercise mode will provide potentially more stress to the cardiopulmonary system so that test specificity and sensitivity are maximized.

Mode selection is made easy when obvious physical limitations are present. For example, when a patient has severe arthritis in both knees, leg exercise modes, such as treadmill walking or cycling, are not warranted. Other examples that may preclude treadmill walking as the mode of choice are postural instability, neuromuscular disease, paraplegia, or stroke. In these cases, leg or arm ergometry may be a viable alternative; however, the relative unfamiliarity most individuals (especially chronic disease patients) have with cycling exercise causes cycling to be a second choice unless necessary. The reason for this is that most individuals do not participate in cycling, and, thus, they may experience local muscular fatigue and must end the test prior to a work rate being achieved that can adequately stress the cardiopulmonary system. The diagnostic value of the test in such instances is reduced. Similar problems are present when arm ergometry is selected as the test mode. Finally, in some circumstances it may also be necessary to select nontraditional exercise modes (See Box 4.2) to evaluate

BOX 4.2: NONTRADITIONAL EXERCISE TESTS

Exercise testing using modes of activity designed to re-create patterns of activity occurring in patients' daily lives is often necessary. These exercise tests are referred to as task-specific tests. They are useful in verifying work capacity for job-related functions and to evaluate symptoms that occur only with specific types of exercise. Jobs that require individuals to carry heavy tools and boxes, get in and out of different body positions repeatedly, climb stairs, walk through viscous material such as water or mud can be simulated in the lab, or the test can be field based. Carrying objects while walking on a treadmill has been an alternative and useful mode of testing for years. Such tests evaluate reproducible exertional symptoms specific to one type of exercise. For example, individuals often complain of exertional symptoms when lifting objects. The activity pattern may not be reproducible in the laboratory, and trying to replicate the symptoms in field testing may be impractical. In such situations, monitoring the actual activity performed in daily life is preferable. This can be accomplished by means of devices such as a Holter monitor that can capture electrocardiographic evidence as symptoms are documented by the individual. Health care personnel should be cognizant of these alternative methods of testing to best understand patients' symptomology in relation to their specific exertional pattern.

the patient, as when task-specific function and symptomology are assessed. In these instances, patients can be made to carry heavy objects, climb stairs, or wear weighted belts. It is often within the therapist's professional discretion to devise such tests to properly assess patients' physiological and symptomatic response. *How would you devise a test if a patient informs you that he/she gets chest pain only when shoveling snow?* Movement tasks may be so unique and symptoms so task specific as to demand that therapists use creativity in devising test procedures and conditions to adequately evaluate their patient.

Various graded exercise protocols have been designed and successfully used during the past half-century. These tests are either continuous or discontinuous, with most of the tests utilizing walking, running, or cycling as the mode of exercise. Generally, there is a strong correlation between $\dot{V}O_{2max}$ values obtained from continuous and discontinuous tests when performed with the same mode of exercise, but the values obtained for cycling are approximately 10% lower than those for treadmill protocols. Discontinuous loading (rest periods interspersed with exercise periods) is used when patients cannot tolerate continued exercise with increasing work intensities. A common example of this is arm ergometer testing. However, when patients can tolerate uninterrupted exercise, continuous loading is chosen. In continuous loading, stages last approximately 2 to 3 minutes each, which is usually enough time for the cardiovascular system to adjust to steady state with each exercise load (stage). Both types of protocols are graded, in that each stage has a metabolic equivalent (MET) value (1 MET = 3.5 $mL{\cdot}kg^{-1}{\cdot}min^{-1}$) assigned to it based on the workload of the stage. That is, these tests begin at one level of exertion or metabolic intensity (i.e., MET level) and advance in different degrees of exertion over time from stage to stage. If the protocol has large increases in intensity between stages, each stage should be longer to allow the cardiovascular system time to adjust to the new workload. This would allow a more precise determination of the cardiovascular responses to a given stage, and the exercise dose is more precisely matched to a physiological response. This is very important to achieve in clinical testing where functional capacity needs to be determined and exercise prescriptions are written.

Another type of continuous protocol is ramp loading. Here, the protocol progresses more rapidly in that each stage is shorter in duration (typically 1 minute). Work intensity on the treadmill or cycle ergometer is changed every minute. For instance, treadmill speed may be held constant with gradual changes in grade (1%–3%) every minute, whereas on the cycle ergometer, power output may change by 5 to 25 watts every minute. The jumps in workload are small, which are tolerated well by patients, but there is no allowance for the attainment of physiological steady state with each stage because stage duration is too short. However, since physiological steady state is not achieved it is harder to define the individual's FAC in terms of workload achieved. Continuous ramp protocols are best used when $\dot{V}O_{2max}$ is being determined by direct measurement.

Purpose of Clinical Exercise Testing

There are three major purposes of clinical exercise testing:

1. Therapeutic application—determines FAC (cardiovascular endurance, $\dot{V}O_{2max/peak}$)
2. Diagnostic application—determines the presence of disease
3. Prognostic application—determines the probable outcome of the disease.

These three general purposes, while distinct, are not mutually exclusive. For example, knowledge of an individual's FAC is useful information for both diagnostic and prognostic purposes. The first application, functional testing, is valuable for activity counseling, exercise prescription, and/or disability assessment. The second application, diagnostic testing, is the initial test of choice to evaluate individuals with at least an intermediate probability of significant coronary artery disease. And in the third application, exercise testing is employed as a tool for prognostic assessment using several indices and the Duke nomogram (Fig. 4.2). Prognosis is related

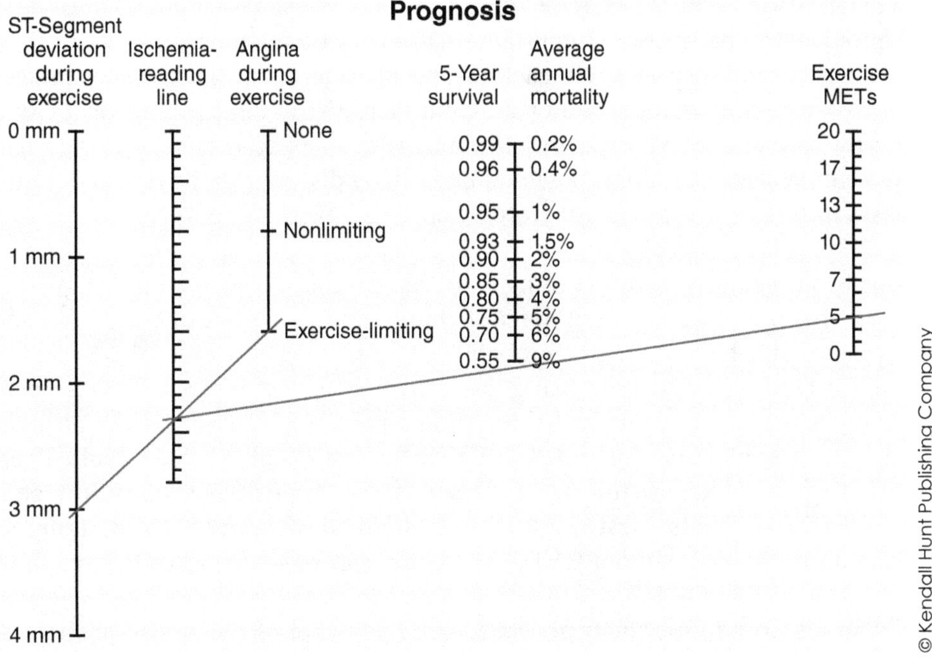

FIGURE 4.2 The Duke nomogram. Patient prognosis can be determined in a process that uses data from an exercise test. ST-segment depression (extreme left scale), angina (middle scale), and functional aerobic capacity in METs (extreme right scale) are determined during exercise testing. The example shows 3-mm ST-segment depression and an anginal episode that was limiting during the test (the test was ended owing to chest pain). These were documented on their respective lines on the nomogram, and a straight line connecting these points is shown. The intersecting point on the ischemia reading line is then connected (with a straight line) to the point signifying the exercise tolerance (5 METs) achieved on the test. This line intersects the prognosis line, which signifies the 5-year survival and average annual mortality rate. In this example, both these qualities are low.

to FAC (measured as $\dot{V}O_{2max}$ or estimated by METs for the work rate performed). In this regard, clinically significant METs for maximal exercise capacity are related to prognosis in the following fashion:

- < 5 METs—poor prognosis; usual limit of functional capacity immediately after myocardial infarction; peak cost of basic activities of daily living
- 10 METs—prognosis with medical therapy as good as coronary bypass surgery

- 13 METs—excellent prognosis regardless of other exercise responses
- 18 METs—elite endurance athletes
- 20 METs—world-class athletes

In general, exercise testing may be used to evaluate coronary artery disease and pulmonary symptoms, to evaluate the effects of cardiopulmonary procedures and the effects of therapy, and to prescribe a safe level of exercise and physical activity for the apparently healthy, asymptomatic population and for individuals with chronic disease.

Sensitivity, Specificity, and Predictive Accuracy of Exercise Testing

The chief diagnostic tool used in exercise testing is the electrocardiogram (ECG). The ECG indicates whether the myocardium is receiving enough O_2 during exercise. Therefore, in exercise testing, the ECG is used to define test outcome as either positive (abnormal) or negative (normal) for ischemia. As is demonstrated further on, the criterion for a positive exercise ECG test is usually an ST segment that is depressed ≥ 1 mm below the **isoelectric** line and that stays depressed for at least 0.08 seconds beyond the J point. However, for the ECG to be effective as a diagnostic tool during exercise testing, an effective exercise protocol must be selected. Matching the exercise protocol to a patient is an important preliminary function.

Both the ECG and the testing protocol impact test specificity and sensitivity. That is to say, exercise testing may be useful in confirming (specificity) and ruling out (sensitivity) disease. The key to successful exercise testing is to stress the cardiopulmonary system sufficiently with an exercise mode that is correctly selected and applied to the patient. When this is done, potential underlying disease may be revealed as indicated by ECG ischemic responses in this way. The exercise protocol and ECG work in concert to maximize test specificity and sensitivity.

Although one of the goals of exercise testing is to help diagnose disease, it is designed to provide not a definitive diagnosis but only an estimate of the probability of the presence of disease. In addition, exercise testing alone cannot establish the estimated probability of disease. There must also be an understanding of the prevalence of CVD in the population being tested before the test is given. This is postulated in Bayes theorem, which states that the posttest probability that a person has disease is the product of the pretest probability of disease presence and the probability that the test result is a true result. There are four possible outcomes to diagnostic exercise testing: (1) True positive—a positive test result in an individual with CVD, (2) False positive—a positive test result in an individual without CVD, (3) True negative—a negative test result in an individual without CVD, (4) False negative—a negative test result in an individual with CVD.

Theoretically, sensitivity and specificity percentages are best applied to population characteristics and not individuals. The ability of the test to detect disease and help the clinician make a correct diagnosis is determined by test sensitivity, specificity, and predictive accuracy. As sensitivity and specificity approach 100%, the ability of the test to discriminate, i.e., differentiate diseased from nondiseased populations, improves. Sensitivity refers to the percentage of patients tested who have CVD and who also test positive. *Can the test detect disease when it is present?* This is the basic question related to sensitivity. Sensitivity, the percentage of CVD patients who produce an abnormal ECG test result, is quantified as follows:

$$\text{Sensitivity} = \text{TP}/(\text{TP} + \text{FN})$$

TP is the true positive (abnormal ECG exercise test in the presence of CVD) and FN is the false negative (normal ECG exercise test in the presence of CVD). Therefore, sensitivity is equal to all those with truly positive tests divided by all those with disease. As you can see, some individuals with disease will test negative. Sensitivity of exercise testing averages about 68% in controlled studies. This means that 68% of those individuals with disease will have a TP exercise ECG and 32% will have an FN exercise ECG. Exercise test sensitivity increases in patients with multivessel disease.

Specificity is the exact opposite of sensitivity because it focuses on healthy subjects who test negative for CVD. Specificity is the ability of the exercise ECG test to correctly exclude disease when it is absent. Another way of saying this is that specificity is equal to all those with truly negative tests divided by all those without disease. Specificity is quantified as follows:

$$\text{Specificity} = \text{TN}/(\text{TN} + \text{FP})$$

TN is the true negative (normal ECG exercise test and no CVD), and FP is the false positive (abnormal ECG exercise test and no CVD). Specificity of exercise testing averages about 77% in controlled studies. This means that 77% of those individuals without disease will have a TN exercise ECG and 23% will have an FP exercise ECG.

To understand the likelihood that any single individual patient has coronary heart disease requires the use of another statistic—predictive accuracy. Predictive accuracy is a measure of how accurately exercise testing identifies the presence or absence of coronary artery disease in patients. Therefore, predictive accuracy applies to both positive and negative tests in the following manner:

$$\text{Positive Tests: Predictive Accuracy} = \text{TP}/(\text{TP} + \text{FP})$$
$$\text{Negative Tests: Predictive Accuracy} = \text{TN}/(\text{TN} + \text{FN})$$

The strength of exercise testing to predict disease depends on the population being tested. If the likelihood of disease in patients is high based on the presence of CVD symptoms (i.e., typical angina), most of the positive tests will be true positives, and not many will be false positives. The converse is also true. When CVD is not likely present, more of the positive tests will be false positives than true positives. Predictive accuracy is reduced in this case. Also, a predictive value is the level of cardiovascular stress attained by the patient during testing. Unless the patient has attained 85% or more of predicted maximal heart rate during the test, a test should not be classified as negative. The reason for this is that ischemic responses do not appear unless the individual is stressed sufficiently. The 85% predicted maximal HR appears to be a reliable threshold to produce negative results if disease is present.

Components of the Stress Test

Conducting the actual test is the same for all protocols and modes of testing, with only minor differences that are mostly related to working the specific ergometer and protocol during the test. If there is any doubt as to the benefit of testing or the safety of testing for a given patient/client and on a given day, the test should not be performed at that time. The pretest sequence requires that a 12-lead ECG be recorded in the supine and exercise postures. The clinician should note any ECG changes between the supine and the exercise position. Resting blood pressure should also be documented in these positions (supine first). Once resting data are collected, the patient can be moved to the testing ergometer, and the test may commence immediately. The 12-lead ECG should be recorded during the last 15 seconds of each stage of the test and at the peak exercise moment. If any arrhythmia is observed, a 3-lead recoding of it should be made of each occurrence. The 3-lead ECG should be continually observed on the monitor during the test. Blood pressure should be measured during the last minute of each stage and verified if necessary. The RPE rating should also be taken from the patient. Other rating scales such as the ones for dyspnea and angina can also be employed for those patients likely to be limited by these symptoms (Fig. 4.3). The recovery or posttest protocol is followed in a sequential fashion:

- Record a 12-lead ECG immediately after exercise (to capture the peak exercise stress point), and then record a 12-lead ECG every 2 minutes until exercise-induced ECG and hemodynamic changes return to baseline
- Blood pressure measures should be made in a like manner, as was previously outlined for the ECG
- As long as symptoms persist after exercise, symptomatic ratings should be obtained using appropriate scales (Fig. 4.3).

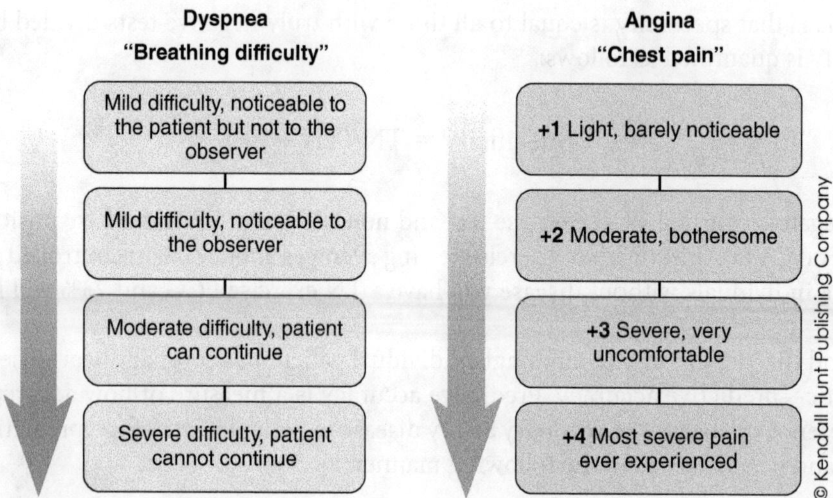

FIGURE 4.3 The dyspnea and angina scales. The two are presented side by side to save space, but one symptom should not be construed as being tied to or caused by the other.

When should the exercise test be terminated? This key question is decided by either the patient, who has the right to terminate the test at any time, or the clinician, who uses clinical judgment to terminate the test when an abnormal finding is presented or when a predetermined end point has been reached. Several medical/physiological indications, grouped according to clinical, hemodynamic, and ECG responses, may arise that will help indicate to the test supervisor that the test should be halted. These include absolute and relative indications for terminating the test:

Absolute Indications

- Drop in systolic blood pressure of ≥ 10 mmHg from baseline blood pressure despite an increase in workload when accompanied by other evidence of ischemia
- Moderate to severe angina (defined as 3 on the standard scale)
- Increasing nervous system symptoms (e.g., ataxia, dizziness, or near syncope)
- Signs of poor perfusion (cyanosis or pallor)
- Technical difficulties monitoring the ECG or systolic blood pressure
- Subject's desire to stop
- Sustained ventricular tachycardia
- ST elevation (≥ 1.0 mm) in leads without diagnostic Q waves (other than V_1 or aV_R)

Relative Indications

- Drop in systolic blood pressure of ≥ 10 mmHg from baseline blood pressure despite an increase in workload in the absence of other evidence of ischemia
- ST or QRS changes such as excessive ST depression (> 2 mm horizontal or downsloping ST segment depression) or marked axis shift
- Arrhythmias other than sustained ventricular tachycardia, including multifocal PVCs, triplets of PVCs, supraventricular tachycardia, heart block, or bradyarrhythmias
- Fatigue, shortness of breath, wheezing, leg cramps, or claudication
- Development of bundle branch block or intraventricular conduction delay that cannot be distinguished from ventricular tachycardia
- Increasing chest pain
- Hypertensive response, that is, systolic blood pressure > 250 mmHg and/or a diastolic blood pressure of more than 115 mmHg

Usually in the clinical arena the test of FAC is symptom limited, in that the end point of the test is dictated by the medical/physiological condition of the patient and not the achievement of $\dot{V}O_{2max}$. Clinical exercise tests should not be halted for an arbitrary criterion such as predicted maximal HR or when 85% of age-adjusted maximal HR has been reached. Rather, what is important is that a true FAC within the patient's symptomatic limitations has been achieved. When viewed this way, FAC can be defined as the peak metabolic/physiological responses and ergometric workload achieved on the test. The clinician should always interpret FAC after considering the signs and symptoms occurring at the termination point. Case Study 4.1 presents results of exercise testing to determine the functional capacity.

CASE STUDY 4.1: Cardiac Bypass Graft Surgery

Stuart (male age 57, weight 81.8 kg, height 172 cm) has a history of coronary artery disease and coronary artery bypass grafts (CABG). He had a history prior to the CABG surgery. He is on dipyridamole, has a body fat of 30 percent, and an age-adjusted maximum HR of 163 bpm. He was given a stress test prior to entering a fitness program. The results are shown below.

Description: Coronary artery disease produces a narrowing of the coronary arteries and restricts the flow of blood to the heart. The purpose of CABG surgery is to correct the situation by improving the flow of blood and O_2 to the heart. Following surgery, Stuart was given a stress test prior to entering a fitness program, as recommended by his physician. The results of his stress test are as follows:

Resting ECG: slight ST-T flattening (no arrhythmias present)
Resting BP: 123/84; Resting HR: 75 bpm
Terminal BP: 170/88; Terminal HR: 135 bpm; Terminal MET: 10.2; Terminal RPP: 230
Terminal RPE: 8; Test terminated due to significant ischemic response, +3 dyspnea, and fatigue.

Bruce Stage	*HR*	*BP*	*MET*	*RPE*	*Comments and Reason for Termination*
1	96 94 96	158/86	**4.7**	3/10 3 4	+2 Dyspnea
2	110 118 118	168/86	**7.1**	4 5 6	+2 Dyspnea, fatigue, ECG showed 1 mm ST/T horizontal depression
3	125 135	170/88	**10.2**	8 8	+3 Dyspnea, fatigue, ECG showed 2.5 mm ST/T horizontal depression

Interpretation: This test is positive for ischemia as ST/T changed from a flattening at rest to 2.5 mm of horizontal depression in the inferior leads at maximal exercise. Angina was not experienced. The return to baseline took 8 minutes. No arrhythmias were present at rest, exercise, or recovery. The physiological responses to exercise were equivocal. HR and systolic BP both increased, and diastolic BP was stable; however, systolic BP failed to increase in a linear fashion from stage 2 to stage 3. Total exercise duration was 8 minutes on the Bruce protocol. The ending stage of Bruce produces a MET response of 10.2 if at steady state. However, Stuart was not at physiological steady state, and, therefore, his functional aerobic capacity (FAC) based on the generalized Bruce equation was 8.9 MET. Therefore, Stuart's FAC is formally documented as 8.9 MET at a HR of 135, BP of 170/88, RPE of 8, and with significant ECG evidence of inferior wall ischemia (without angina) and symptoms of dyspnea and fatigue. Peak workload was 3.4 mph @ 14% grade. Stuart will likely not be cleared to enter the fitness program until the ischemic response to exercise is rectified. He is clearly more suited for a clinical exercise program such as phase III cardiopulmonary rehabilitation.

Chapter Questions

1. Distinguish between the therapeutic and medical purposes of exercise testing.
2. What does test sensitivity mean in relation to clinical exercise testing, and how can one increase the sensitivity of an exercise test?

PART TWO

ELECTROCARDIOGRAPHY BASICS

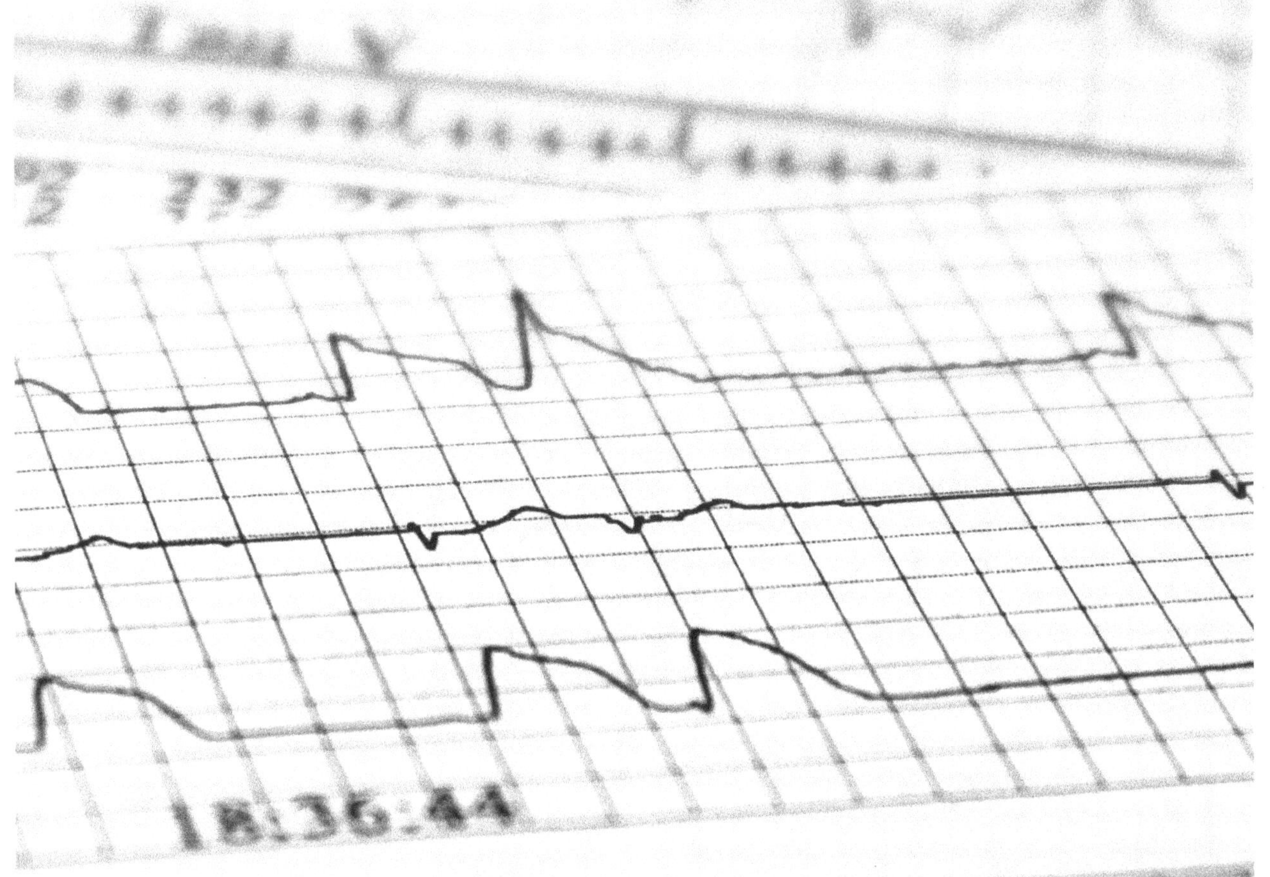

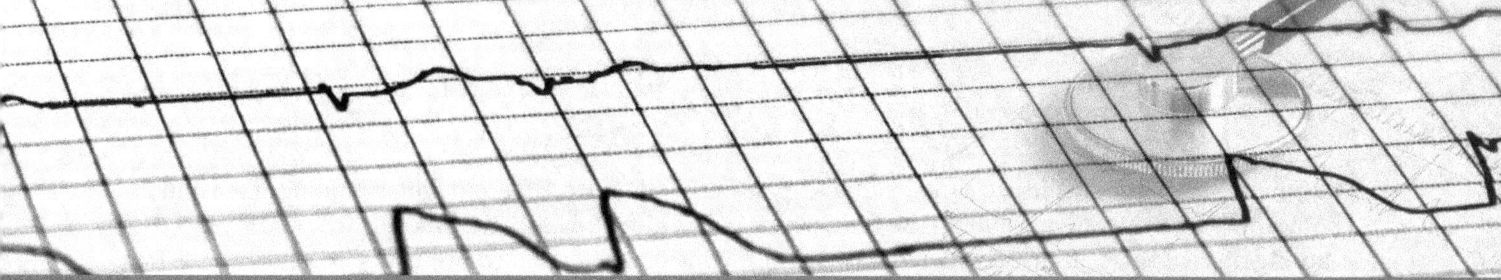

CHAPTER 5

Introduction to the Electrocardiogram

The electrocardiogram is one of the most useful diagnostic tests and is easy to perform routinely in the assessment of patients with chest pain. It has become a cornerstone for diagnosing cardiac ischemia and rhythm disturbances.

CONTENT OUTLINE

- ECG Graph Paper
- The Standard 12-Lead ECG
  - Basic Waveforms
  - Heart Rate
    - Dark Line Method
    - 1500 Method
    - 6-Second Method
  - Development of the Standard 12-Lead ECG
    - Limb Leads
    - Chest Leads
- Normal Sinus Rhythm
  - The P Wave
  - PR Interval
  - QRS Complex
  - ST Segment
  - T Wave
  - U Wave
  - QT Interval
  - TP Interval
- Artifact
- Chapter Questions

The nineteenth century witnessed a tremendous expansion of our knowledge and understanding of the human body and how it operates, including the functioning of the human heart. The **electrocardiogram** (ECG), a recording of the heart's electrical activity, was one of the major scientific advancements to contribute to our understanding of the human heart. Although the first ECG was recorded in 1877 by Augustus Waller, it would be in 1903 that the Dutch physiologist Dr. Willem Einthoven, building on the work of Waller and others, was credited with the invention of the first electrocardiograph machine. Einthoven's first machine (Fig. 5.1), weighing in at over 600 pounds, required the patient to sit with both arms and the left leg in separate buckets of saline solution. It took five technicians to operate it. However, as the precursor to the modern ECG machine, it was to revolutionize the diagnosis of heart disease.

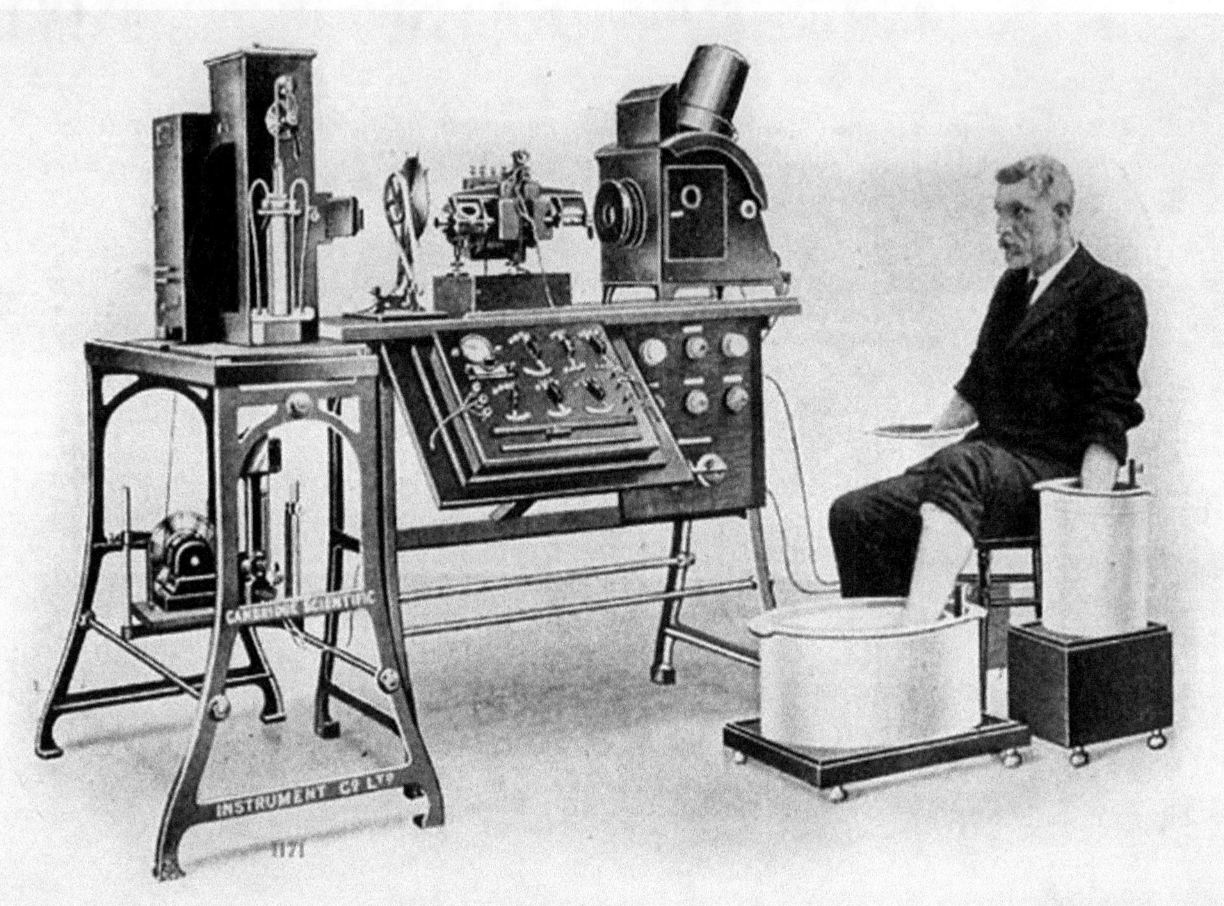
CAMBRIDGE SCIENTIFIC
INSTRUMENT Co LTD
PHOTOGRAPH OF A COMPLETE ELECTROCARDIOGRAPH, SHOWING THE MANNER IN WHICH THE ELECTRODES ARE ATTACHED TO THE PATIENT, IN THIS CASE THE HANDS AND ONE FOOT BEING IMMERSED IN JARS OF SALT SOLUTION

FIGURE 5.1 Dr. Willem Einthoven's electrocardiograph machine.

Source: https://commons.wikimedia.org/wiki/File:Willem_Einthoven_ECG.jpg

Einthoven's first ECG machines were made in Germany, where "kardio" is the word for heart. Hence, the original abbreviation was EKG. In the United States, ECG is the more commonly used abbreviation, but both are still in common use.

Einthoven's buckets acted as **electrodes** that conducted the electrical current from the skin's surface to the device. These three electrodes were used to produce **Einthoven's Triangle**, a principle still employed today and to be discussed later in this chapter. Modern ECG machines utilize small electrodes placed on the patient's skin at specific locations. **Lead** wires are attached to the electrodes, which then transmit the electrical activity to the ECG machine. The electrical activity is displayed on an **oscilloscope** or printed on graph paper. The end of each lead wire is labeled with two letters designating to which electrode each lead should be attached. For example, LL stands for left leg and RA for right arm. Figure 5.2 displays the standard 12-lead electrode placement. This chapter focuses on the formation of the ECG leads and the characteristics of the normal ECG.

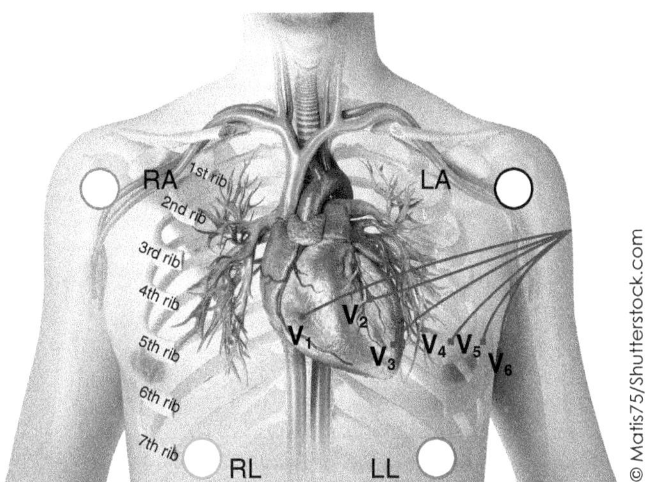

FIGURE 5.2 Standard 12-lead electrode placement.

ECG Graph Paper

Most ECGs are printed onto standardized graph paper. Understanding how the graph paper is configured and the speed at which the machine records the ECG tracing is imperative for accurately interpreting the ECG.

The graph paper consists of a series of 1-mm^2 (1 mm wide and 1 mm tall) small boxes, which normally appear thin and light on the ECG graph paper. Large boxes are 25 mm^2 in area (5 mm wide and 5 mm tall) and are bounded by thicker and darker lines. Thus, one large box contains 25 small boxes. Figure 5.3 depicts the standard graph paper configuration. This allows the ECG waveforms to be measured vertically and horizontally. The amplitude (vertical direction) of the ECG waveforms is measured in millimeters. Because the paper travels through the machine at a standard speed, horizontal measures of the waveforms are in time. At a standard paper speed of 25 mm/s, one small box is 0.04 s long, whereas one large box is 0.20 s long.

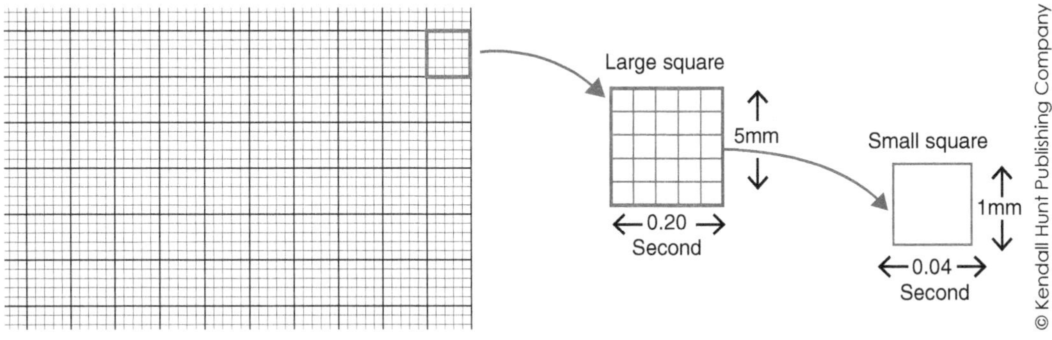

FIGURE 5.3 ECG graph paper. Each small box is 1 mm2. Each large box is 25 mm2. At a standard paper speed of 25 mm/s, each small box is 0.04 s long and each large box 0.20 s.

Though the standard paper speed is 25 mm/s, most ECG machines can operate at two different speeds, 25 mm/s or 50 mm/s. The reason for the second speed setting is that sometimes waveforms can appear too cramped together to clearly view them at standard speed. The faster speed setting spreads out the waveforms, making them easier to visualize and make accurate measurements. However, all measurements taken at this speed must be halved so that comparisons to standard measurements can be made. For example, if a waveform is measured as 0.08 s in length at 50 mm/s, the same waveform at 25 mm/s would be 0.04 s.

A **calibration mark** should be printed at one end of each standard 12-lead ECG printout. It may appear at either the beginning or the end of each recording. The standard **calibration signal** is 10 mm high and 5 mm wide (0.2 s long), depicting that 10-mm signal strength represents 1 mV and that paper speed is the standard 25 mm/s. The calibration signal can either be doubled or cut in half to better interpret the ECG. If ECG waveforms are too big and run into each other on the 12-lead ECG, reducing the calibration signal to 0.5 mV (5 mm high) decreases the waveform size by half. Likewise, if ECG waveforms are too small to adequately view, doubling the calibration signal to 2.0 mV (20 mm high) doubles the waveform size, making them easier to see. Like changes in paper speed, waveform amplitudes measured at half calibration must be doubled to obtain standard measures, whereas those measured at double calibration must be halved to achieve standard measures. If the calibration marks appear 0.4 s (2 large boxes wide), this indicates that a 50 mm/s paper speed was used. These variations in calibration marks are depicted in Figure 5.4.

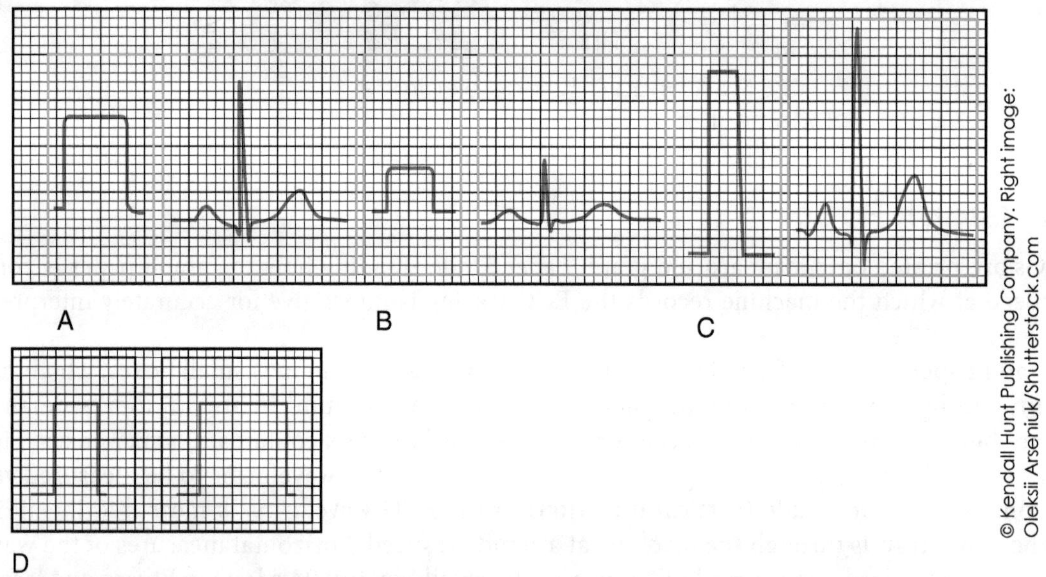

FIGURE 5.4 ECG calibration. **A**, standard. **B**, half. **C**, double calibration marks. **D**, on left, is calibration marks for paper at 25 mm/s and on right for 50 mm/s. Both are using the same amplitude of 10 mm/mV.

The Standard 12-Lead ECG

The standard 12-lead ECG printout is depicted in Figure 5.5. The 12-lead ECG printout is 12 seconds long and contains views of all 12 leads, which are most typically arranged in four columns of three leads with one or more full 12 s **rhythm strip**(s) at the bottom. The first column contains the **bipolar limb leads** (I, II, and III); column two contains the unipolar limb leads (aV_R, aV_L, aV_F); column three contains the first three chest leads (V_1, V_2, V_3); and column four contains the last three chest leads (V_4, V_5, V_6). Leads are separated horizontally by vertical lines called lead dividers. Lead dividers should never be used in ECG interpretation. The rhythm strip displayed most often is of lead II. One should use the rhythm strip to determine heart rate and rhythm (discussed later).

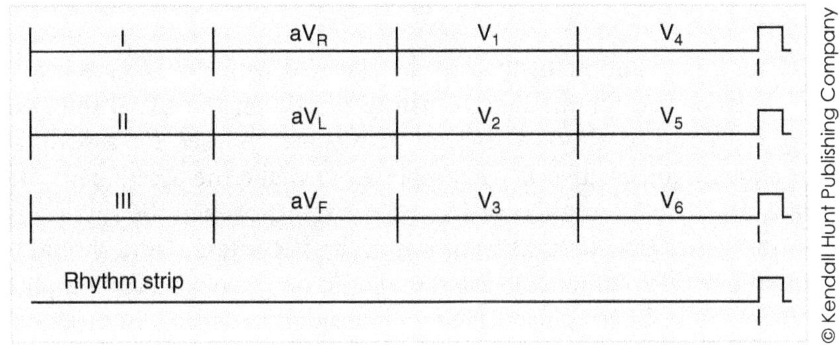

FIGURE 5.5 Standard 12-lead printout configuration. Leads are arranged in four columns of three leads each. Vertical column dividers separate leads. At the bottom is one or more rhythm strips, most commonly of lead II. Calibration marks are displayed either at the beginning or at the end of the 12-lead printout, in this case at the end.

Basic Waveforms

The waveforms traced on the ECG are due to the heart's electrical activity (Fig. 5.6). An ECG lead consists of both a negative end and a positive end. When there is no electrical activity a flat line is traced, the isoelectric line (sometimes called the baseline). **Positive deflections** are waveforms traced above the isoelectric line and occur owing to a wave of electrical activity moving directly in line from the negative pole to the positive pole of a lead. A **negative deflection** occurs below the baseline and is produced by a wave of electrical activity moving directly in line from the positive pole to the negative pole of a lead. Lastly, **biphasic deflections** are waveforms that have both positive and negative portions. A special subset of biphasic deflections are **equiphasic deflections,** which have equal positive and negative portions.

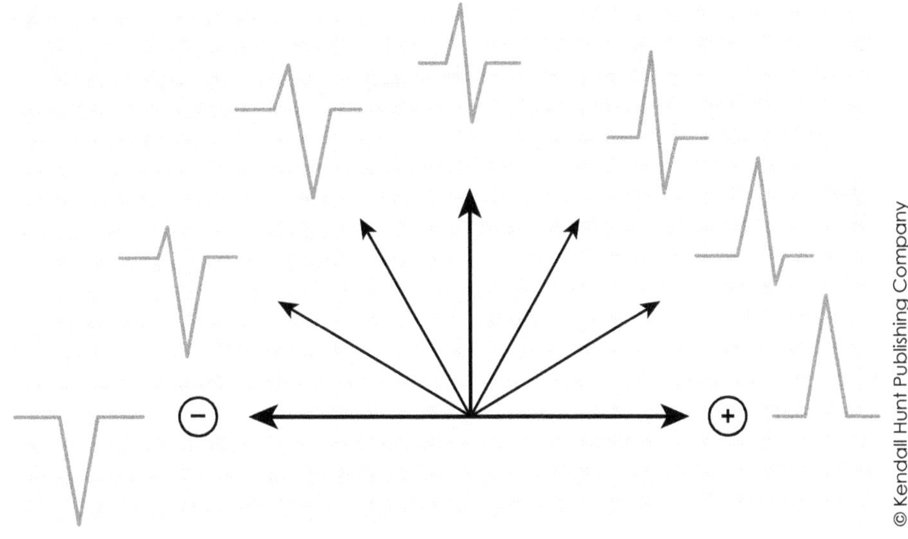

FIGURE 5.6 Types of ECG deflections. Positive deflections are created when a wave of depolarization flows directly toward the positive pole of a lead. Negative deflections are created when a wave of depolarization flows directly away from the positive pole (toward the negative pole) of a lead. Biphasic deflections are created when a wave has both positive and negative portions. An equiphasic deflection has equal positive and negative portions. The biphasic deflections that are more toward the positive pole of the lead have larger positive than negative portions, and conversely for those more toward the negative pole.

Heart Rate

One of the most basic, yet important, items that can be assessed with the ECG is heart rate (HR). There are three common methods employed for the determination of HR on the ECG: the **Dark Line Method**, the **1500 Method**, and the **6-Second Method**. A rhythm strip is always used for assessing HR because rhythm strips usually contain enough consecutive ECG complexes to make the assessment. Before choosing which method to use, determine if there is a **regular** or **irregular rhythm**. When the rhythm is regular, the distance between all R waves is the same. This distance is known as the **RR interval** and should be measured from the most prominent point on one QRS complex to the same point on the next QRS complex. When that distance is different, the rhythm is said to be irregular. There will be small variations in distance between consecutive R waves. A good rule of thumb to follow is if the difference between the shortest RR interval and the longest RR interval is more than 2 small boxes, the rhythm should be considered irregular.

Dark Line Method. The first method commonly used to assess HR on the ECG is the Dark Line Method. This method can be used only with a regular rhythm and usually provides only a rough approximation of the HR. This method is best used in settings in which a close estimate is sufficient, such as during exercise to determine whether an individual is working within their **target HR** range. To use this method, one begins by locating an R wave that falls on a dark line on the ECG paper. That point is used as our starting point. Each subsequent dark line to the right is labeled with a value that indicates its corresponding HR. The first bold line after the selected R wave is labeled 300, the next 150, then 100, 75, 60, 50, 43, 38, and so on. For example, as in Figure 5.7, if the subsequent R wave falls exactly four dark lines away from the starting point, the HR is exactly 75 bpm. Or, as happens most of the time, when the subsequent R wave falls in between the dark lines, an estimation of HR can be made. In Figure 5.8, the subsequent R wave falls between the 4th and the 5th dark lines after the starting point. In this case, the HR can be said to be between 75 and 100 bpm. Because each dark line is 0.2 s in duration at standard paper speed, then:

$$60 \text{ s/min} \div 0.2 \text{ s/beat} = 300 \text{ beats per minute (bpm)}$$
$$60 \text{ s/min} \div 0.4 \text{ s/beat} = 150 \text{ bpm}$$
$$60 \text{ s/min} \div 0.6 \text{ s/beat} = 100 \text{ bpm, etc.}$$

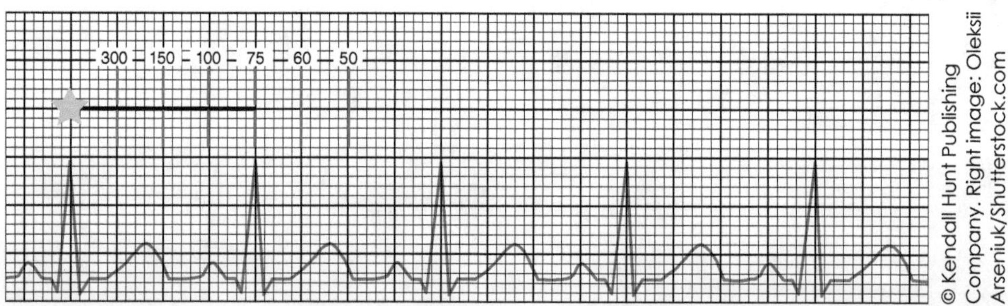

FIGURE 5.7 Dark line method. The peak of each R wave falls exactly on a dark line in this rhythm strip, with each R wave being four dark lines apart. Applying the dark line method, the HR is determined to be 75 bpm.

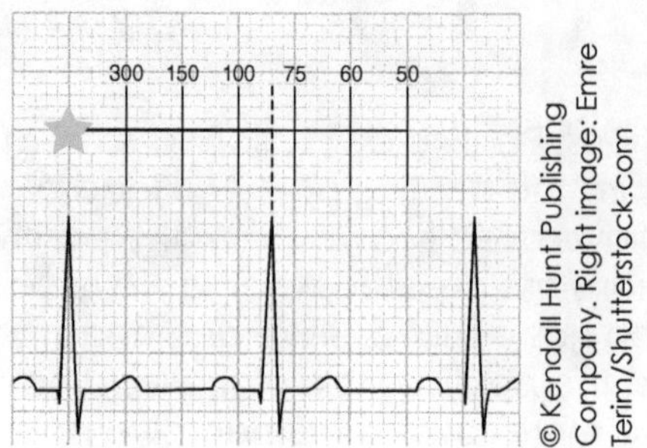

FIGURE 5.8 Dark line method. Label the first R wave as the starting point, as indicated here with a star. Then apply your numbers to subsequent dark lines. The next R wave falls in between the 3rd and 4th dark lines after the starting dark line. Thus, the HR is said to be between 75 and 100 bpm.

Similarly, **rate calculators** are available that allow more accurate and quicker determination of HR. A rate calculator, displayed in Figure 5.9, is often either affixed to the ECG machine for quick reference or laminated and handily available to hold up to the ECG tracing for a speedy measurement. It is more accurate because it has all the HR values for the thin lines identified as well as for the dark lines.

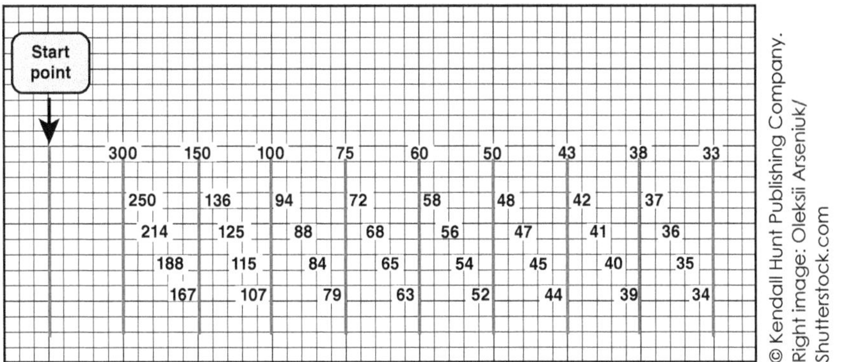

FIGURE 5.9 Rate calculator. The calculator labels not only the HR demarcations for the dark lines but also all lines in between, as can be seen. The rate calculator can be held up to the ECG printout to easily and quickly determine HR.

Note that though we have described how to assess **ventricular rate**, one can use the same method to assess **atrial rate**. When assessing atrial rate, one would use the peak of the P waves instead of the peak of the R waves. Atrial rate can also similarly be determined using the other methods described next.

1500 Method. The next and the most accurate method of assessing HR is the 1500 Method. This method is also used only with a regular rhythm. On the ECG paper, there are 1500 small squares in one minute (60 s/min ÷ 0.04 s/small square = 1500 small squares/min). To employ this method, simply count the number of small squares between consecutive R waves (RR interval). For example, if it is determined that there are 20 small boxes between consecutive R waves, divide 1500 by 20 to get a HR of 75 bpm (Fig. 5.10). Although this method is the most accurate, the major disadvantage of it is that it requires a calculation to be made.

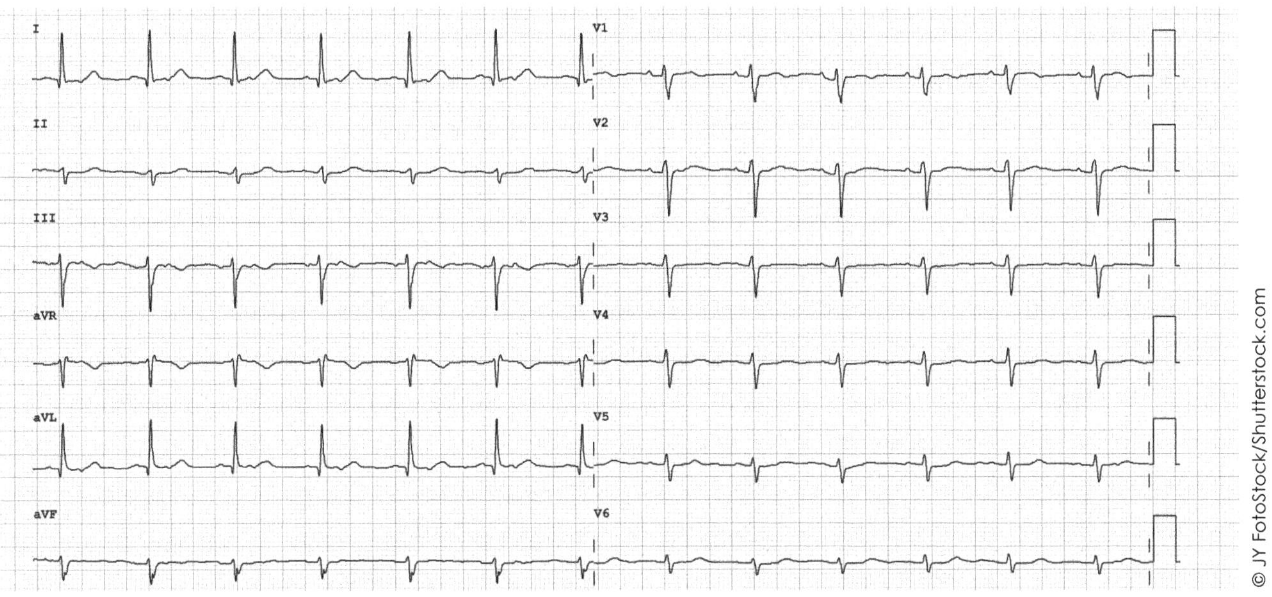

FIGURE 5.10 Example of a12 lead ECG showing normal sinus rhythm. In the 1500 method find the R wave that is directly on top of a dark line (Lead III for example). There are 20 small boxes between consecutive R waves. 1500 / 20 = 75 bpm.

6-Second Method. The third and final method is the 6-Second Method. This is the only method that can be used to estimate HR when the rhythm is irregular. It can also be used with regular rhythms but is not as accurate. To use this method, one simply counts the number of QRS complexes present in a 6-second area of the ECG tracing. After counting the number of QRS complexes present within 6 seconds, multiply that by 10 to get the number of QRS complexes (and, therefore, beats) per minute (Fig. 5.11).

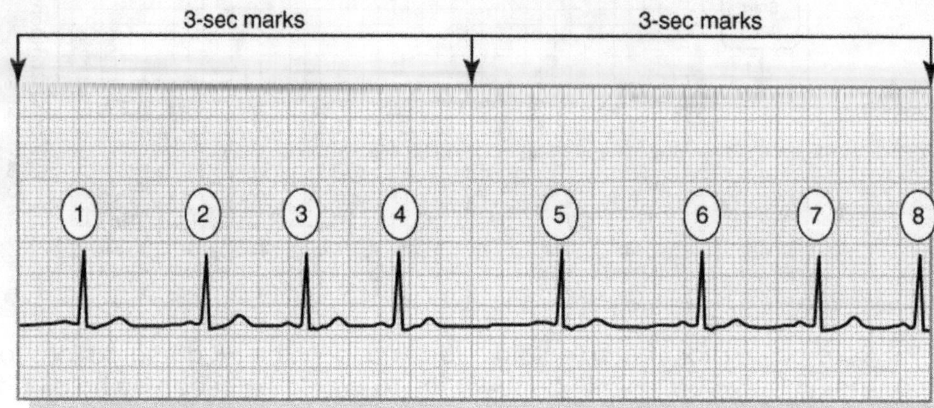

There are 8 cardiac cycles within this six-second strip. Therefore, the HR = 80 bpm (8 cycles × 10 seconds)

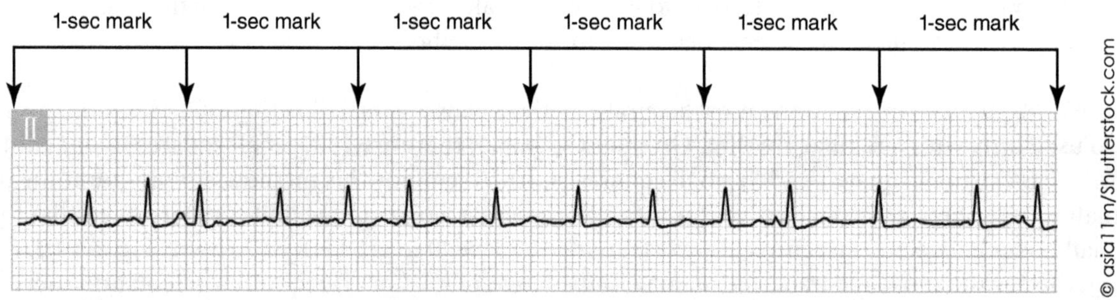

FIGURE 5.11 Six-second method. This entire rhythm strip is 6 seconds long. 14 cardiac cycles occur within 6 seconds on this rhythm strip. Since there are ten 6-second time periods within one minute. $14 \times 10 \approx 140$ bpm.

Most ECG paper has small hash marks at the top or bottom of the ECG paper to indicate 3-second blocks of time. In this case, two 3-second blocks would make up 6 seconds. However, not all ECG tracing paper is marked in 3-second blocks. Sometimes, it may have 1 second marks or 2 second marks, or even no marks. A fail-safe method of ensuring that a 6-second block of time on the ECG is being measured is to count 30 large boxes, which is equal to 6 seconds ($6 \text{ s} \div 0.2 \text{ s/large box} = 30$ large boxes). If your paper does have hash marks, 3 second marks contain 15 large boxes, 2 second marks contain 10 large boxes, and 1 second marks contain 5 large boxes.

The concepts employed for the 6-Second Method could be used for different time intervals. For example, you could count the number of QRS complexes in a 12-second interval and multiply the result by 5 instead of 10. Six seconds is most commonly used for convenience.

Development of the Standard 12-Lead ECG

As previously mentioned, Dr. Willem Einthoven is the Dutch physiologist who developed the principles used in the modern ECG. He defined the specific points on the body for electrode placement for measuring the heart's electrical activity. He used 10 electrodes to record the 12-lead ECG: 6 **limb leads** (3 bipolar and 3 unipolar) and 6 **chest** (precordial or ventral) **leads**.

Limb Leads

Four electrodes are placed to develop the six limb leads: right arm (RA), left arm (LA), right leg (RL), and left leg (LL). Although originally placed on the extremities by Einthoven, the electrodes are much more commonly placed on the torso today, as depicted in Figure 5.2. The right leg (RL) electrode always serves as an electrical ground and is therefore not used to measure any electrical activity. The other three electrodes form the bipolar limb leads (leads I, II, and III) in what is known as Einthoven's Triangle (Figs. 5.12 and 5.13).

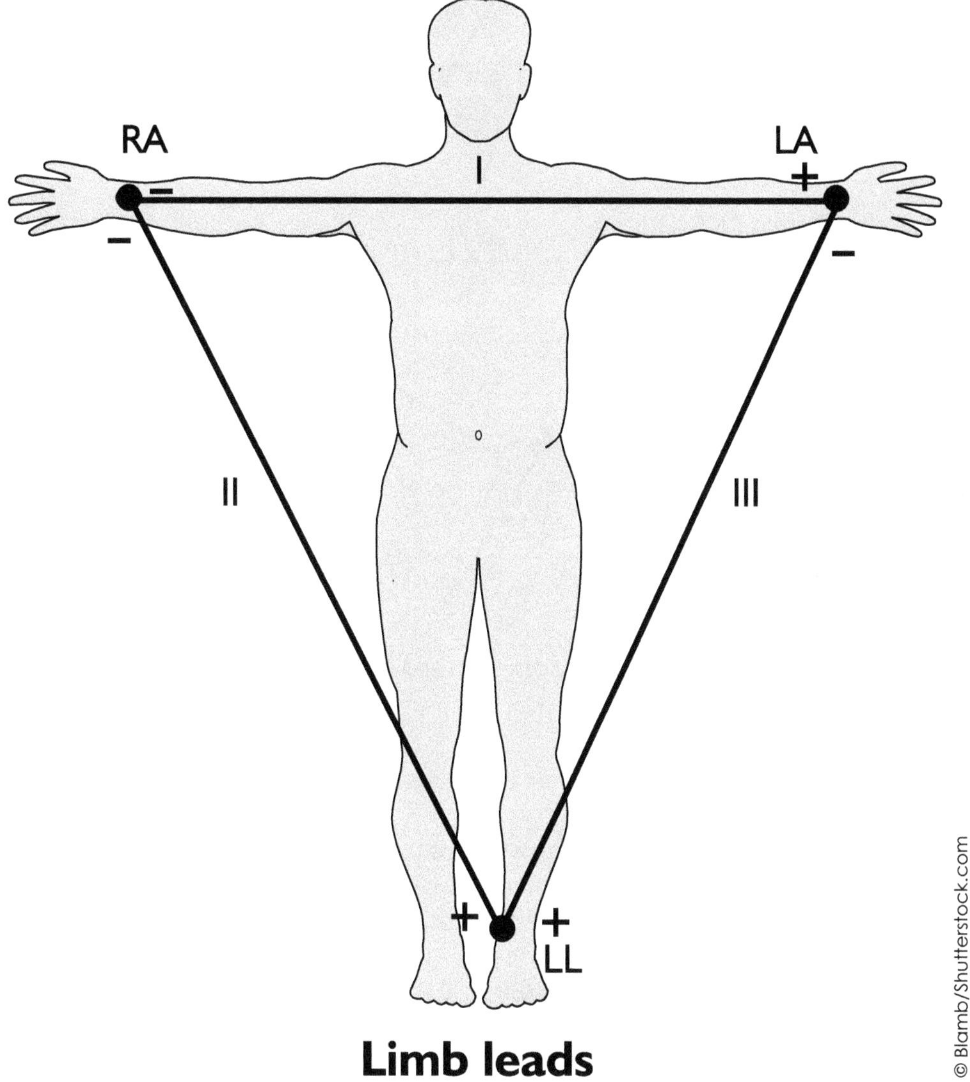

FIGURE 5.12 Einthoven's Triangle. In lead I, the left arm (LA) electrode is the positive pole and the right arm (RA) electrode is the negative pole. In lead II, the left leg (LL) electrode is the positive pole, and the right arm (RA) electrode is the negative pole. In lead III, the left leg (LL) electrode is the positive pole, and the left arm (LA) electrode is the negative pole.

Leads I, II, and III are bipolar because electrical activity is recorded between two electrodes, with one electrode serving as the positive pole of the lead and the other as the negative pole of the lead.

Lead I employs the LA electrode as the positive pole of the lead and the RA as the negative pole. Therefore, Lead I measures electrical activity from the negative pole (RA) to the positive pole (LA). The positive pole of each lead is the direction from which we view the heart. Thus, the positive pole of each lead is considered as the eye or camera viewpoint looking at the heart's electrical activity. Another way to consider this is that the

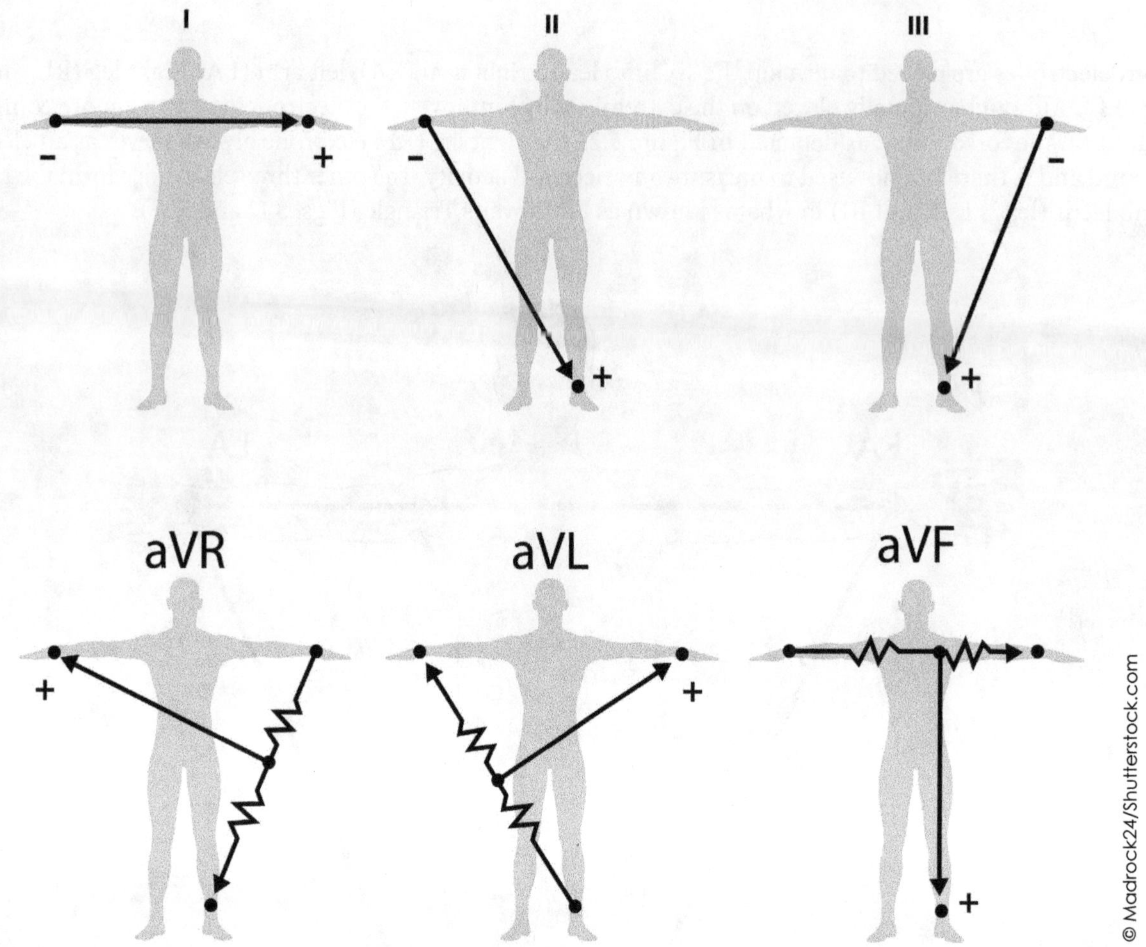

FIGURE 5.13 Limb Leads. Each limb lead is depicted separately.

electrical activity measured at the RA electrode is subtracted from the electrical activity measured at the LA electrode (LA − RA).

Lead II employs the LL electrode as the positive pole of the lead and the RA as the negative pole. Therefore, Lead II measures electrical activity from the negative pole (RA) to the positive pole (LL). The electrical activity measured at the RA electrode is subtracted from the electrical activity measured at the LL electrode (LL − RA).

Lead III employs the LL electrode as the positive pole of the lead and the LA as the negative pole. Therefore, Lead III measures electrical activity from the negative pole (LA) to the positive pole (LL). The electrical activity measured at the LA electrode is subtracted from the electrical activity measured at the LL electrode (LL − LA).

In Einthoven's equation, I + III = II. This means that the electrical activity in lead I plus the electrical activity in lead III is equal to the electrical activity in lead II. Let's prove it!

Lead I = LA − RA, Lead II = LL − RA, Lead III = LL − LA

When Lead I and Lead III are added, the LA placements cancel out, leaving LL − RA, which is lead II.

$$\begin{array}{l} \mathrm{I} = \cancel{\mathrm{LA}} - \mathrm{RA} \\ \underline{\mathrm{III} = \mathrm{LL} - \cancel{\mathrm{LA}}} \\ \mathrm{II} = \mathrm{LL} - \mathrm{RA} \end{array}$$

This means that the sum of the amplitudes of the R waves in leads I and III is equal to the amplitude of the R wave in lead II (Fig. 5.14). If this is found not to hold true, the most likely problem is in the electrode placements. Thus, a good practice is to make sure electrode placements are accurate before assessing the ECG.

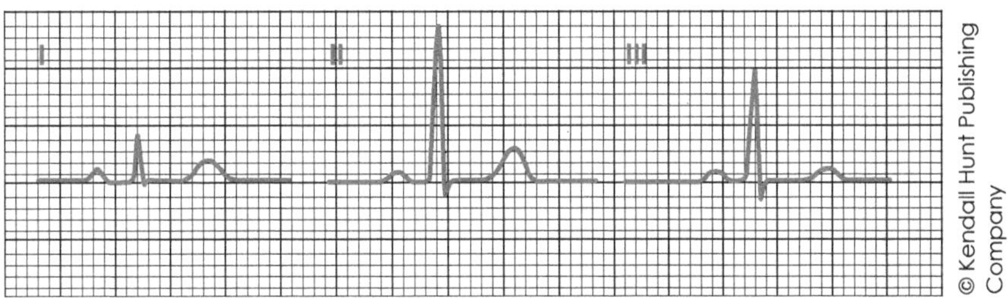

FIGURE 5.14 The amplitude of the R wave in lead I is 4 mm and in lead III is 10 mm. 4 mm + 10 mm = 14 mm. This is equal to the amplitude of lead II.

The **unipolar limb leads** are also known as the **augmented voltage leads** (or augmented vector leads) because they are developed through a combination of leads. Again, like with the bipolar limb leads, the electrodes RA, LA, and LL are used to create these leads. Each electrode serves as the positive pole of one of the leads, while the combination of the other two serves as the negative pole, augmenting the signal strength from the measuring electrode.

Lead aV_F (pronounced augmented voltage foot lead) is measured from the LL electrode to its negative pole, which is the combination of the LA and RA electrodes. **Lead aV_L** is measured from the LA electrode to its negative pole, which is a combination of the RA and LL electrodes. **Lead aV_R** is measured from the RA electrode to its negative pole, which is a combination of the LA and LL electrodes. See Figures 5.13 and 5.15 for a depiction of the unipolar limb leads.

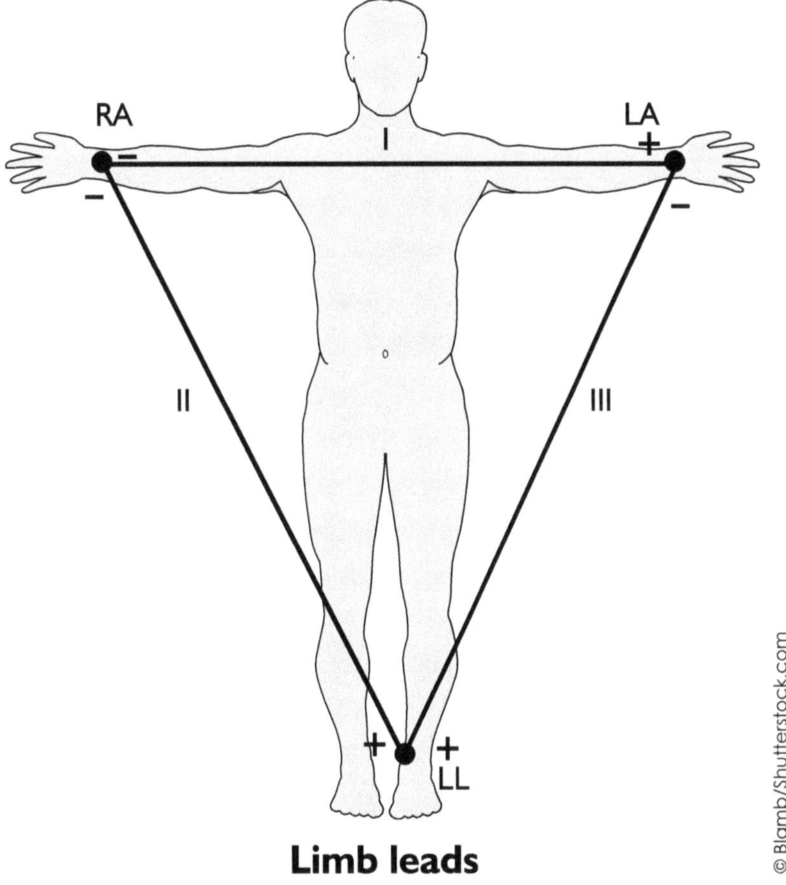

FIGURE 5.15 The unipolar limb leads or augmented voltage limb leads. The positive pole of aVF is the left leg (LL) electrode, whereas the negative pole is a combination of the right arm (RA) and left arm (LA) electrodes. The positive pole of aVL is the left arm (LA) electrode, whereas the negative pole is a combination of the right arm (RA) and left leg (LL) electrodes. The positive pole of aVR is the right arm (RA) electrode, whereas the negative pole is a combination of the left arm (LA) and left leg (LL) electrodes.

The six limb leads measure electrical activity of the heart in the **frontal (coronal) plane.** The **hexaxial reference system** is a diagram that shows the relationship of the six limb leads in the frontal plane (Fig. 5.16). In this system, the circle is divided into 30° segments. By convention, labeling degree marks starts at 0° on the right and proceeds in a clockwise fashion until the 180° mark at the left. The top hemisphere is labeled in a counterclockwise direction using negative degrees. Typically, only the positive pole of each lead is labeled on the hexaxial reference system, and it is implied that the negative pole is 180° away from the positive pole. For example, the positive pole of lead I is at 0° and the negative pole at 180°.

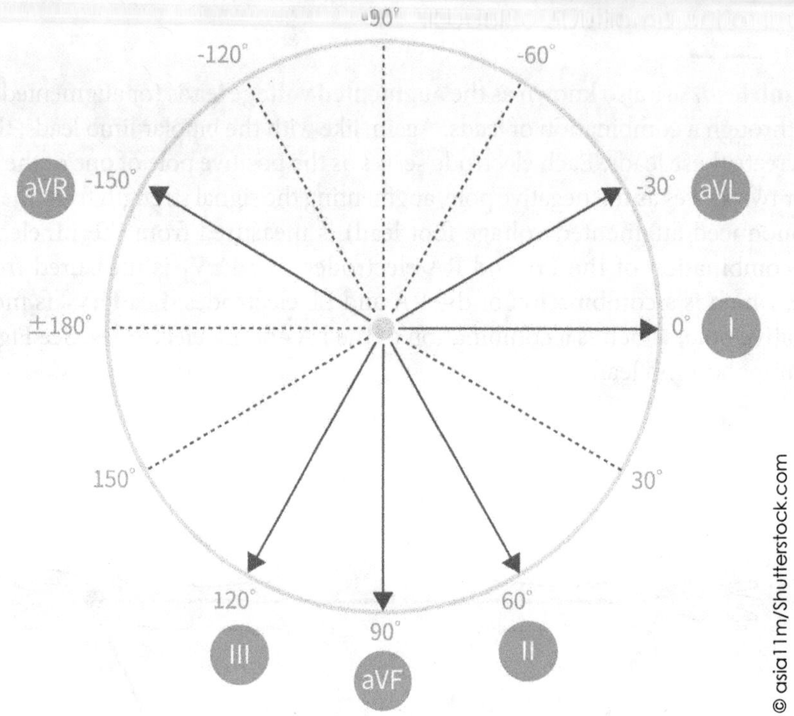

FIGURE 5.16 Hexaxial reference system. The circle is centered at the AV node and is split into 30° segments. The positive pole of each lead is labeled. The negative pole of each lead is 180 away from its positive pole.

The negative degrees convention for labeling the top hemisphere can be confusing. Negative degrees do not necessarily refer to the negative poles of leads. Note that the positive poles of leads aV_R and aV_L are at -150° and -30°, respectively, whereas their negative poles are at +30° and +150°, respectively. In the next chapter, this system is used to determine the heart's mean electrical axis in the frontal plane.

Chest Leads

Unlike the limb leads, **chest** (ventral or precordial) **leads** examine the heart's electrical activity in the **horizontal** (transverse) **plane.** The positive poles of each lead are at the chest locations for **lead V_1, V_2, V_3, V_4, V_5,** and **V_6,** and the negative poles are all a single imaginary point in the center of the heart, usually said to be positioned at the AV node (or an imaginary point in the center of the heart). The electrocardiograph calculates this point. However, a discussion of how it does so is beyond the scope of this text. The positioning of each electrode is displayed in Figure 5.2. Figure 5.17 shows the chest leads in the horizontal plane. The ECG leads V_1 and V_2 view the heart more from the right in the horizontal plane. Leads V_3 and V_4 view the heart from an anterior perspective. Leads V_5 and V_6 view the lateral aspect of the heart.

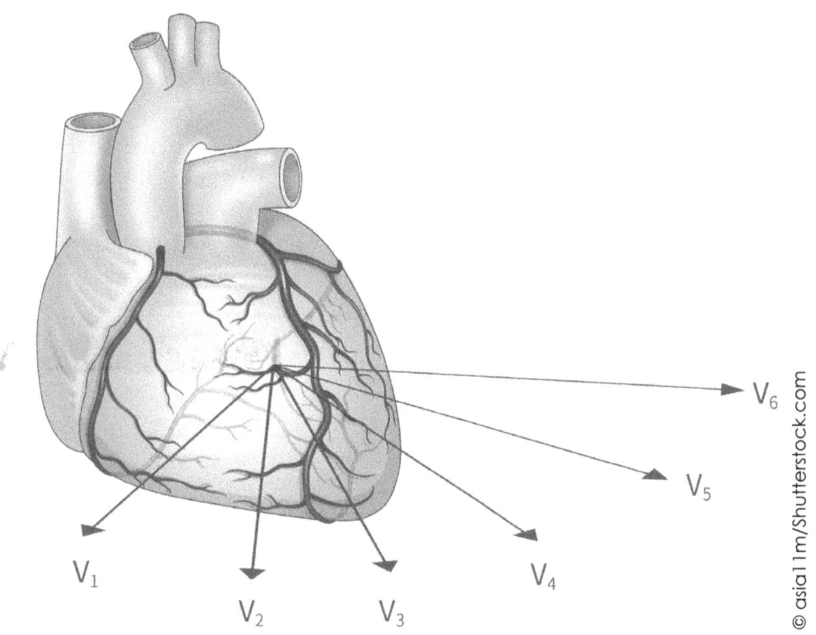

FIGURE 5.17 Chest leads in the horizontal plane. The positive pole of each lead is its electrode, and the negative pole is an imaginary point at the center of the heart, usually said to be located at the AV node.

Normal Sinus Rhythm

Normal sinus rhythm (NSR) is the established rhythm at rest when the heart is functioning properly. In a normal heart, the net vector of the depolarization wave is downward and to the left, toward the apex of the heart. This is within the region known as the **normal axis** (NA) or **normal axis deviation** (NAD), mostly in line with the positive pole of lead II. Thus, the QRS complex in lead II must be positive, and lead aV_R must be negative. Every QRS complex must be preceded by a P wave (1:1 ratio of P to QRS). The heart rhythm must be regular, and the HR must be between 60 and 100 bpm. The length of all intervals must be within normal limits, and all waveforms must be of normal morphology and dimension and be identical in every cycle. Each interval and waveform are depicted in Figure 5.18.

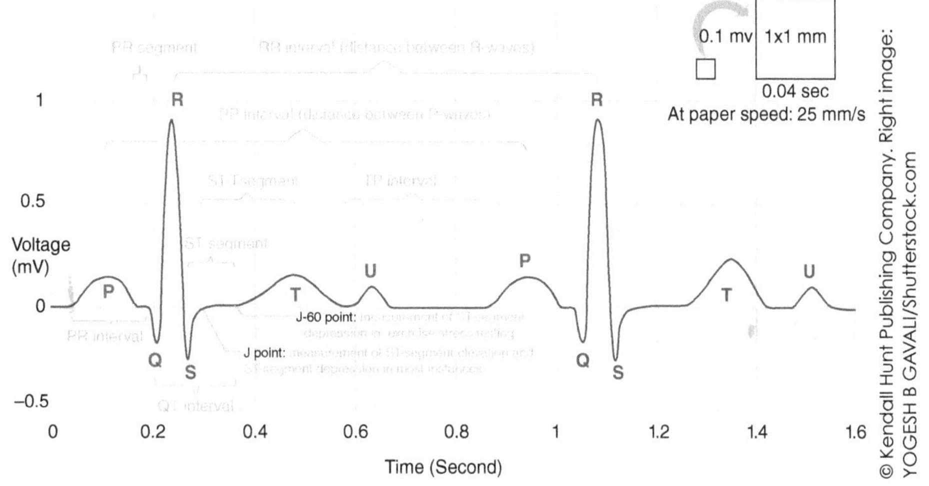

FIGURE 5.18 Basic waveforms and intervals of the ECG.

The P Wave

The **P wave** occurs because of atrial depolarization, which normally originates from the SA node and proceeds to the AV node. The P wave should be a positive deflection in all leads except aV_R, which is a negative deflection. If the reverse is true (aVR is positive and lead II is negative), this indicates that the origin of the rhythm was outside of the SA node and most likely occurred in the AV node. When the AV node is the pacemaker, it is referred to as a **junctional rhythm.**

Normal limits for the size of the P wave are a height of < 2.5 mm (2.5 small boxes) and a duration of 0.06 to 0.10 seconds (1.5–2.5 small boxes; Fig. 5.19). When the P wave is of a different shape (tall and peaked, wide and notched or humped, or biphasic), it is abnormal and most often indicates the presence of some sort of **chamber enlargement.** Additionally, the **PP interval** can be measured to assess the atrial rate. Like the ventricles, the atria should exhibit regularity and a rate of between 60 and 100 bpm. Invariably, the atrial rate should be identical to the ventricular rate in NSR.

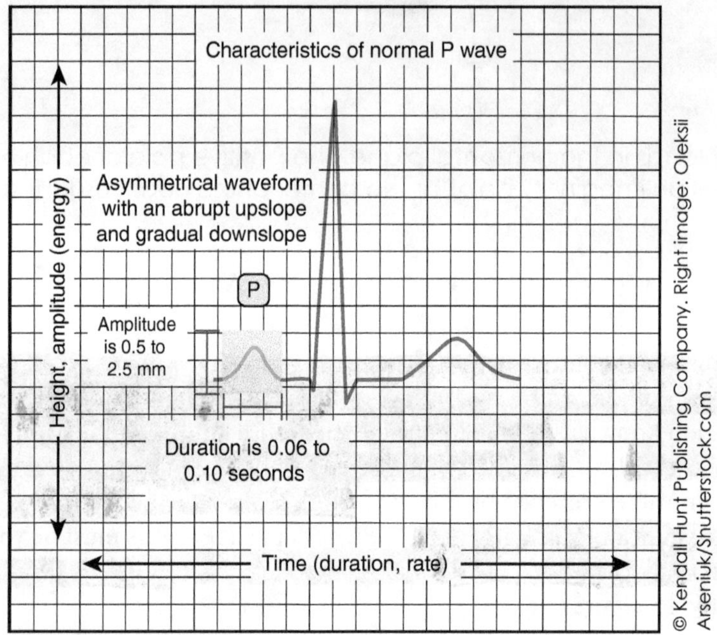

FIGURE 5.19 The normal P wave. The P wave depicted here is approximately 1.25 mm tall and 0.10 s long and is very slightly asymmetrical, with a steeper upslope than downslope.

PR Interval

The PR interval (PRI) commences at the beginning of the P wave and terminates at the start of the QRS complex, as seen in Figure 5.20. The PRI includes both the P wave and the PR segment. It should be between 0.12 and 0.20 s in duration. Short PRIs often occur with **premature atrial complexes** (PAC) in which the beat originates from somewhere above the AV junction but outside of the SA node. Long PRIs most commonly occur in **atrioventricular blocks.** In AV blocks, the electrical impulse has some degree of difficulty passing through the AV junction to the ventricles. The PRI is the time required for the impulse to travel from its area of initiation at the SA node to the AV node to the point where the signal is transferred to the ventricles at the AV bundle (Bundle of His). It represents the time from the initiation of atrial depolarization to the onset of ventricular depolarization. Atrial contraction, and therefore the atrial kick, chiefly occurs during the PR segment. The **PR segment** is nearly always isoelectric, except in certain conditions such as **pericarditis.**

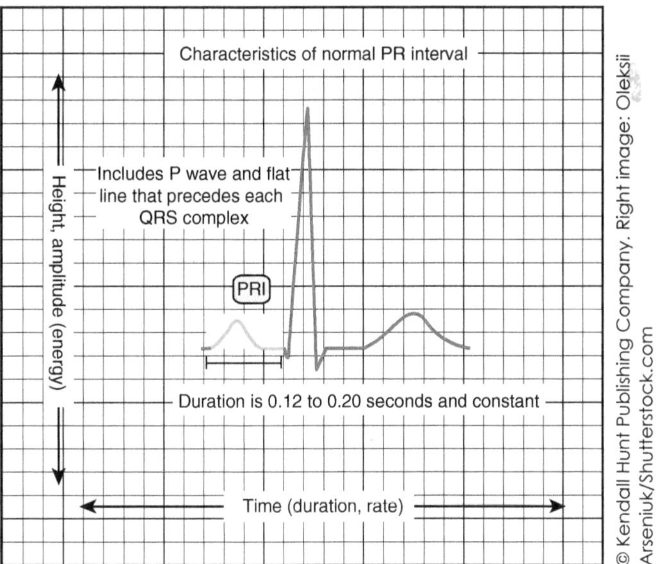

FIGURE 5.20 The normal PR Interval (PRI). The PRI depicted here is approximately 3.75 small boxes or 0.15 s long.

QRS Complex

Ventricular depolarization produces the **QRS complex**, with the larger, more muscular left ventricle exerting dominance. Because of this dominance, the QRS complex to a large degree measures the electrical activity of the left ventricle. The QRS complex is measured from the beginning of the complex (Q or R) to the end of the complex (R or S) and should be 0.06 to 0.10 s (1.5–2.5 small boxes) long (Fig. 5.21). The most common irregularity seen in QRS complexes is an abnormal width, occurring in a variety of conditions. When measuring the QRS complex, begin where the complex begins to deviate from the isoelectric line at the end of the PR segment and end at the point where the complex transitions into the ST segment. Particularly, the ending point is sometimes hard to locate exactly, especially when ST segment elevation or depression is present. Usually, however, one can locate a small inflection point, indicating a change in electrical flow and the end of the QRS complex. Often, this is better seen in one lead than in another. Compare several leads to make the best determination of QRS complex duration.

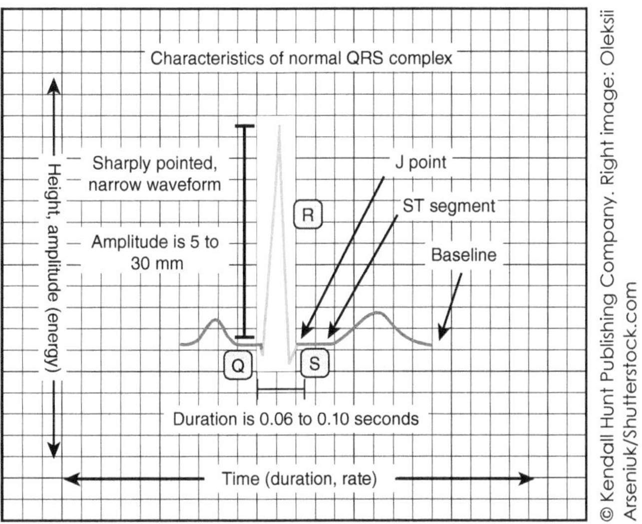

FIGURE 5.21 The normal QRS complex. The QRS complex depicted here contains all three parts (Q, R, and S), is approximately 0.08 s long, and the R wave is approximately 11 mm tall, whereas the S wave dips nearly 1 mm below the baseline for a net 10-mm amplitude for this QRS complex (11 mm − 1 mm = 10 mm).

Regarding the composition and nomenclature of the QRS complex, if the initial deflection is negative, it is a Q wave. It is normal to have either a small Q wave or no Q wave present in the QRS complex, depending on which lead is being viewed. Q waves that are > 0.03 s in duration and/or greater than 1/3 of the amplitude of the R wave are abnormal (Fig. 5.22) and indicative of a past **myocardial infarction** (MI). Any positive deflections of the QRS complex are called R waves. Most, but not all, QRS complexes contain an R wave. Commonly, the R wave is the most prominent part of the QRS complex. Some QRS complexes contain more than one R wave, as occurs in some **bundle branch blocks** (BBB). When there is a second R wave, it is designated R′ (pronounced R prime) (Fig. 5.23). Any negative deflection of the QRS complex seen after an R wave is an S wave. Likewise, more than one S wave can sometimes occur, and the second receives an S′ (pronounced S prime) designation. Sometimes, a combination of lowercase and uppercase letters may be used to indicate the amplitudes of the waves. When the combination is utilized, a lowercase letter denotes an amplitude of < 3 mm. Uppercase letters denote amplitudes > 3 mm (e.g., qRs, RsR′, or rR′). No matter which components are present, the entire complex can always be referred to as the QRS complex.

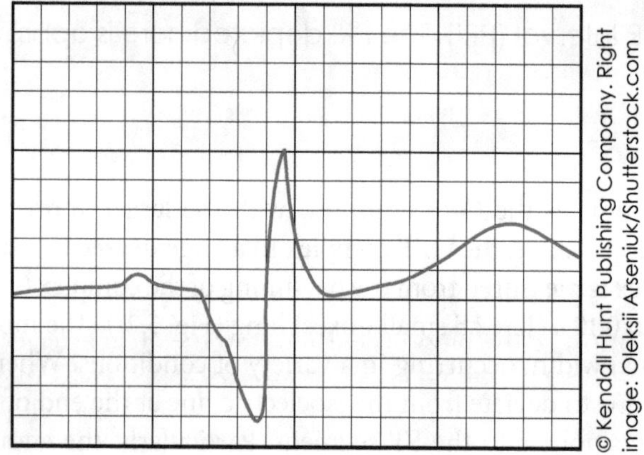

FIGURE 5.22 Significant (abnormal or pathological) Q waves. A Q wave greater than 0.03 s wide or greater than 1/3 the height of the R wave is considered significant. Significant Q wave is a sign of a previous (old) myocardial infarction (MI).

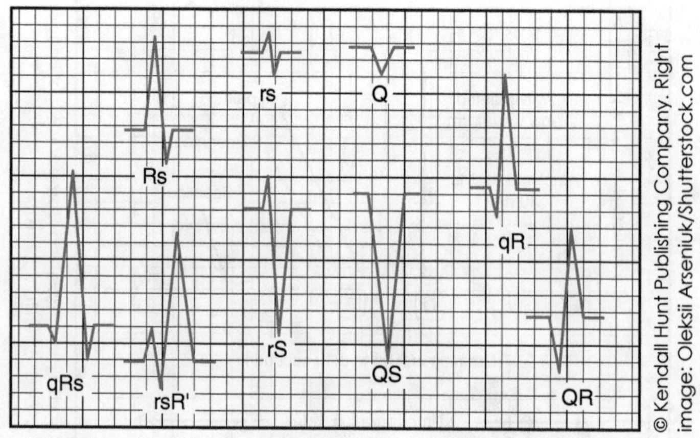

FIGURE 5.23 Examples of QRS complex nomenclature. Waves less than 3 mm in amplitude are labeled with a lowercase letter, and waves greater than 3 mm in amplitude are labeled with an uppercase letter.

As previously discussed, the QRS complex signifies ventricular depolarization. Because the left bundle branch (LBB) is located closer to the bundle of His than the right bundle branch (RBB), the impulse reaches the LBB first, therefore initiating septal depolarization in a left to right fashion. From there, the ventricles depolarize from the septum outward, with the ventricles depolarizing nearly simultaneously, but the left slightly ahead of the right. The larger, more muscular left ventricle is electrically dominant and draws the net wave of depolarization leftward. A Q wave normally results owing to depolarization of the interventricular septum, whereas R and S waves are indicative of near simultaneous left and right ventricular depolarization.

The amplitude of the QRS complex is highly variable, normally ranging anywhere from 5 to 30 mm. Shorter or taller QRS complexes do not always indicate pathology. Tall R waves are usually characteristic of **ventricular hypertrophy**. The amplitude of the chest leads is often higher than that of the limb leads because the chest leads lie closer to the heart. Additionally, QRS complexes are typically of larger amplitude in men than women and likewise in younger than older individuals.

The QRS complex varies from one lead to the next because each lead views the heart from a different angle. In leads I, II, III, aV_F, V_5, and V_6, the QRS complexes are primarily positive. In leads aV_R, aV_L, V_1, and V_2, they are primarily negative, whereas leads V_3 and V_4 are primarily more biphasic. These trends will be of value when assessing the ECG for the presence of certain conditions.

ST Segment

The **ST segment** (Fig. 5.24) is normally a time during which there is no electrical activity in the heart between ventricular depolarization (QRS complex) and ventricular repolarization (T wave). Thus, the ST segment is normally isoelectric. It is measured from the end of the QRS complex to the beginning of the T wave. The ST segment occurs during phase 2 (plateau) of the action potential. As depolarization has already occurred, myocardial contraction has begun, and the ST segment typically correlates with the time right after the opening of the semilunar valves when most of the blood is ejected into the great arteries producing the stroke volume. Refer to the Wiggers Diagram (Fig. 1.9), which depicts a large drop in ventricular volume occurring during the ST segment.

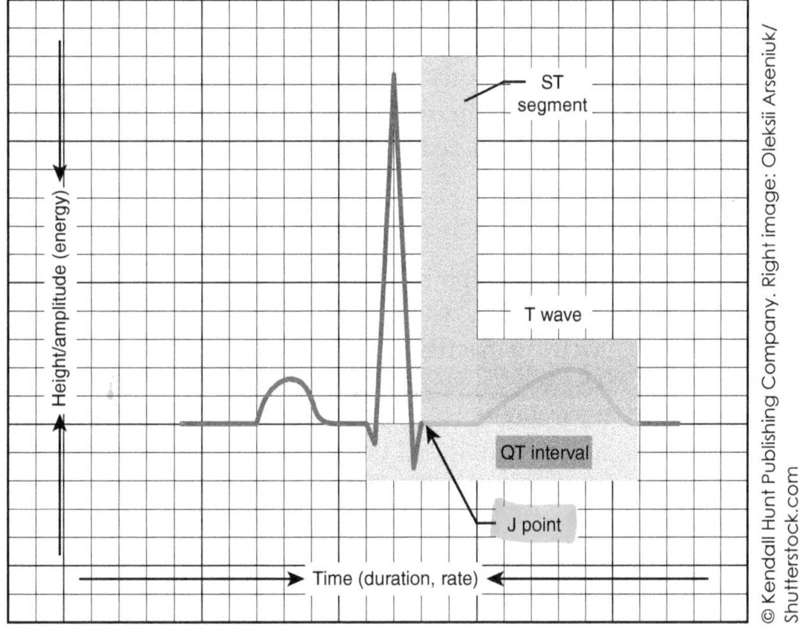

FIGURE 5.24 The ST segment. The ST segment begins at the end of the QRS complex, in this case at the end of the S wave, and ends at the beginning of the T wave. It is normally isoelectric.

The ST segment can be elevated or depressed (Fig. 5.25) in various conditions. **ST segment depression** is indicative of the electrical impulse moving slower than normal through the myocardium. ST depression can indicate the presence of myocardial ischemia, an old MI, ventricular hypertrophy, and BBB. **ST segment elevation** is a current of injury indicative of **acute myocardial infarction** (AMI). ST segment elevation can be seen in some other conditions or even as a normal variant in some individuals.

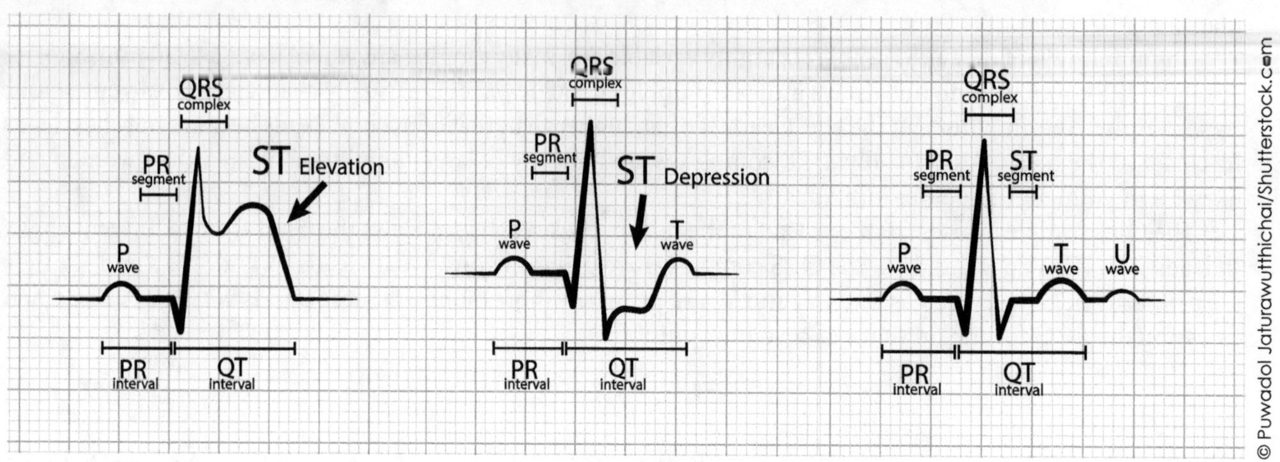

FIGURE 5.25 The normal ST segment is flat and isoelectric as opposed to an ST segment that is elevated and one that is depressed.

If the ST segment is not isoelectric, how is the location of the isoelectric line determined? The two places that should nearly always be isoelectric are the PR segment and the **TP interval** (distance from the end of the T wave to the beginning of the P wave of the next cardiac cycle). Both areas are of value to pinpoint the baseline, but the PR segment is the more stable indicator. Note, however, that the presence of certain conditions, such as pericarditis, can affect the PR segment. Once the isoelectric line is determined, the **J point** (the point where the QRS complex ends and the ST segment begins) can be located. The J point should be isoelectric but can often deviate from the isoelectric line. Recent research has suggested using the **J-60** or **J-80 points** instead because there is less likelihood of myocardial electrical potential differences at these time frames than at the J point itself. These points are located 60 and 80 ms, respectively, after the J point. Ordinarily, 1 mm or greater deviation of the J point from isoelectric is considered abnormal.

T Wave

The **T wave** is produced on the electrocardiograph by ventricular repolarization and occurs as the ventricles begin to relax. Isovolumetric relaxation coincides with the end of repolarization (Fig. 1.9). As the T wave ends, the ventricles return to diastole and electrical inactivity until the beginning of the next QRS complex.

The T wave should normally follow the same direction as the QRS complex (Fig. 5.26). That is, if the QRS complex is positive in a lead, the T wave should be positive in that lead. If the QRS complex is negative in a lead, the T wave should be negative in that lead. Recall that when a wave of depolarization moves toward the positive pole of a lead, it produces a positive deflection. When a wave of repolarization moves away from the positive pole of a lead (i.e., toward the negative pole), it will also produce a positive deflection. If a T wave is encountered that is in the opposite direction from the QRS complex (inverted T wave) in more than one lead, it likely indicates pathology. Isolated inverted T waves are commonly seen in aV_R and less frequently in leads III, aV_F, or aV_L.

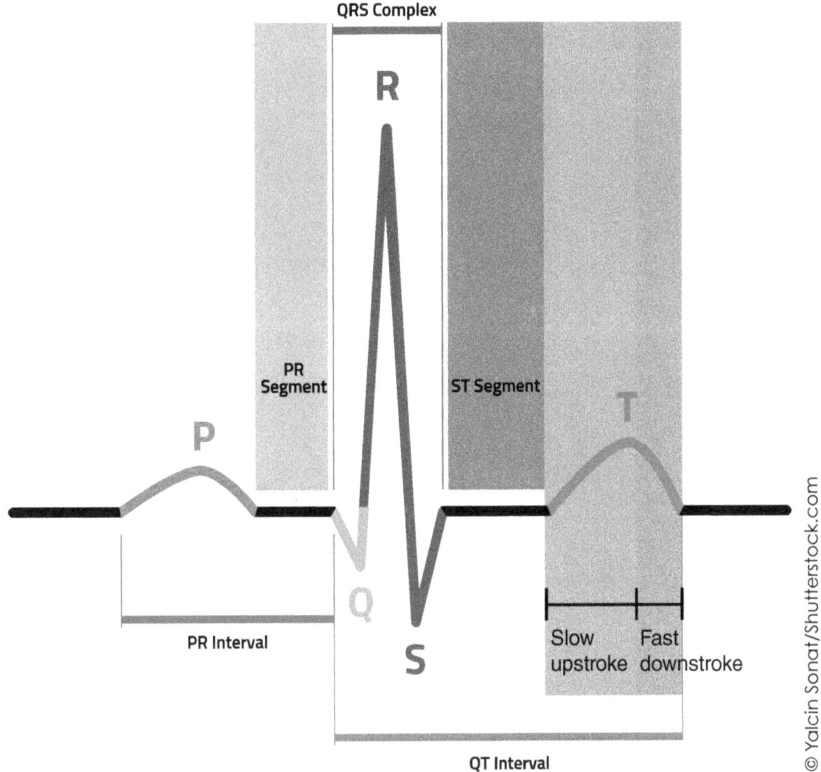

FIGURE 5.26 T wave. Note the slow upstroke and faster, more abrupt downstroke of the T wave.

T waves are normally asymmetrical with a more gradual upstroke and sharper downstroke, although T waves in females are somewhat more symmetrical than in males. Most commonly, symmetrical T waves are pathological. Peaked or "tented" T waves are considered abnormal, as are also "notched" or "humped" T waves. T wave amplitude is typically no greater than 5 mm in the chest leads and 10 mm in the limb leads.

U Wave

U waves are not commonly present, but can sometimes be noted as a last, small, rounded deflection after the T wave (Fig. 5.27). Although the source of the U wave is not known, it is thought to be caused by the terminal stages of ventricular repolarization such as repolarization of the Purkinje fibers or papillary muscles. A normal ECG either does not exhibit or has a small U wave. If a U wave is prominent or abnormally shaped, it is considered abnormal, as witnessed in the case of **hypokalemia**.

QT Interval

The **QT interval** spans the beginning of the QRS complex to the completion of the T wave. Physiologically, it represents the entirety of ventricular electrical activity. The QT interval varies with HR. Slower HRs have longer QT intervals, whereas faster HRs have shorter ones. Thus, formulae have been devised to correct the QT interval for HR (QTc). A normal QTc is < 0.44 s and less than half the RR interval. Elongated QT intervals increase the risk of a rhythm, known as **Torsades de Pointes (TdP)**, which increases the risk of sudden cardiac death. Several causes of elongated QT intervals are discussed elsewhere in this text.

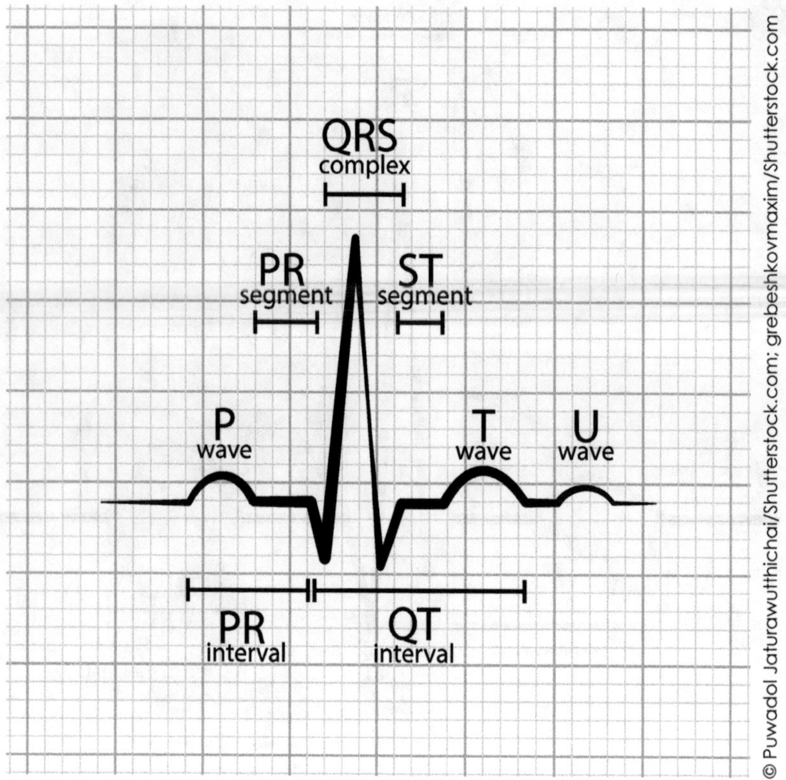

FIGURE 5.27 The U wave, sometimes appears as a last small wave after a T wave. It is thought to represent the terminal stages of ventricular repolarization.

TP Interval

As briefly mentioned earlier, the TP interval is the time from the end of the T wave to the beginning of the P wave of the next cardiac cycle (the time in between heartbeats). During this time, both the atria and the ventricles are electrically inactive and in diastole. Thus, the TP interval should be isoelectric. Passive filling of the ventricles occurs during this time frame, as noted on the Wiggers Diagram (Fig. 1.9) through the increase in ventricular volume.

■ Artifact

Artifacts are tracings on the ECG that are not a result of the heart's electrical activity (Fig. 5.28). The presence of artifact makes it difficult to properly interpret the ECG. Thus, the goal is to always take the necessary precautions to minimize the appearance of artifact on ECG tracings. There are three primary types of artifact: muscle artifact, movement artifact, and electromagnetic interference artifact. Muscle artifact appears on the ECG as a high-frequency, low-amplitude irregular distortion of the isoelectric line. They may be caused by: (1) tense muscles or shivering, (2) poor skin preparation for electrode placement, (3) loose, poorly placed, or dried out electrodes, (4) loose, worn out or poorly connected lead wires, (5) or a malfunctioning ECG machine. In contrast to muscle artifact, movement artifact (a.k.a. wandering baseline) appears as a low-frequency, high-amplitude distortion of the isoelectric line and occurs because of patient movement, deep breathing, or changes in acceleration of a moving vehicle. Finally, electromagnetic interference is caused by interference by nearby electrical sources such as improperly grounded electrical equipment or the nearby use of radios. Artifact can be minimized by taking commonsense measures such as ensuring proper electrode preparation and placement, minimizing the use of nearby electrical equipment, and minimizing patient movement.

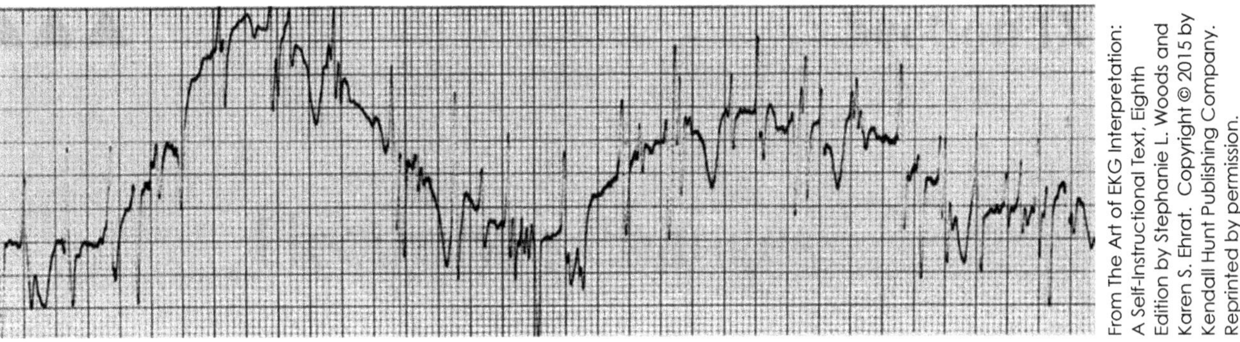

FIGURE 5.28 Example of artifact on an ECG strip.

How can one differentiate artifact from waveforms originating from the heart? In most cases, there is little to no regularity or consistency to artifact, whereas cardiac electrical activity is typically patterned in some form or fashion. The main exception to this is sources of electromagnetic interference that emit energy at a regular frequency.

As we will see later in this text, some life-threatening dysrhythmias have chaotic waveforms that appear similar to artifact. However, even those chaotic dysrhythmias typically repeat themselves in a pattern. Always remember, however, to compare your ECG interpretation to the clinical status of the patient. For example, a cardiac electrical rhythm known as **ventricular fibrillation** does not result in cardiac output. Therefore, the patient is unconscious, not breathing, and pulseless. If the ECG seems to show ventricular fibrillation but the patient is awake and alert, then the interpretation is incorrect and what is being observed is likely artifact.

Chapter Questions

1. True/False, the QRS complex shows ventricular contraction. Support your answer.
2. Using the ECG rhythm strip at the bottom of the 12-lead ECG pictured below, determine the HR using the methods presented in the chapter.

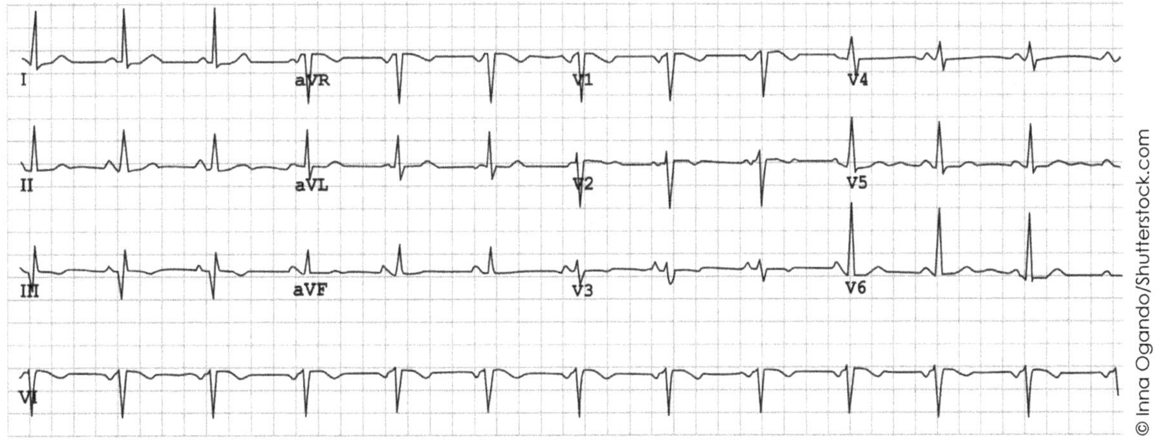

3. How do the frontal plane leads differ from the horizontal plane leads?

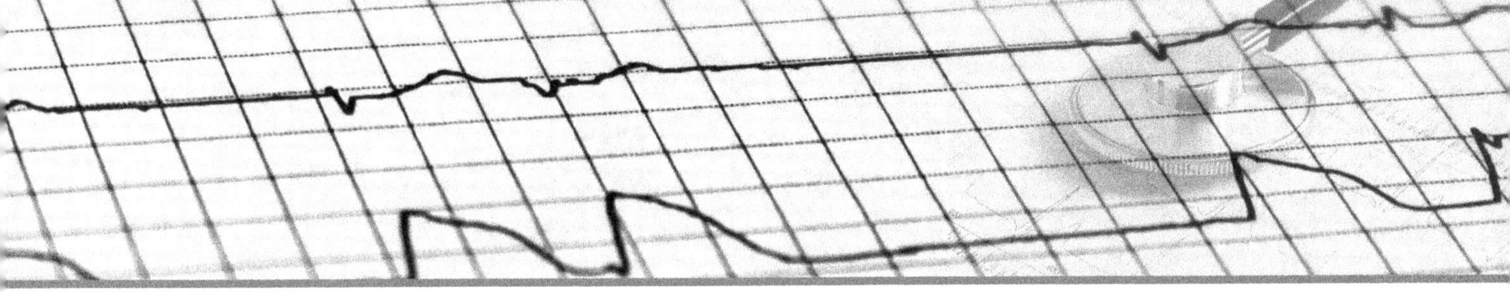

CHAPTER 6

Determination of Electrical Axis

The mean electrical axis is the average of all the instantaneous mean electrical vectors occurring sequentially during depolarization of the ventricles. Assessment of the heart's electrical axis is an integral part of ECG interpretation.

CONTENT OUTLINE

- Instantaneous Vectors
- Mean QRS Axis
- Determination of Mean QRS Axis
  - Two-Lead Method (Quadrant Method)
  - Hexaxial Reference System Method (Degree Method)
- Causes of Axis Deviation
  - Left Axis Deviation (LAD)
  - Right Axis Deviation (RAD)
  - Extreme Axis Deviation (EAD)
- Chapter Questions

Before embarking on a discussion of electrical axis in this chapter, recall from Chapter 5 the development of the leads, particularly the limb leads, and their placement in the hexaxial reference system (Fig. 5.16) and how deflections are created (Fig. 5.6). It is clinically useful to determine electrical axis, because various heart pathologies affect how the electrical impulse is conducted throughout the myocardium and the magnitude of the voltage of those electrical impulses. Axis determination can aid in the confirmation of a diagnosis or can help rule out the presence of some conditions to help narrow the search for a correct diagnosis. Although the clinical focus is on pathologic causes of an abnormal heart axis, other factors that influence the axis include the heart's size and position within the chest as well as the patient's body size and position.

Instantaneous Vectors

As waves of depolarization and repolarization of the cardiac fibers occur throughout the myocardium, many small electrical currents, known as **instantaneous vectors**, are created in many different directions simultaneously (Fig. 6.1). The average of all these instantaneous vectors at any given moment is the mean instantaneous vector recorded by the ECG. The direction and magnitude of the mean instantaneous vector is called the **mean electrical axis** of the heart and is depicted as the large arrow in Figure 6.1. Axis is defined in the frontal plane only. Most commonly, we look at the mean electrical axis of the QRS complex, because it is more clinically significant. However, we can also determine the mean axis of atrial depolarization, called the **P axis**. The P axis, however, is rarely determined and will not be covered in this text.

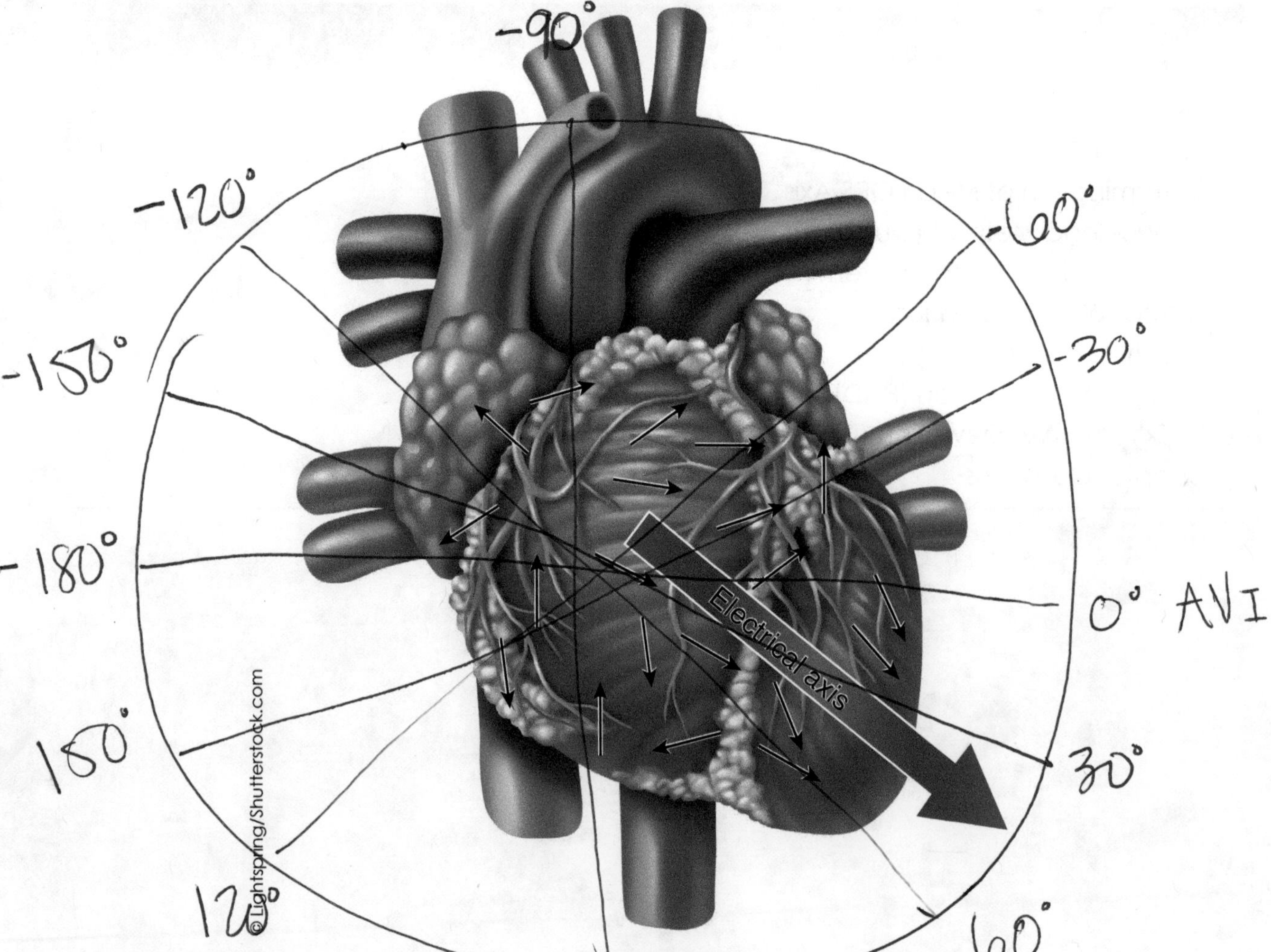

FIGURE 6.1 The waves of depolarization throughout the heart produce many instantaneous vectors in many different directions. The ECG records the average of all instantaneous vectors as the mean electrical axis. In the normal heart, the mean electrical axis is downward and to the left, as shown by the large arrow.

Mean QRS Axis

In a normal heart, as discussed in Chapter 1, the origin of the electrical impulse is the SA node. From the SA node, the impulse travels throughout the atria and to the AV node. It pauses briefly at the AV node and is then transmitted to the bundle of His in the ventricles and on to the right and left bundle branches in the interventricular septum, then outward throughout the ventricles via the Purkinje fibers. Owing to the significantly larger mass of the left ventricle, the vectors there are larger and longer lasting than those of the right ventricle, drawing the mean electrical axis leftward. Therefore, the normal mean electrical QRS axis points downward and to the left across the precordium.

Determination of Mean QRS Axis

Recall that the mean electrical axis is viewed only in the frontal plane. Thus, axis determination involves only the bipolar limb leads (I, II, III) and the unipolar limb leads (aV_F, aV_L, aV_R). Figure 6.2 depicts the hexaxial reference system drawn over the patient's chest, the center of the circle positioned at the AV node with the six bisecting lines representing the six limb leads. This circle can also be partitioned into quadrants. A normal heart has an axis that falls within the lower left-hand quadrant between 0° and 90°. This is referred to as normal axis (NA) or normal axis deviation (NAD). The four quadrants are aligned as follows:

- 0° and 90° is normal axis (NA)
- 90° and 180° is **right axis deviation (RAD)**
- 0° and −90° is **left axis deviation (LAD)**
- −90° and + 180° is **extreme axis deviation (EAD)** (also known as extreme right axis deviation, indeterminant axis, northwest axis, or no man's land)

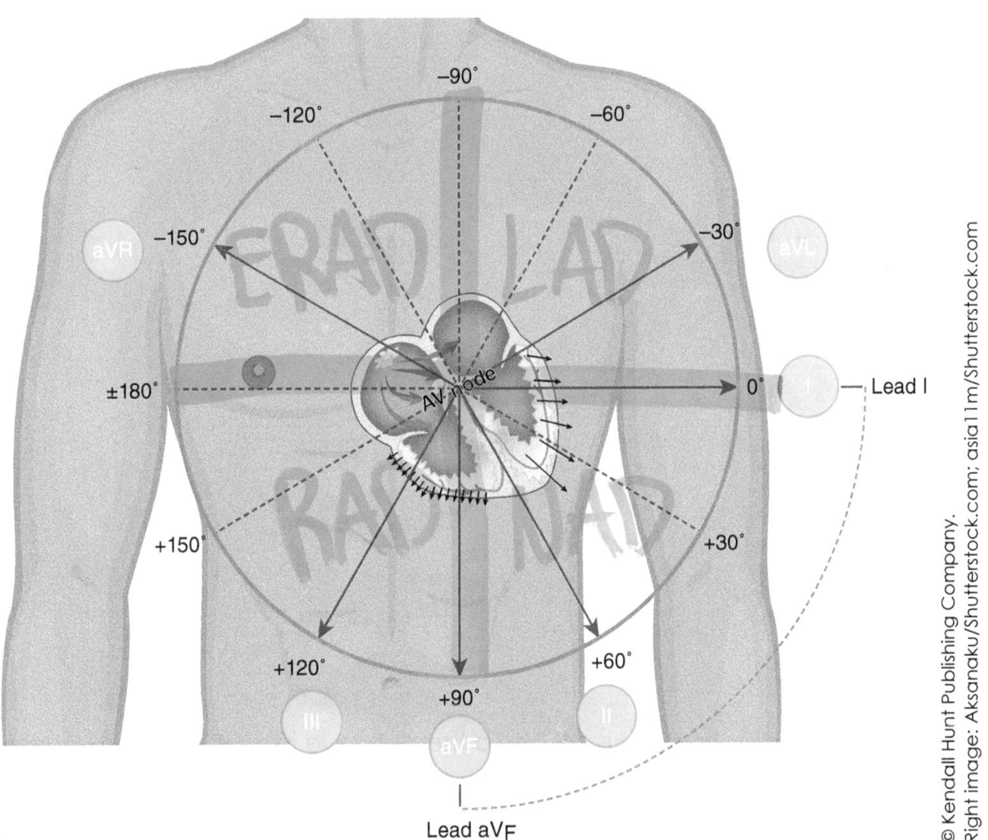

FIGURE 6.2 The hexaxial reference system depicts the directions of the six limb leads in the frontal plane by using a circle with its center positioned at the AV node.

There are two methods that can be employed to determine the electrical axis: Two-Lead Method (also referred to as the Quadrant Method) and the Hexaxial Reference System Method (also known as the Degree Method). The two-lead method will only tell us which quadrant the axis falls within, and this information is sufficient in many cases, but the Hexaxial Reference System Method provides a more accurate measure of the axis.

Two-Lead Method (Quadrant Method)

The Two-Lead Method uses leads I and aV_F to determine which quadrant the heart's mean electrical axis falls within. These two leads are employed because they split the circle into quadrants, with lead I running horizontally and aV_F vertically. If lead I has a QRS complex that is more positive than it is negative, the mean electrical axis must lie closer to the positive pole of lead I than to the negative pole. If lead I has a QRS complex that is more negative than positive, the mean electrical axis must lie closer to the negative pole of that lead (Fig. 6.3). Similarly, if lead aV_F has a QRS complex that is more positive than negative, the mean electrical axis lies closer to the positive pole of lead aV_F than to its negative pole. If lead aV_F has a QRS complex that is more negative than positive, the mean electrical axis is closer to the negative pole of aV_F (Fig. 6.4). Putting these two together, the mean electrical axis can be localized to one of the four quadrants (Fig. 6.5):

- Leads I and aV_F are positive; the axis is within NA
- Lead I is positive and aV_F is negative; the axis is within LAD
- Lead I is negative and aV_F is positive; the axis is within RAD
- Leads I and aV_F are both negative; the axis is within EAD

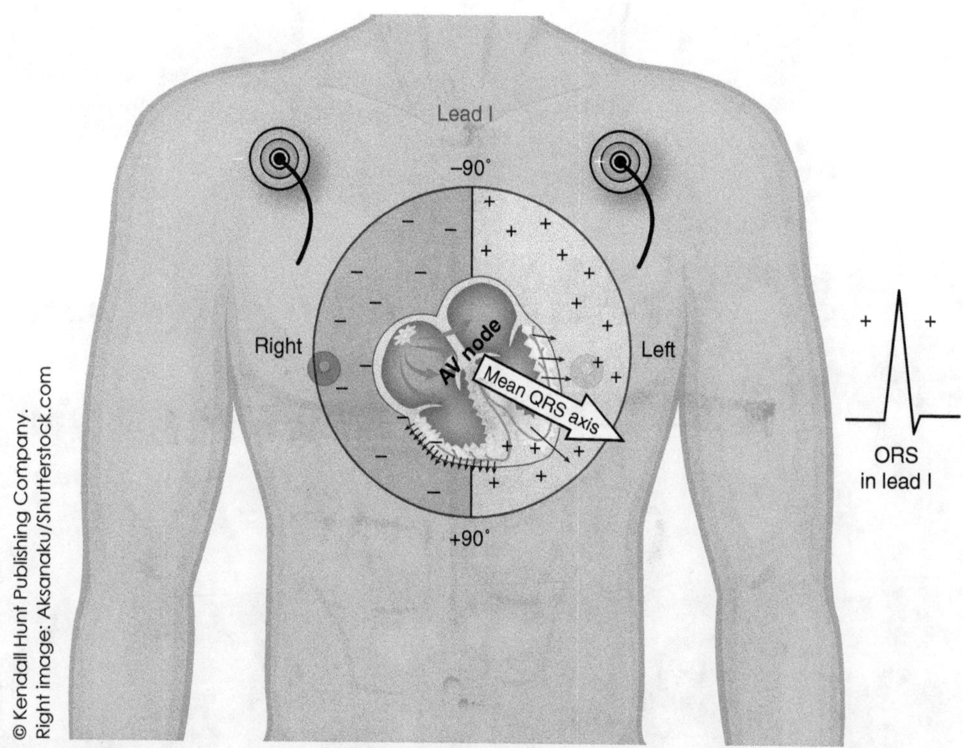

FIGURE 6.3 The positive pole of lead I is at 0° and the negative pole at 180°. When lead I has a more positive QRS complex, the mean QRS axis must be located somewhere on the right half of the circle. When lead I has a more negative QRS complex, the mean QRS axis must be located somewhere on the left half of the circle.

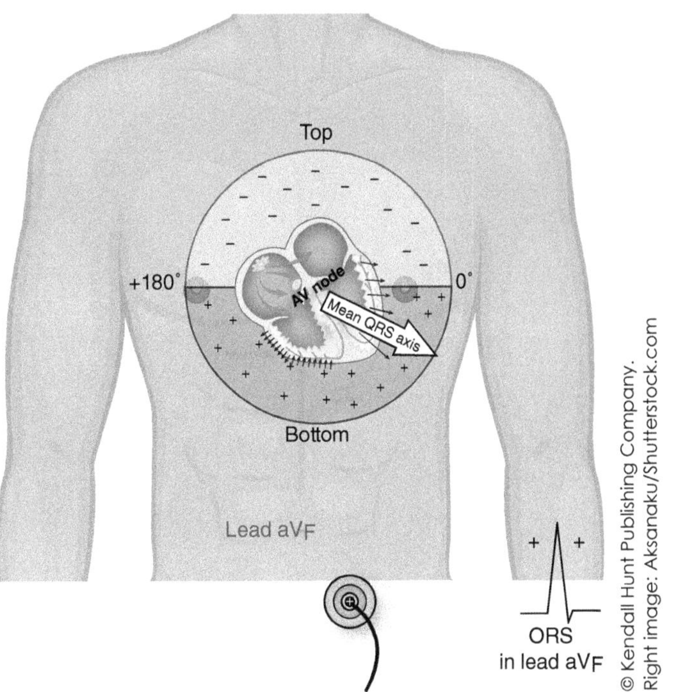

FIGURE 6.4 The positive pole of lead aV_F is at 90° and the negative pole at −90°. When lead aV_F has a more positive QRS complex, the mean QRS axis must be located somewhere on the bottom half of the circle. When lead aV_F has a more negative QRS complex, the mean QRS axis must be located somewhere on the top half of the circle.

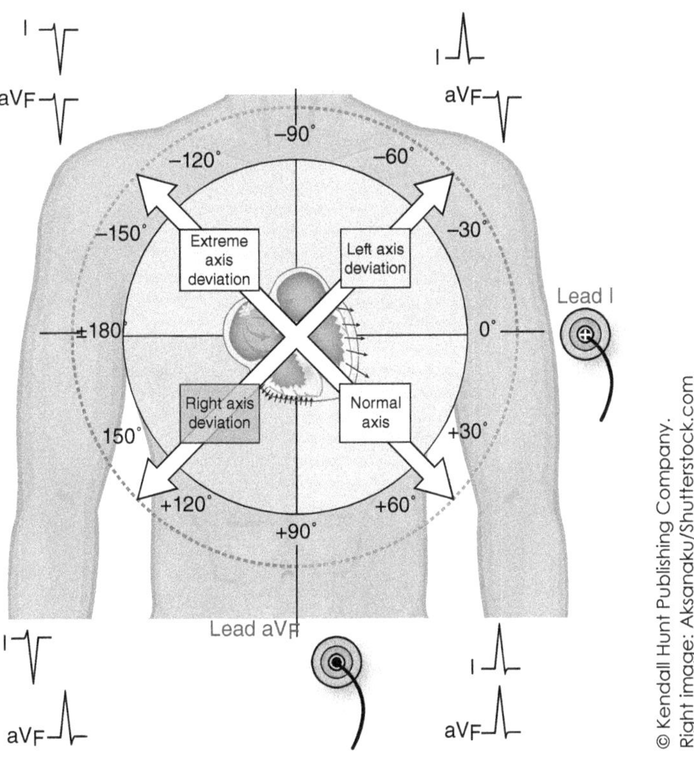

FIGURE 6.5 Two-Lead Method of Axis Determination. With the use of both leads I and aVF, the quadrant in which the mean electrical axis lies can be located. If both leads I and aVF are positive, the mean electrical axis is normal. If lead I is positive and lead II is negative, the axis is in the LAD quadrant. If lead I is negative and lead aVF is positive, the axis is in the RAD quadrant. If both leads I and aVF are negative, the axis is in the EAD quadrant.

Hexaxial Reference System Method (Degree Method)

The Two-Lead Method is easier and quicker, but the Hexaxial Reference System Method yields a much more accurate axis determination. Additionally, it can be used even when the QRS complex in leads I or aV_F is not clearly positive or negative. There are a couple of ways in which this method can be used. First, identify the lead possessing the greatest voltage. This will be the lead that is either the tallest or the deepest. The axis is most in line with that lead. If the lead with the greatest voltage has a mostly positive deflection (tallest lead), the axis is toward the positive pole of that lead. If the lead with the greatest voltage has a mostly negative deflection (deepest lead), the axis is toward the negative pole of that lead. Second, identify the lead whose QRS complex is most equiphasic (equal deflections above and below the isoelectric line). The most equiphasic lead is approximately perpendicular to (90° away from or at a right angle to) the mean electrical axis. For example, if lead II is most equiphasic, then the axis is most in line with the axis of lead aV_L, which is perpendicular to lead II. Then look at the QRS complex of the perpendicular (90°) lead. If the QRS of that lead is more positive, then the axis is toward the positive pole of that lead. If the QRS of that lead is more negative, then the axis is toward the negative pole of that lead. For example, if aVL (our 90° lead) has a positive deflection, the axis is approximately −30° and if negative, approximately 150°. Figure 6.6 shows examples of using these methods to determine the mean electrical axis.

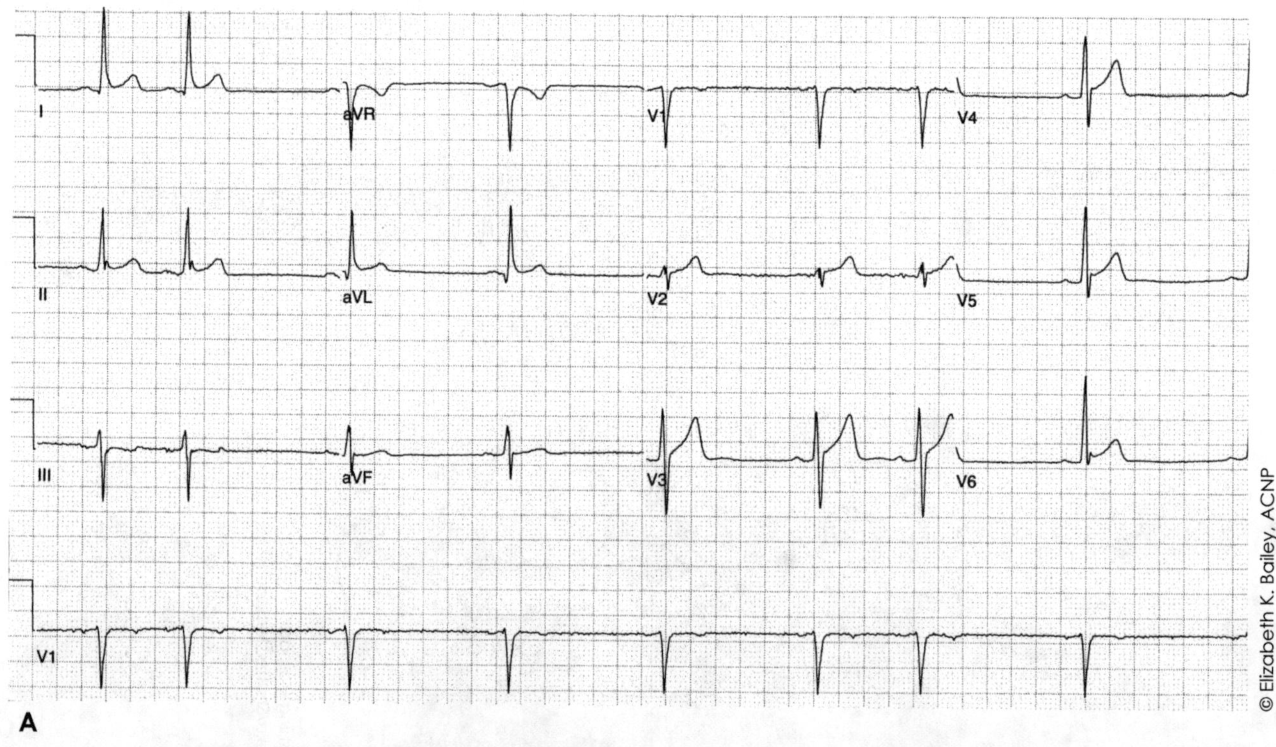

FIGURE 6.6 Examples using the hexaxial reference system method to determine mean QRS axis. **A**—Using the voltage criteria with the hexaxial reference system. Lead I has the greatest voltage, so the axis of this heart is most in line with lead I. Lead I contains a primarily positive deflection, so the axis is estimated to be near the positive pole of I (at 0°), which is in the NAD quadrant (remember that the NAD quadrant typically is said to extend ± 15 degrees past the 0°–90° borders of the quadrant). Using the equiphasic criteria with the hexaxial reference system. Lead aVF is most equiphasic, therefore the axis of this heart is approximately 90° away from lead aVF, which is lead I. Lead I has a primarily positive QRS, so the axis is estimated to be at the positive pole of lead I (at 0°), which is in the NAD quadrant.

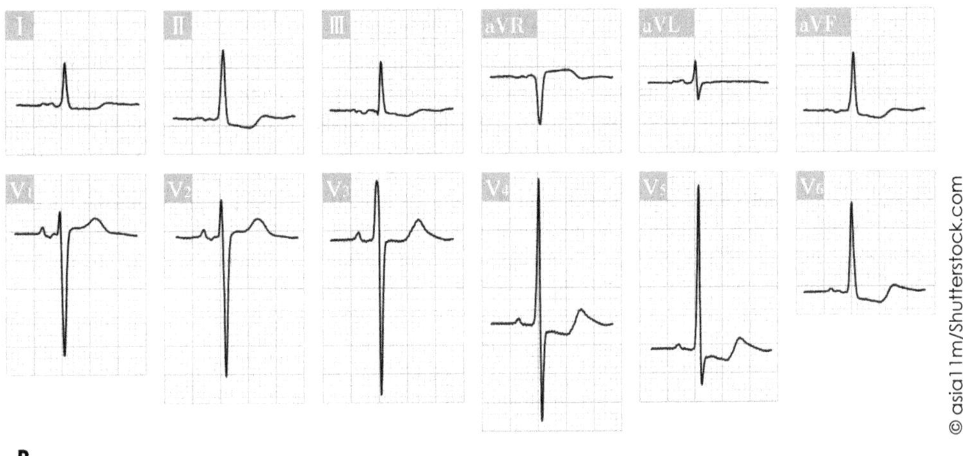

© asia11m/Shutterstock.com

B

B—Using the voltage criteria with the hexaxial reference system. Lead II has the greatest voltage, so the axis of this heart is most in line with lead II. Lead II contains a primarily positive deflection, so the axis is estimated to be near the positive pole of II (at 30°), which is in the NAD quadrant. Using the equiphasic criteria with the hexaxial reference system. Lead aVL is most equiphasic, and the axis of this heart is therefore approximately 90° away from lead aVL, which is lead II. Lead II has a primarily positive QRS, so the axis is estimated to be at the positive pole of lead II (at 30°), which is in the NAD quadrant.

Causes of Axis Deviation

Now that we have learned how to determine the electrical axis, let's turn our attention to a discussion of causes of alterations in the axis from normal.

Left Axis Deviation (LAD)

In LAD, the axis is shifted much more laterally than normal. Causes can be both pathologic and nonpathologic. Nonpathologic causes of LAD include normal variants, a "horizontal heart," or an athletic heart. A "horizontal heart" most commonly occurs in obesity and pregnancy. Whether because of high levels of abdominal fat or the presence of a fetus in the abdomen, the heart is pushed upward owing to increased abdominal pressure, causing the heart to sit more horizontally and shifting the electrical axis leftward. Also, if respirations are exaggerated, as occurs during exercise or in some pulmonary conditions, during the expiratory phase, as the diaphragm moves upward, the heart moves more horizontally. In the athletic heart, both left-sided chamber size and muscle mass increase as an adaptation owing to the increased demands of chronic exercise. The increased left-sided myocardium draws the axis leftward.

Pathologic causes of LAD include left bundle branch block, left anterior hemiblock, left ventricular hypertrophy, Wolfe-Parkinson White syndrome, ventricular ectopic rhythms, hyperkalemia, emphysema, atrial septal defects, some pacemakers, and inferior wall myocardial infarction (MI). During an MI, some of the myocardial tissue dies. The dead area does not depolarize. Therefore, the vectors on the reciprocal area of the heart are dominant, and the axis points away from the area of infarct. The lateral leads are reciprocal to the inferior leads. Thus, an inferior MI tends to cause LAD.

Right Axis Deviation (RAD)

As with LAD, causes of RAD may be either nonpathologic or pathologic in origin. RAD may appear as a normal variant. Whereas LAD can be noted in a "horizontal heart," RAD is common in a "vertical heart." A "vertical heart" is seen commonly in children and tall, slender individuals and sometimes during the inhalation phase of exaggerated breathing.

As with LAD, there are also quite a few pathologic causes of RAD. However, the most common causes of pathologic RAD stem from pulmonary conditions such as chronic obstructive pulmonary disease (COPD), pulmonary embolism, emphysema, pulmonary stenosis, pulmonary hypertension, and emphysema. Other pathologic causes of RAD include right bundle branch block (RBBB), left posterior hemiblock (LPH), right ventricular hypertrophy (RVH), Marfan Syndrome, and anterior and/or lateral wall MIs. Additionally, reversal of the right and left arm electrodes will result in RAD, so lead connections should always be checked.

Extreme Axis Deviation (EAD)

Unlike LAD and RAD, EAD does not occur as a normal variant but is seen only if lead transposition occurs and in a few pathologic conditions. EAD is rare, and lead transposition is the most likely cause. Thus, if EAD is noted, it is always a good idea to check your lead connections. The pathologic causes of EAD include emphysema, hyperkalemia, some pacemakers, and ventricular tachycardia.

Chapter Questions

1. Explain why a normal ventricular axis is downward and to the left.
2. Name the causes of a "horizontal" heart and a "vertical" heart?
3. Explain how lead transposition results in EAD on the ECG.
4. Why is the mean electrical axis approximately perpendicular to the most equiphasic of the limb leads?

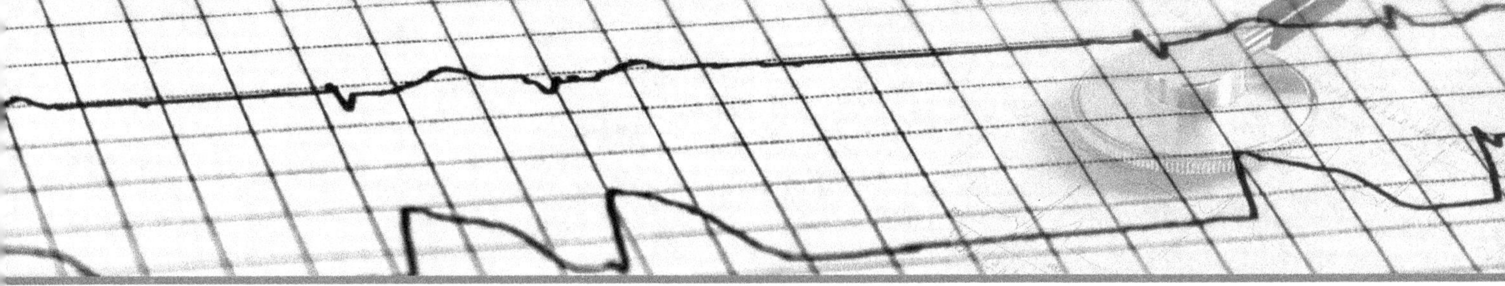

CHAPTER 7

Myocardial Enlargement

As with any muscle, if forced to work too hard, the heart can enlarge. This enlargement may be either pathologic (with degraded function) or physiologic (with enhanced function) depending on the nature of the imposed chronic stress.

CONTENT OUTLINE

- Right Atrial Enlargement
- Left Atrial Enlargement
- Ventricular Hypertrophy
  - Right Ventricular Hypertrophy
  - Left Ventricular Hypertrophy
- Hemodynamic and Mechanical Stressors in Left Ventricular Hypertrophy
- Chapter Questions

Hypertrophy refers to an enlargement of cell size. In terms of cardiac enlargement, dilation is said to occur when the heart muscle lengthens and hypertrophy when it thickens. Dilation results from volume overload, whereas hypertrophy results from pressure overload. Both cardiac dilation (eccentric hypertrophy) and hypertrophy (concentric hypertrophy) can occur owing to physiologic or pathologic causes. When pathologic, both can be detrimental to function. Although both dilation and hypertrophy can and do occur in the atria or ventricles, the atria primarily dilate while the ventricles hypertrophy. Both are discussed in this chapter along with classic ECG changes accompanying each: P wave changes when assessing atrial enlargement and QRS complex and ST-T changes when assessing ventricular hypertrophy.

When the myocardium experiences a volume overload, whether from a physiologic cause like endurance training or a pathologic cause such as valvular disease, the fibers lengthen. Thus, sarcomeres are added in series (myofibrils get longer). Conversely, when there is a high afterload, the fibers thicken to increase contractility. New myofibrils are added to muscle fibers with the addition of sarcomeres in parallel (see Fig. 7.1).

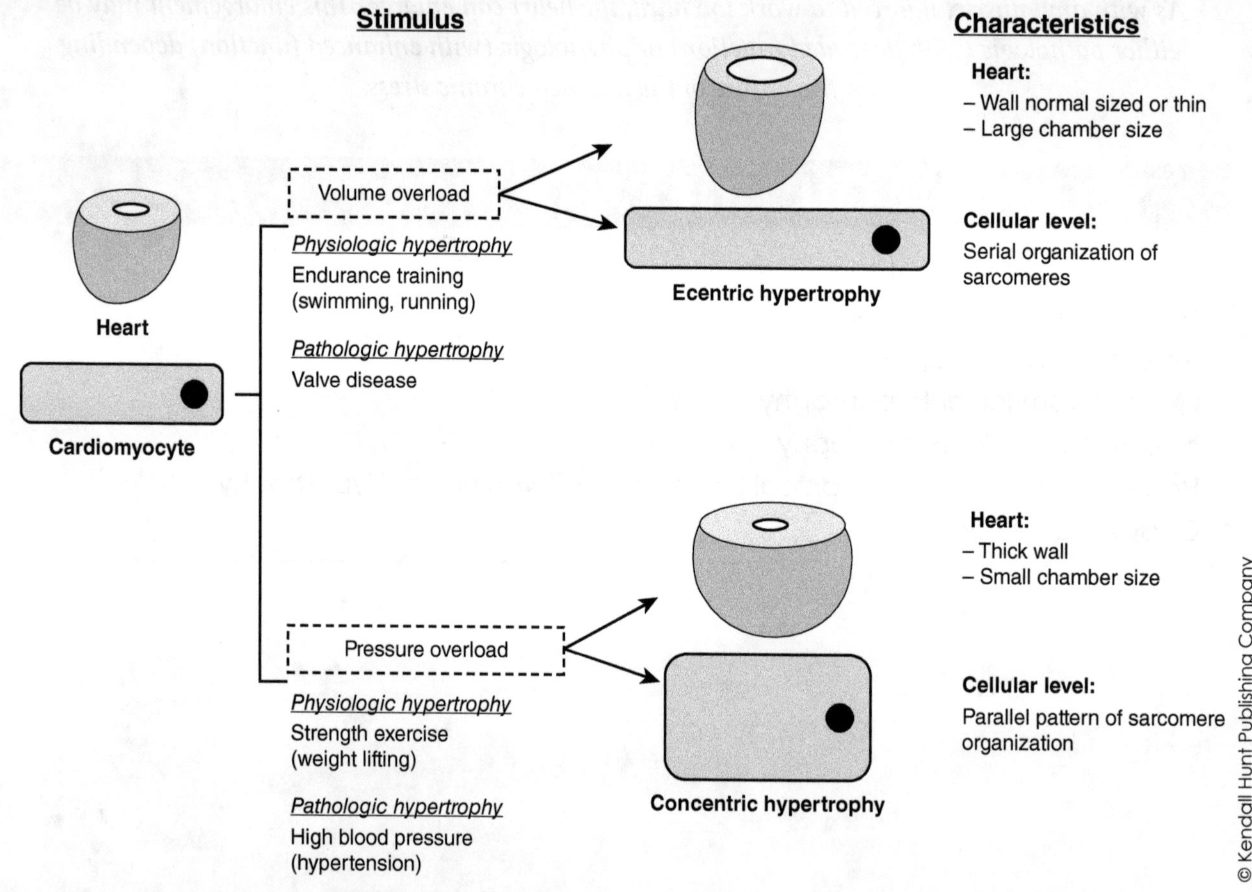

FIGURE 7.1 The mechanisms whereby the left ventricle structurally remodels according to the mechanical and hemodynamic stimuli placed on it.

Right Atrial Enlargements

Recall that the normal P wave is no more than 0.1 seconds long and no more than 2.5 mm in amplitude. Because the right atrium depolarizes slightly before the left, the first portion of the P wave represents right atrial depolarization, whereas the latter portion represents left atrial depolarization (Fig. 7.2). The best ECG leads for assessing atrial enlargements are leads II (and often the other inferior leads—III and aVF) and V_1. Lead II is usually most parallel to the net wave of depolarization through the atria, and therefore records the largest deflections, and is best for visualizing changes in atrial depolarization. V_1 is positioned directly over the right atrium and normally produces a biphasic P wave.

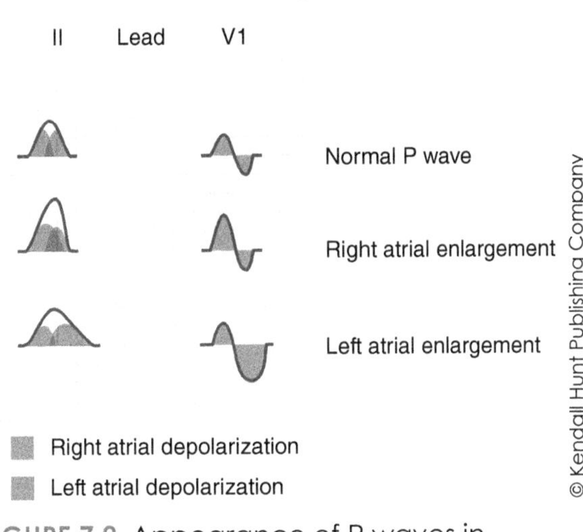

FIGURE 7.2 Appearance of P waves in leads II and V_1 in normal, RAE, and LAE.

As we learned in chapter 1 (Fig. 1.2), the right heart provides the driving force for the pulmonary circuit. The most common causes of right heart dysfunction involve abnormalities in the lungs. Other causes include congenital heart defects and pulmonary and tricuspid valve dysfunction. In chronic pulmonary conditions, we often see **hypoxemia**. Different from the systemic circulation where hypoxemia leads to vasodilation, hypoxemia in the lungs causes vasoconstriction. This is a protective mechanism to prevent ventilation and perfusion mismatch (V/Q mismatch). Once vasoconstriction occurs in the lungs, the pressure in the lungs and thus the right side of the heart increases. The right side of the heart is a low-pressure system in relation to the left side of the heart. This increase in pressure in the right side of the heart can quickly lead to dysfunction even with small increases in pressure. Right ventricular hypertrophy (RVH) often precedes right atrial enlargement (RAE).

RAE causes an increased electrical dominance of the right atrium over the left, resulting in a tall P wave (> 2.5 mm) in lead II (and commonly III and aVF), although the width is usually normal. The abnormal P wave in RAE is often referred to as **P pulmonale** because RAE is most commonly a manifestation of pulmonary disease (Fig. 7.3). Additionally, V_1 (and often V_2) usually has a biphasic P wave that is normally equiphasic (Fig. 7.4). In the presence of RAE, the first, positive portion of the P wave (produced by right atrial depolarization) is larger in area (> 1 mm^2) than the terminal, negative portion (produced by left atrial depolarization).

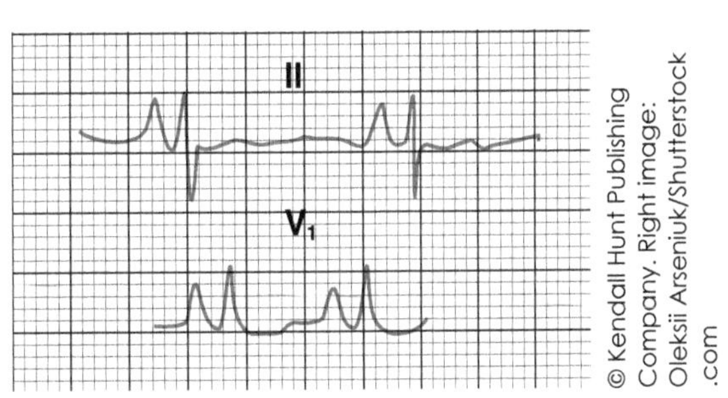

FIGURE 7.3 Peaked P waves are seen in Leads II and V_1. This finding is known as **P pulmonale**, commonly seen in RAE.

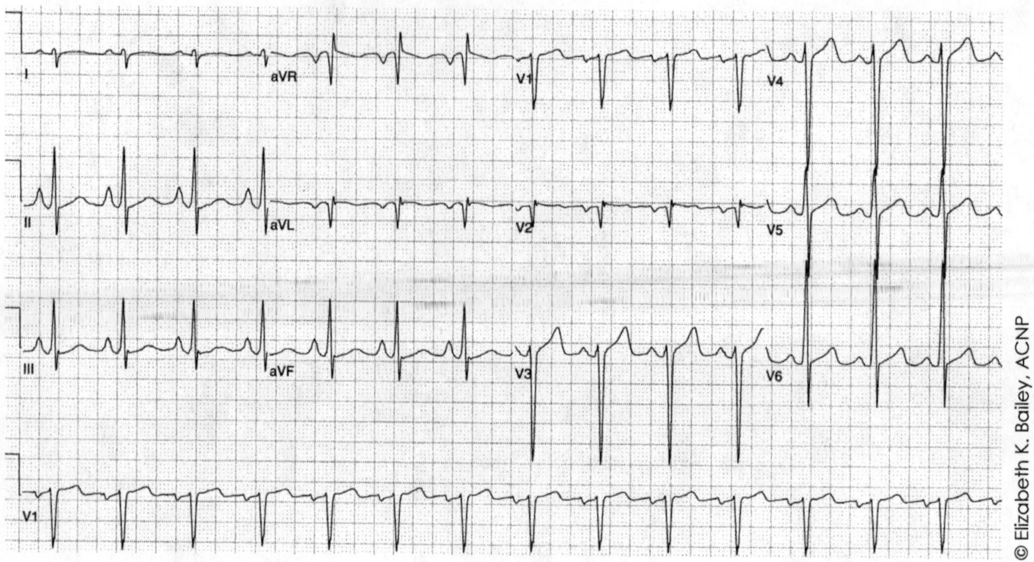

FIGURE 7.4 A 12-lead ECG depicting RAE in a 32-year-old Black male. Note the biphasic P waves in leads V_1 and V_2 and the tall, peaked P waves in the inferior leads.

Left Atrial Enlargement

Left atrial enlargement (LAE) can be caused by multiple pathophysiologic factors, including, but not limited to, aortic and mitral valve disease (both stenosis and regurgitation), poorly controlled hypertension, which results in left ventricular hypertrophy, cardiomyopathies, and coronary artery disease. As with RAE, LAE is manifested on the ECG by P wave abnormalities in the same leads (Fig. 7.2). Left atrial depolarization normally occurs slightly after right atrial depolarization. Thus, LAE prolongs the total time for atrial depolarization, resulting in a P wave greater than 0.10 seconds' duration. Figure 7.5 shows an example of LAE. The height of P waves in LAE can be normal or increased in amplitude. The long P wave often has a "notched" or "hump" shape. This finding is called **P mitrale** and was first described in those with rheumatic mitral valve disease.

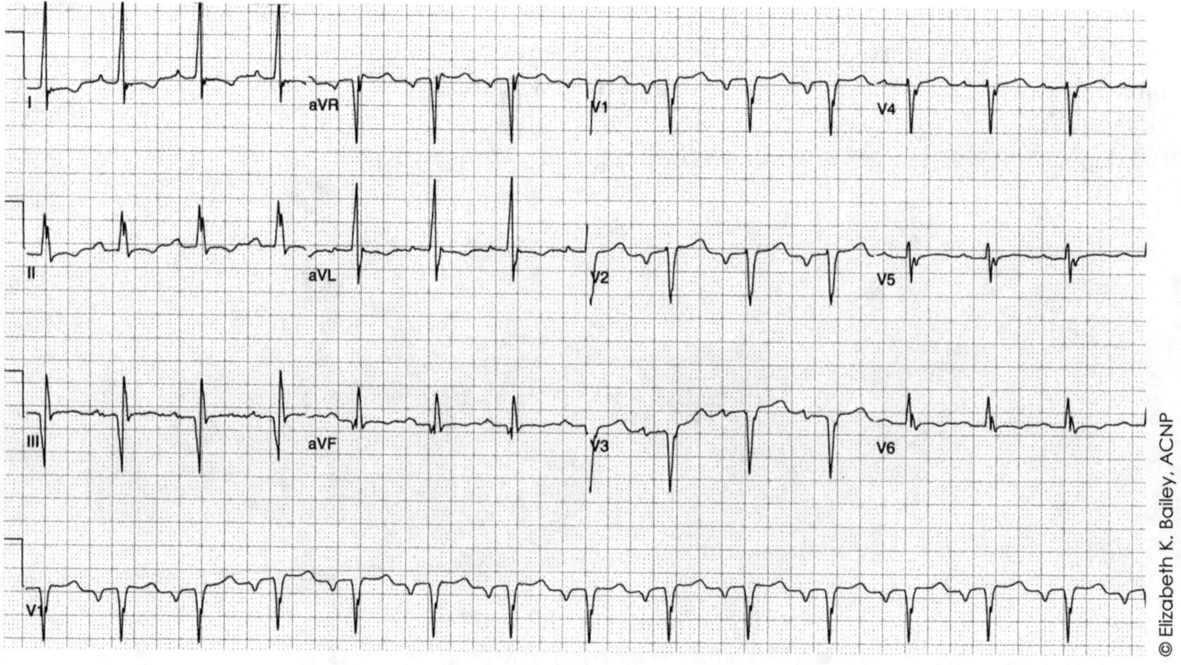

FIGURE 7.5 A 12-lead ECG depicting LAE in a 67-year-old White male. Note the wide P waves seen across several leads and the negative P waves in leads V_1 and V_2.

The second P wave finding in LAE is the biphasic P wave with an initial positive deflection followed by a negative deflection (Fig. 7.6, Lead V_1). From an anatomic standpoint, the left atrium lies posterior to the right atrium. Therefore, when the left atrium experiences the delayed depolarization seen in LAE, there is a negative deflection of the P wave. In LAE (lead V_1 and often V_2), the terminal negative portion of the P wave is larger in area (> 1 mm^2) than the initial positive portion.

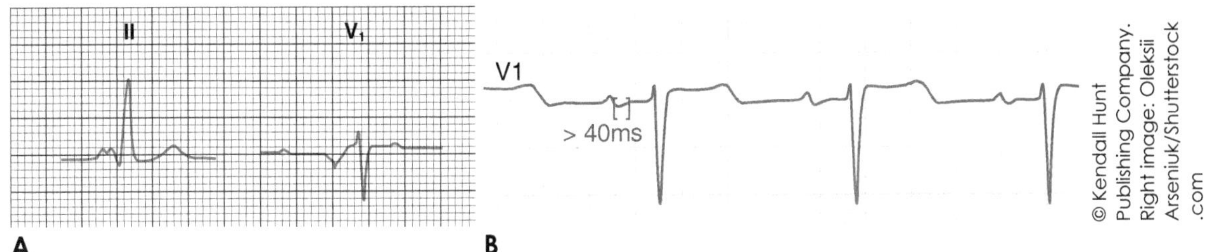

FIGURE 7.6 In **A**, the "hump"-shaped P wave seen in Lead II is also known as *P mitrale*. Notice the negative deflection of the P wave in V_1. In **B**, the P wave terminal portion is > 40 ms duration in V_1. These findings are commonly seen in LAE.

Ventricular Hypertrophy

Whereas atrial enlargement predominantly affects the P wave, ventricular hypertrophy affects the QRS complex and often the ST segment and T wave, particularly in the chest leads. The normal pattern of waveforms in V_1–V_6 can be seen at the top of Figure 7.7. In the normal heart, depolarization of the left ventricle occurs slightly before the right. Depolarization of the right ventricle normally causes an rS pattern with a small positive R wave and a larger negative S wave in V_1 and V_2. This is because of the spread of depolarization away

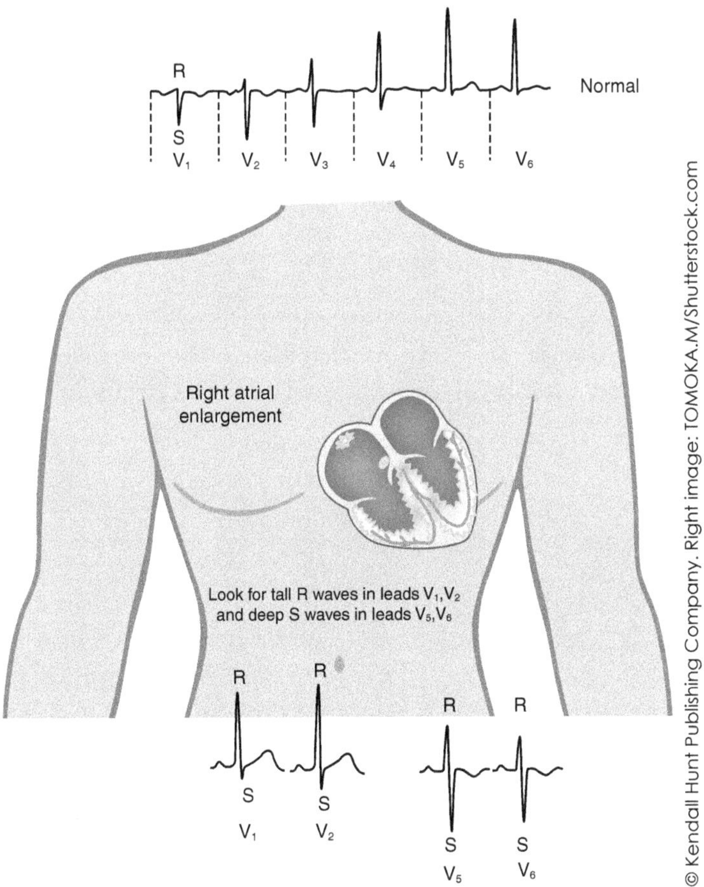

FIGURE 7.7 Normal pattern of QRS complex in V_1–V_6 (top) and as seen in RVH pattern (bottom).

from the right ventricle and toward the larger left ventricle. Conversely, the left-sided chest leads, V_5 and V_6, are normally most in line with the wave of ventricular depolarization, producing a QRS with a tall R and a small S. Ventricular hypertrophy affects this pattern. Additionally, secondary repolarization abnormalities frequently appear in the affected area. If depolarization is abnormal, repolarization will often also be abnormal. Recall that repolarization is seen in the ST-T complex. Repolarization of an enlarged ventricle causes what is often called a ventricular strain pattern (Fig. 7.8) on the affected side. These abnormalities include down-sloping ST segment depression, which usually merges nearly imperceptibly into an inverted (opposite direction of the R wave) T wave.

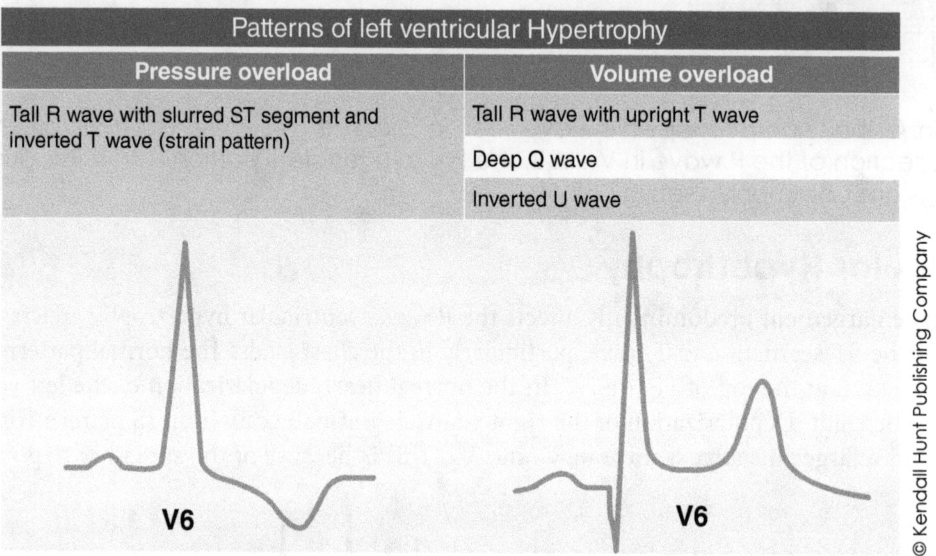

Patterns of left ventricular Hypertrophy	
Pressure overload	**Volume overload**
Tall R wave with slurred ST segment and inverted T wave (strain pattern)	Tall R wave with upright T wave
	Deep Q wave
	Inverted U wave

FIGURE 7.8 The strain pattern differs with the nature of the stress imposed on the heart (i.e., pressure overload or volume overload). Note the down-sloping ST segment merges into the inverted T wave in the pressure overload pattern.

Right Ventricular Hypertrophy (RVH)

As mentioned earlier, RVH is often caused by chronic hypoxemia and results in pulmonary hypertension (see Case Study 7.1). Common causes include chronic obstructive pulmonary disease (COPD) and advanced interstitial lung diseases.

CASE STUDY 7.1.

Mr. Smith is a 76-year-old man who presented to his doctor with progressive shortness of breath. He is a past smoker and was previously diagnosed with COPD. After an initial improvement with inhaler therapy, his dyspnea worsened. He also had new onset of peripheral edema in his lower extremities.

His chest X-ray is shown in the following figures. The PA image (Figure A) shows enlargement of the pulmonary arteries (see arrowheads) and a prominent right heart border (see short arrow). The lateral image (Figure B) shows the lack of a retrocardiac space, which is due to enlargement of the right ventricle (see block arrow).

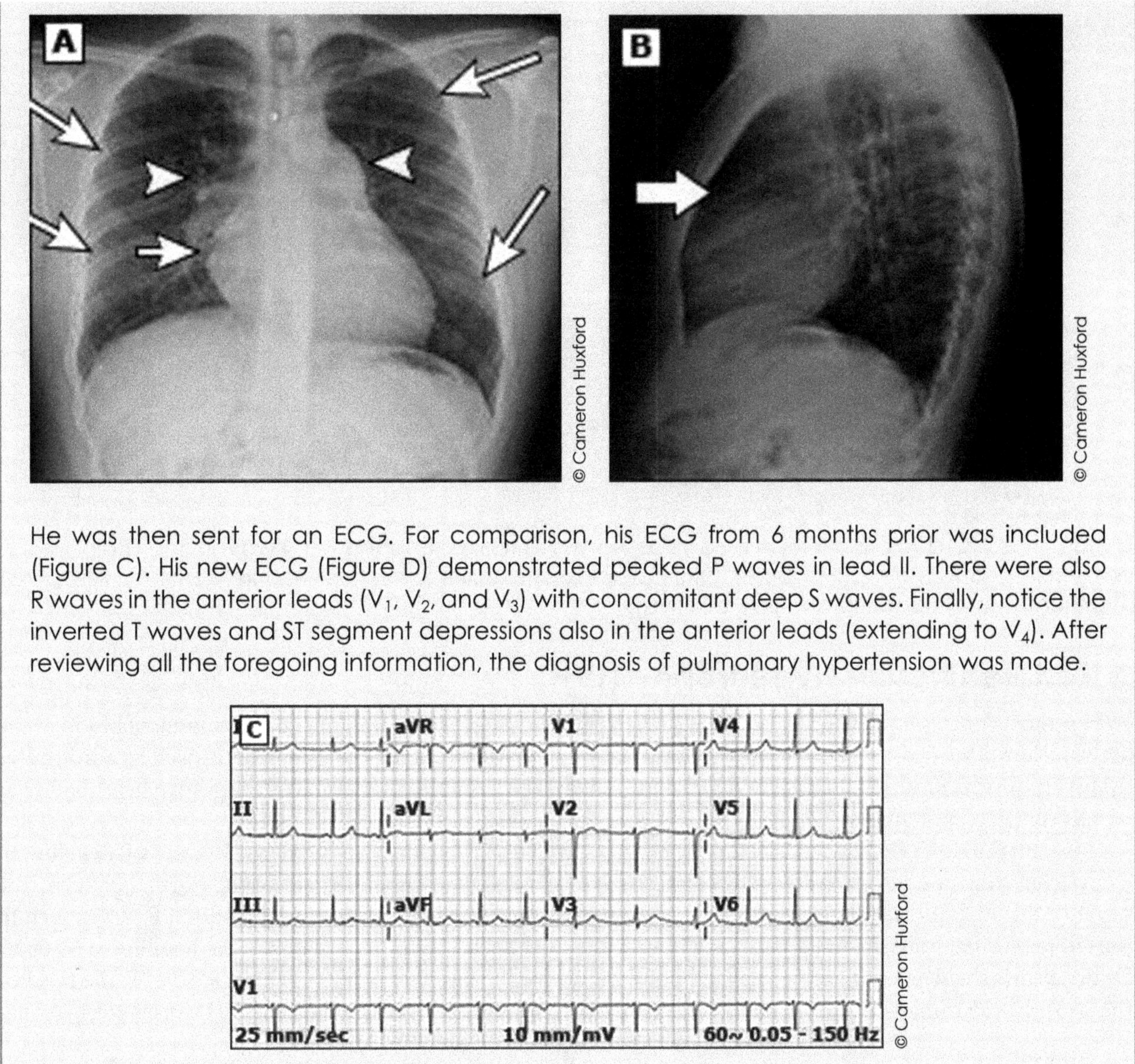

He was then sent for an ECG. For comparison, his ECG from 6 months prior was included (Figure C). His new ECG (Figure D) demonstrated peaked P waves in lead II. There were also R waves in the anterior leads (V_1, V_2, and V_3) with concomitant deep S waves. Finally, notice the inverted T waves and ST segment depressions also in the anterior leads (extending to V_4). After reviewing all the foregoing information, the diagnosis of pulmonary hypertension was made.

D
aVR
V1
V4
II
aVL
V2
V5
III
aVF
V3
V6
V1
25 mm/sec
10 mm/mV
60~ 0.05 - 150 Hz
© Cameron Huxford

In RVH, the normal V_1–V_6 pattern changes owing to the thickened right ventricular wall. Tall R waves are seen in the right-sided chest leads, V_1 and V_2 (R to S ratio > 1.0), and much more biphasic QRS complexes in the left-sided chest leads, V_5 and V_6 (R to S ratio is much closer to 1.0 or maybe < 1.0). There is also a strain pattern in leads V_1 and V_2 (may also be seen in the inferior limb leads—II, III, and aVF). Additionally, if RVH is severe, it may cause a shift of the electrical axis to RAD (lead I is positive and aVF is negative). Figure 7.9 shows a patient with RVH.

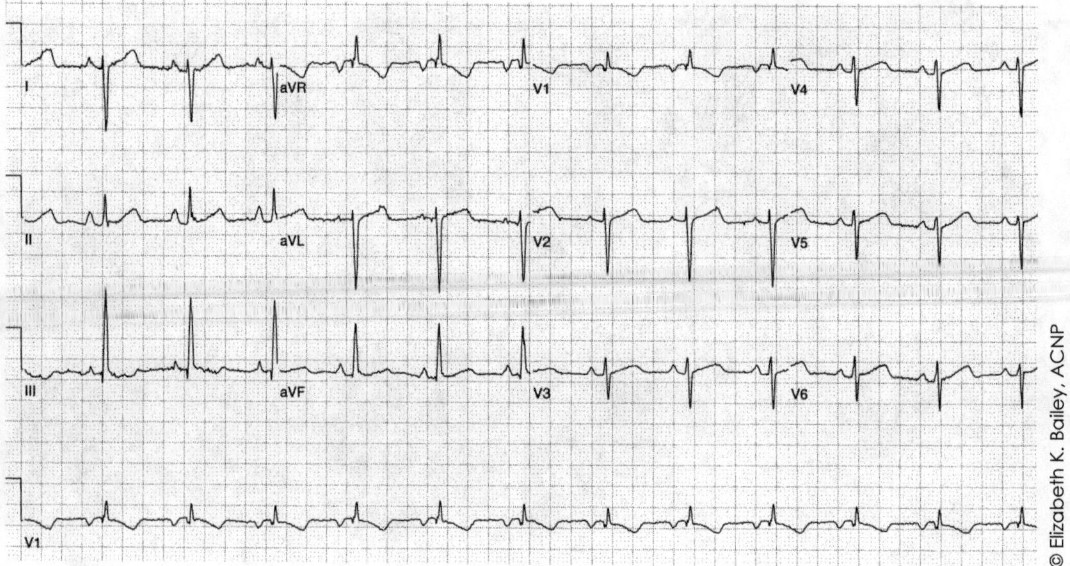

FIGURE 7.9 ECG depicting RVH in a 60-year-old White male. Note the tall R waves and strain pattern in V_1 and the more biphasic QRS complexes (deeper S than normal) in V_5 and V_6. Also, RAD is present (lead I negative and aVF positive).

Left Ventricular Hypertrophy (LVH)

LVH is most commonly caused by pathologic changes that increase the pressure or the volume of blood in the left ventricle. This is often seen in those with poorly controlled systemic hypertension as well as aortic valve dysfunction (specifically, aortic stenosis). The presence of LVH increases the risk of congestive heart failure as well as ventricular arrhythmias.

As with RVH, LVH shows characteristic changes in the QRS complex of the ECG. Whereas RVH showed a deviation from the normal V_1–V_6 QRS pattern, LVH produces an enhancement of the normal pattern. The negative S waves normally noted in the right precordial leads are deeper than usual, and tall R waves seen in the left precordial leads are taller than usual. As a rule, if the sum of the S wave below the baseline in V_1 or V_2 (whichever is the deeper of the two) plus the R wave above the baseline in V_5 or V_6 (whichever is the taller of the two) is $>$ 35 mm, then LVH is likely (Fig. 7.10). Also, like RVH, repolarization in LVH causes a ventricular

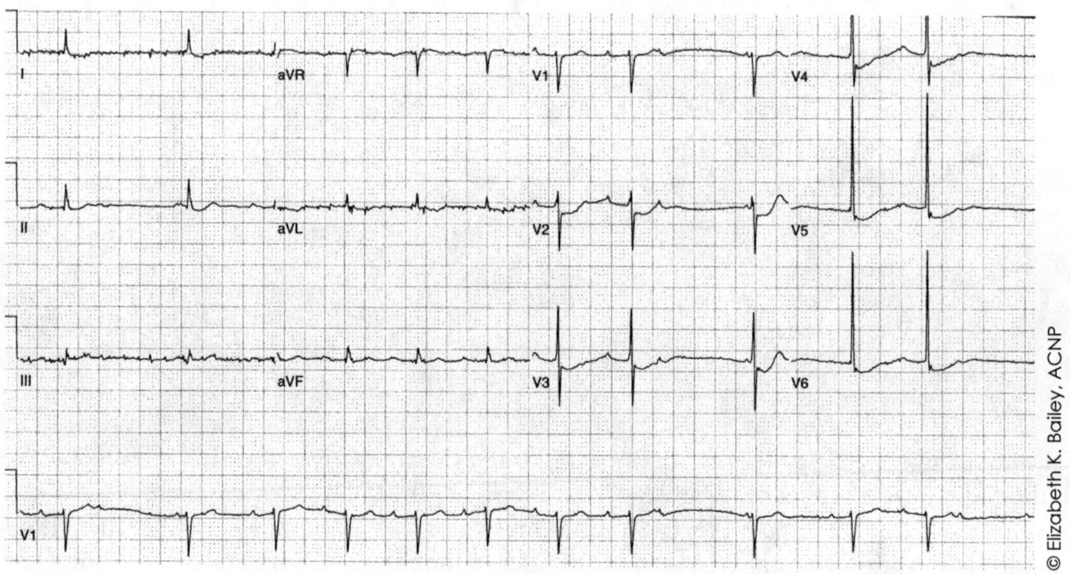

FIGURE 7.10 The 12-lead ECG of a 95-year-old Black female depicting LVH with strain. Note the tall R waves in the left chest leads and the strain pattern (repolarization abnormality).

TABLE 7.1 The Romhilt–Estes Point Scoring System.

ECG Changes	*Points*
Any limb lead R wave or S wave > 2 mV or SV1/SV2 ≥3 mV or RV5/RV6 ≥3 mV	3
ST-T abnormality, no digitalis therapy/with digitalis therapy	3/1
LA abnormality	3
LAD	2
Intrinsicoid deflection in V_5/V_6 > 50 mV	1
QRS duration > 90 msec	1

A score of ≥5 indicates definite LVH with 4 points being probably LVH.

strain pattern. This time, however, the affected side is the left side and therefore manifests in V_5 and V_6 (and sometimes the high lateral leads—I and aVL). Some amount of LAD (lead I is positive and lead aVF is negative) is also often present in LVH. Although LAD by itself is not useful in diagnosing LVH, it can assist in the diagnosis of LVH in the presence of other criteria. Several other diagnostic criteria have been developed for the detection of LVH (Table 7.1).

Hemodynamic and Mechanical Stressors in Left Ventricular Hypertrophy (LVH)

Table 7.2 presents the mechanisms implicated in the two basic forms of left ventricular hypertrophy. Hypertrophy of the myocardial tissue is an important compensatory mechanism for an increased **pressure** or **volume overload** imposed on the heart and provides the mechanical adjustment necessary to overcome the

TABLE 7.2 Summary of characteristics for the hypertrophy patterns (concentric and eccentric) and hemodynamic mechanisms influencing pathologic and physiologic LVH.

	Pathologic LVH		*Physiologic LVH*	
	Concentric	*Eccentric*	*Concentric*	*Eccentric*
Stimulating Hemodynamic Mechanisms	Increased Pressure (afterload)	Increased Volume (preload)	Increased Pressure (afterload)	Increased Volume (preload)
Potential Etiology of Stimulus	Hypertension, Aortic Stenosis	Valvular Disease	Resistance Exercise Training	Endurance Exercise Training
Ventricle Morphology	Parallel addition of new myofibrils (wall thickening), frequently with myocyte necrosis and increased fibrosis	Series addition of sarcomeres (wall dilation and thinning), frequently with myocyte necrosis	Parallel addition of new myofibrils (wall thickening) with increased capillary density	Series addition of sarcomeres (chamber volume enlargement)
Ventricular Mechanics	Diastolic dysfunction with stiffness and decreased contractility	Decreased contractility often associated with side-to-side slippage of **myocytes**	Normal or enhanced contractility and myocardial efficiency	Normal or enhanced contractility and myocardial efficiency
Ventricular Function	Abnormal	Abnormal	Normal	Normal or Supranormal
Potential to Regress	No	No	Yes	Yes

extra burden. Hypertrophy resulting from uncomplicated hypertension and characterized by normal left ventricular function would fit a model stating that left ventricular mass is a continuous variable with no threshold. LVH, then, may initially be a beneficial adaptive response for the cardiovascular system that could progress into a maladaptive condition that increases the risk of cardiovascular morbid events.

There is also evidence to suggest that rather than quantity of mass, it is the quality of the cellular components as well as the function of the hypertrophied myocardium that poses the risk of a cardiovascular morbid event. The functional performance or efficacy and the oxygen delivering capacity of the hypertrophied left ventricle, together with the reversibility of LVH once the overload is removed, have led to its classification as either pathologic or physiologic. These classifications are also defined by the nature of both the imposed load and the resulting myocardial adaptations. Each type possesses different mechanical, structural, and biochemical properties, thereby separating them into two distinctly different states. Figure 7.1 condenses the pertinent information from Table 7.2.

Chapter Questions

1. Determine the enlargement and/or hypertrophy patterns in the following ECG.

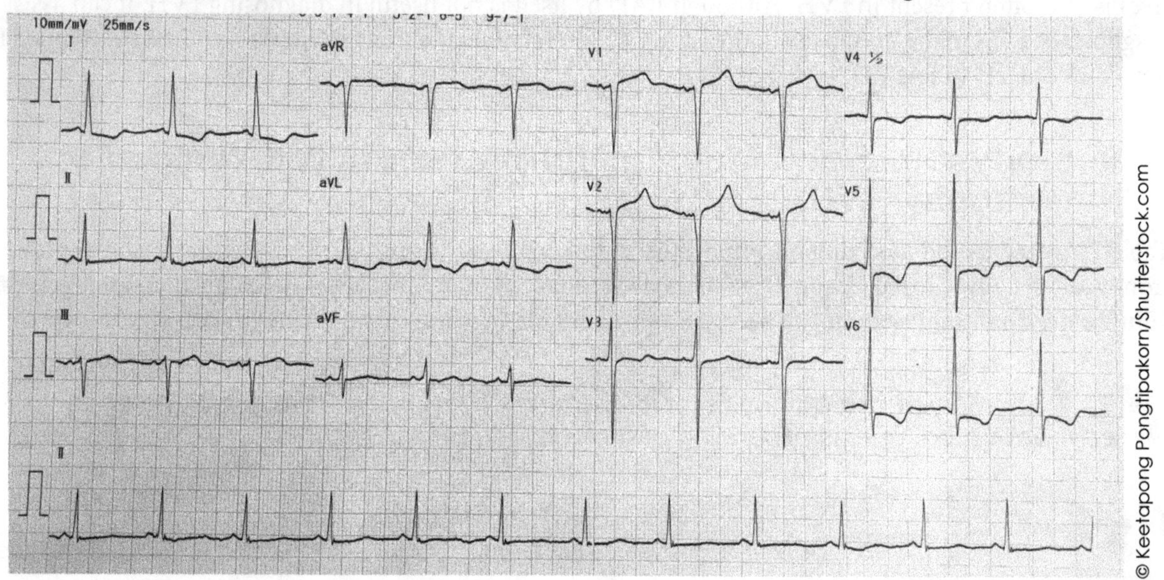

2. Compare and contrast the mechanisms by which the atria enlarge and the ventricles hypertrophy.

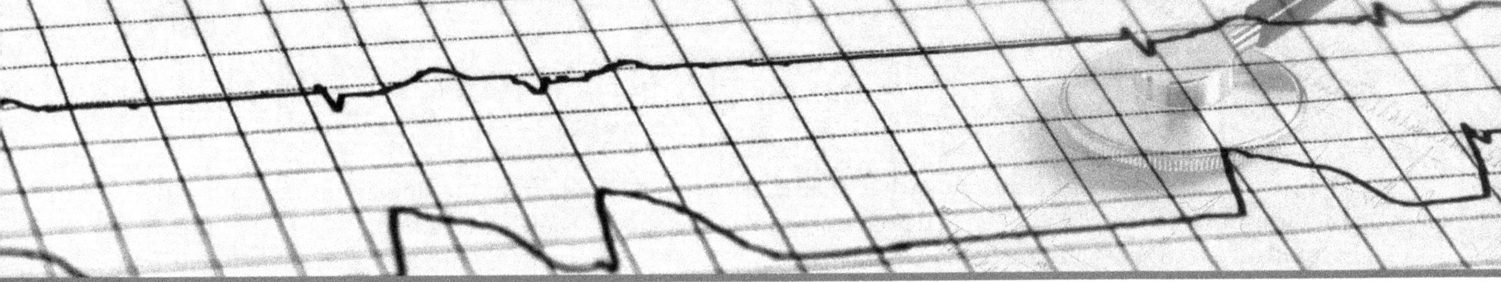

CHAPTER 8

Bundle Branch Blocks

Bundle branch block is a condition in which there is a delay along the pathway that electrical impulses travel to make the heart's ventricles fire. In the presence of bundle branch blocks, it is sometimes harder for the heart to pump blood efficiently through the body.

CONTENT OUTLINE

- Right Bundle Branch Block (RBBB)
- Left Bundle Branch Block (LBBB)
- Hemiblocks
- Bifascicular and Trifascicular Blocks
- Chapter Questions

The activation of the ventricles occurs when the electrical transmission from the sinoatrial (SA) node arrives at the atrioventricular (AV) node and propagates down the bundle branches (Fig. 8.1). Prior to this, the atria have already been activated, but because atrial tissue is not continuous with ventricular tissue there is only one normal route for the electrical signal to penetrate the **cardiac skeleton**. That route is through the AV node and the bundle of His, collectively called the AV junction, and, finally, down each bundle branch to activate the ventricles.

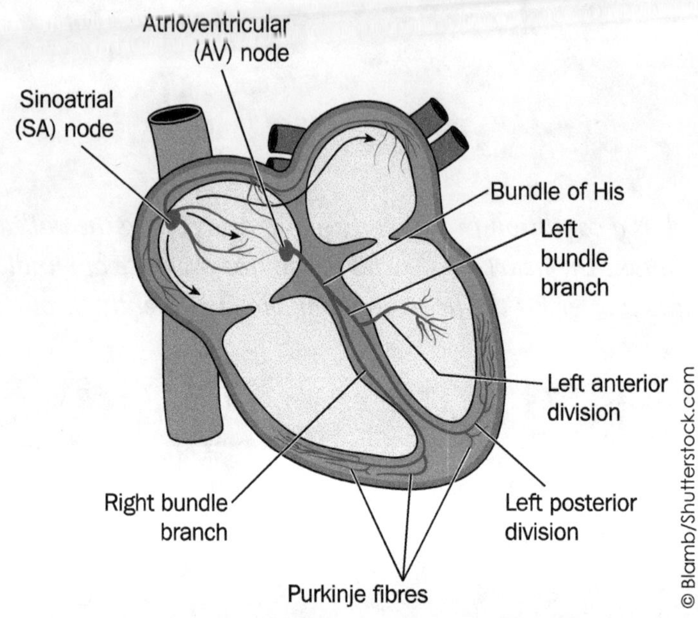

FIGURE 8.1 The normal intraventricular conduction system. The bundle of His divides into the left bundle branch and right bundle branch. The left bundle branch divides into anterior, posterior, and, in some cases, median fascicles.

Normally, the left side of the interventricular septum is activated first and then the ventricles are activated via the left and right bundle branches. The process is quick, usually taking about 100 ms. This quick activation assures a "tight" QRS complex with a normal width of less than or equal to 100 ms (two and a half small boxes on the electrocardiogram [ECG] graph paper). The activation pattern can be interrupted at any point beginning at the AV node, which results in a prolonged (wider than normal) QRS width. For bundle branch block, ventricular activation is always in either of the two bundle branches. The designation, block, is misleading, but it is the terminology that has been used historically, and it is still in use. A better term, arguably, is conduction disturbance because most of these "blocks" are delays in the transmission of the depolarization wave down the bundle branch, which slows but doesn't block electrical conduction.

Right Bundle Branch Block (RBBB)

A conduction disturbance somewhere in the right bundle branch delays the stimulation of the right ventricle, resulting in a wide QRS complex. Further, there is a tell-tale morphological change in the QRS complex resulting from this right bundle branch delay. This resultant change in the shape of the QRS complex can be predicted by first considering the normal activation process of the right and left ventricles.

The first part of the ventricles to be depolarized is the interventricular septum. The stimulation occurs from the left wall of the septum to the right wall by a branch of the left bundle—the left middle (septal) fascicle (Fig. 8.1). This activation vector (Fig. 8.2A1) results in a small r wave deflection (the septal r) in the right chest lead. This depolarization vector (left to right) is aimed at lead V_1. At the same time, the vector depicted in picture A of Figure 8.2 fires away from the left chest lead, producing a small septal q wave in lead V_6. Since this activation pattern involves a left-to-right firing sequence by a portion of the left bundle branch, RBBB will not affect the septal phase of ventricular stimulation.

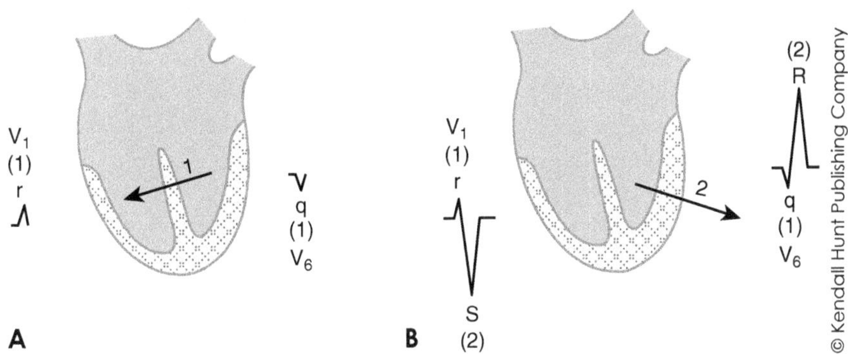

FIGURE 8.2 Normal right and left ventricular activation pattern. **A** depicts the first part of ventricular depolarization proceeding from the left septal wall to the right (vector 1) and the ECG inscriptions produced in V_1 and V_6. The arrow represents the left to right orientation of vector 1. **B** shows the last part of ventricular depolarization. The left ventricle with its more substantial vector (2) points to the left chest lead V_6. Left ventricular activation inscribes a deep S wave in V_1 and a tall R wave in V_6. **B** shows the final form the ECG tracing takes at the end of normal ventricular activation. The QRS complexes are normal width.

Following septal stimulation, there is the near simultaneous depolarization of the left and right ventricles (Fig. 8.2B). The schematic drawing of the left ventricle indicates a much more muscular left ventricle, making it electrically dominant over the right ventricle. This is easily seen in the size of the left ventricular S wave in V_1 and the left ventricular R wave in V_6 (Fig. 8.2B), with the predominant vector (Fig. 8.2B2) leftward pointing. The electrical discharge from the right ventricle is normally "buried" here.

This normal activation sequence is shown again in Figure 8.3A and B. However, in RBBB there is a delay in the total time needed for stimulation of the right ventricle. The conduction "block" is somewhere along the RBB. The delay, once released, produces an R′ wave in V_1, signifying the late right ventricular depolarization. This late activation of the right ventricle also shows up in V_6 as a wide S wave (Fig. 8.3C). Therefore, in RBBB the left ventricle completely depolarizes while right ventricular depolarization is continuing. This is signified in Figure 8.3 C3 as a third vector pointing at V_1 (producing the late R wave, designated as R′) and away from V_6 (producing the S wave). This third vector represents a rightward spread of a delayed and slow right ventricular depolarization.

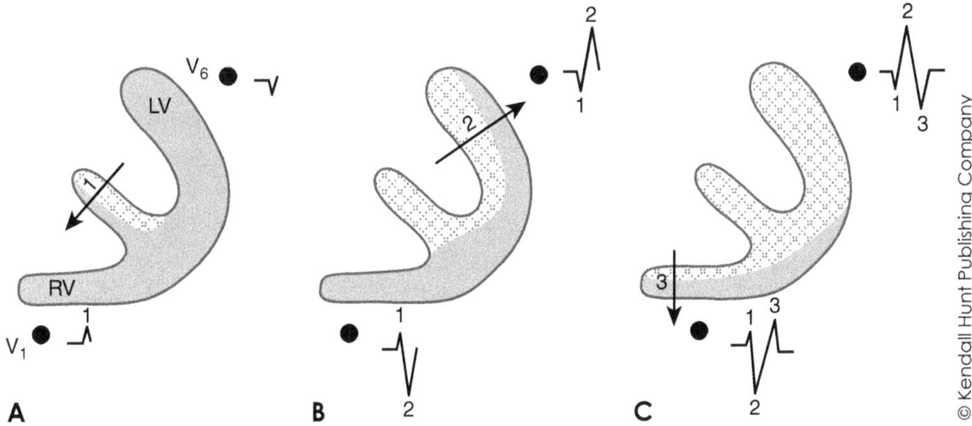

FIGURE 8.3 Stepwise sequence of ventricular depolarization in right bundle branch block.

Therefore, in RBBB there is a distinct pattern of an rSR′ complex in V_1 and a qRS (broad S) complex in V_6. The broad S is sometimes referred to as a slurred S. These are the two best leads in which to view these characteristic ECG changes, leading to a definitive interpretation of RBBB. Figures 8.4, 8.5 and 8.6 present three 12-lead ECG tracings showing the typical RBBB pattern. Also shown in Figures 8.4 and 8.5 is a typical associated pattern in RBBB, namely, T wave inversion (a strain pattern). An inverted T wave in V_1 is a secondary change in RBBB and involves no inference of abnormalities associated with primary ST-T changes common to ischemia or a drug effect. Additionally, Figure 8.6 presents a patient with incomplete RBBB. In complete RBBB, the QRS width is ≥ 0.12 sec in duration. Incomplete RBBB shows the same abnormal QRS pattern in leads V_1 and V_6 but with a duration between 0.1 and 0.12 s. In other words, the delay in the propagation of right ventricular stimulation is not as great.

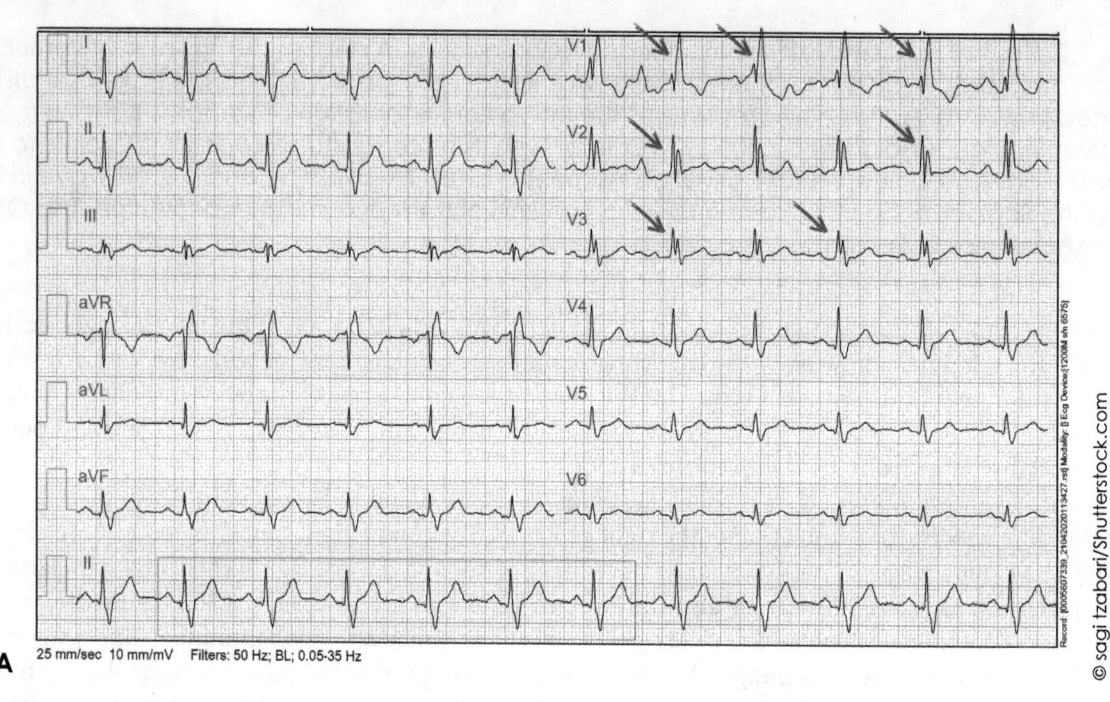

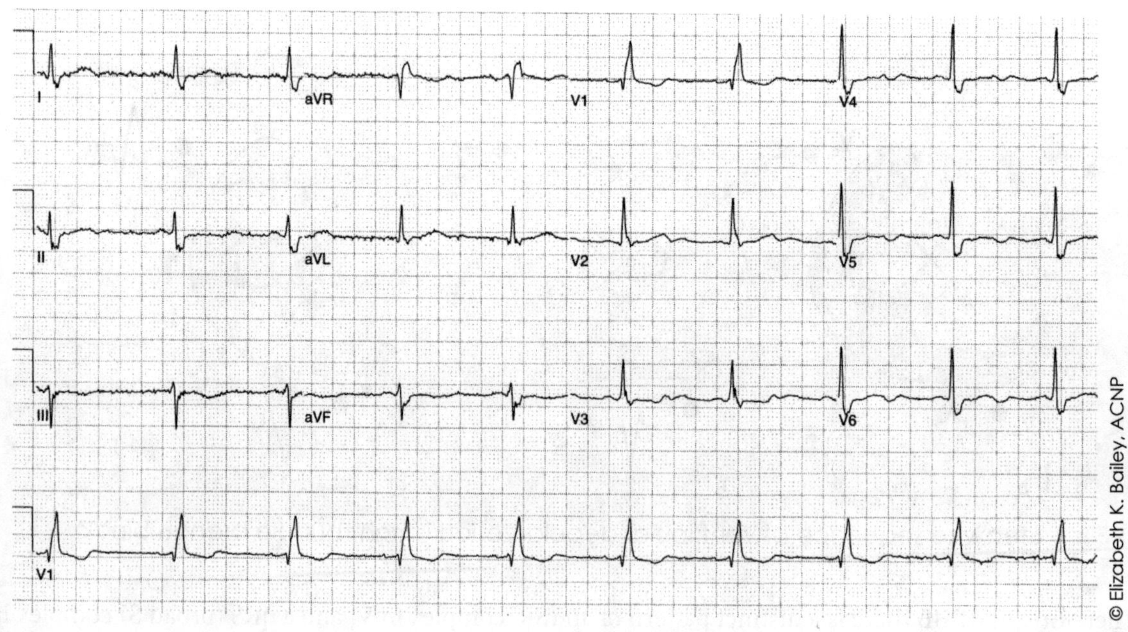

FIGURE 8.4 **A** is an abnormal 12-lead ECG showing RBBB with the rSR' pattern (arrows) in leads $V_{1\text{-}3}$ and slurred S waves in leads $V_{4\text{-}6}$. **B** is the 12-lead ECG of a 90-year-old White male with RBBB and LAD.

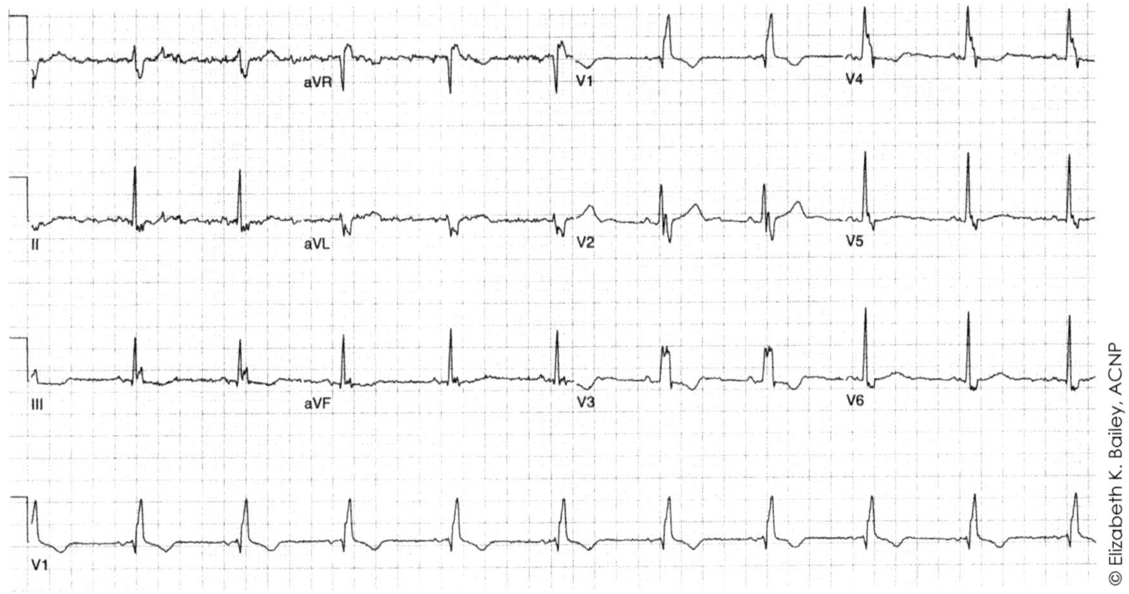

FIGURE 8.5 Abnormal 12-lead ECG in an 88-year-old female patient. The ECG shows normal sinus rhythm with RBBB.

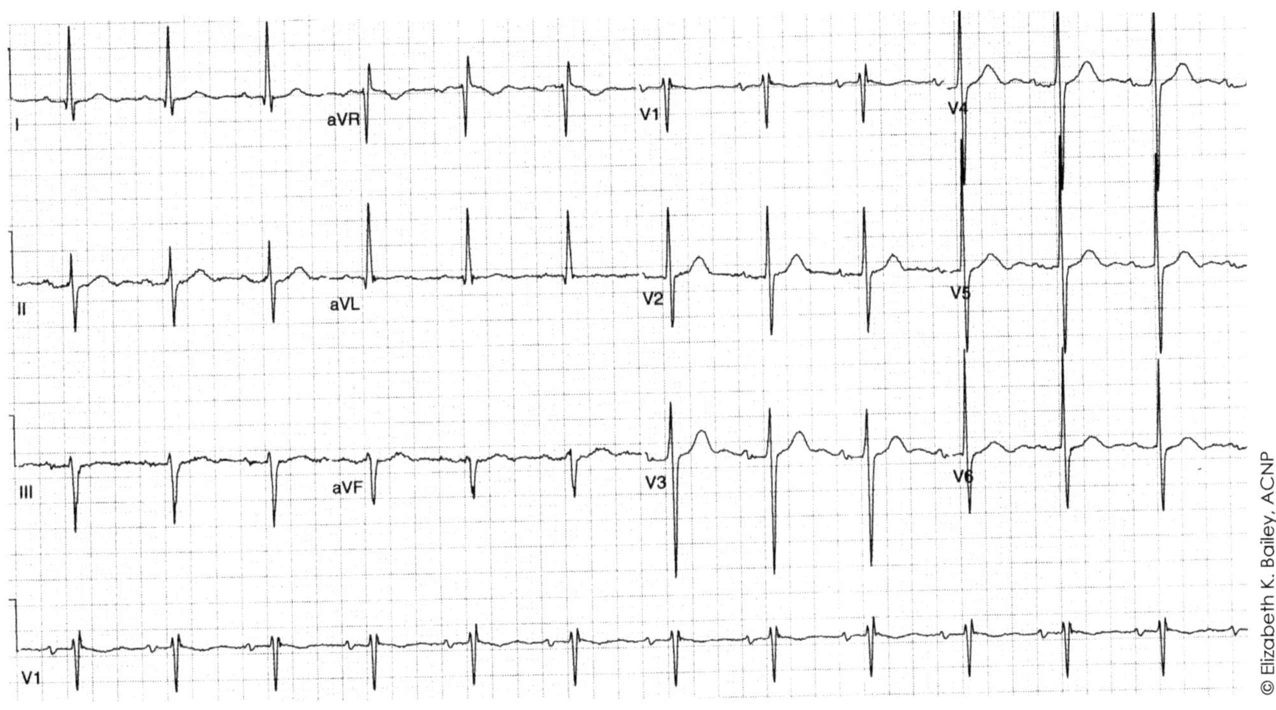

FIGURE 8.6 Abnormal 12-lead ECG in a 70-year-old male patient. The ECG shows normal sinus rhythm, left axis deviation, and incomplete RBBB. RBBB can be complete or incomplete. In incomplete RBBB, the QRS duration is between 0.1 and 0.12 s.

What is the significance of RBBB on an ECG? RBBB is usually an incidental finding, meaning that the ECG would have been carried out for another reason. However, in the presence of symptoms like chest pain or shortness of breath or syncope, it might signify underlying heart or lung disorders such as the following:

- Long-standing right heart failure
- Myocardial infarction (heart attack)
- Congenital heart conditions (hole in the heart)
- Long-standing lung conditions affecting the right side of the heart
- Pulmonary embolism (clot in the lung)

RBBB seen in elderly individuals without heart problems could be attributable to degenerative changes in the right bundle branch as a normal consequence of aging.

Left Bundle Branch Block (LBBB)

All conductance delays through the bundle branches produce widened QRS complexes. With a delay in the LBB, the pattern produced is different than that seen by a delay in the RBB. At the outset of this discussion, it is important to note that the main distinction between the two is as follows: RBBB mainly affects the terminal phase of ventricular activation, whereas LBBB affects the early phase.

Septal activation normally commences in a left to right vector as the left bundle branch depolarizes (Fig. 8.2A and Fig. 8.3A). This vector produces in V_1 a small septal r wave and a septal q wave in V_6. LBBB reverses the septal vector in ventricular sequential depolarization by switching the vector from rightward to leftward (Fig. 8.7A). This occurs as a direct consequence of the delay in depolarizing the left wall of the interventricular septum. Instead, the right wall is depolarized first and in the opposite direction (Fig. 8.7A). This change in the activation sequence of LBBB has several consequences. First, the total time for left ventricular depolarization is prolonged, resulting in wide QRS complexes because the right and left ventricles are no longer fired in a near simultaneous fashion. This is shown in Figure 8.7B. There is a wide, entirely negative complex in V_1 and a wide, entirely positive complex in V_6. In each case, the complexes are sometimes shown as notched at their points (QS wave in V_1 and the R wave in V_6). Summarizing, in LBBB the entire stimulation sequence is reoriented from right to left (toward V_6) with the dominant left ventricle firing late. The morphology of the QRS complex is therefore radically different than that shown during normal ventricular activation shown in Figure 8.2. Figure 8.8 shows a 12-lead ECG with LBBB. Just as secondary T wave inversion occurs in RBBB, so too can they occur in LBBB, usually seen in leads with tall R waves (the left precordial leads) as a characteristic of LBBB. LBBB can also be incomplete, in which case the QRS complexes are between 0.1 and 0.12 s wide.

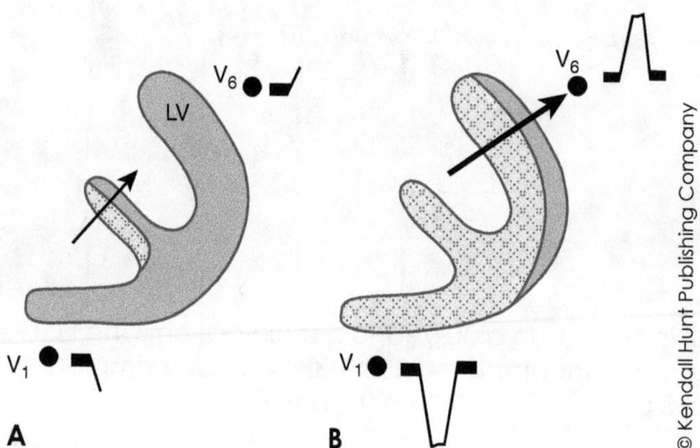

FIGURE 8.7 Stepwise sequence of ventricular depolarization in left bundle branch block.

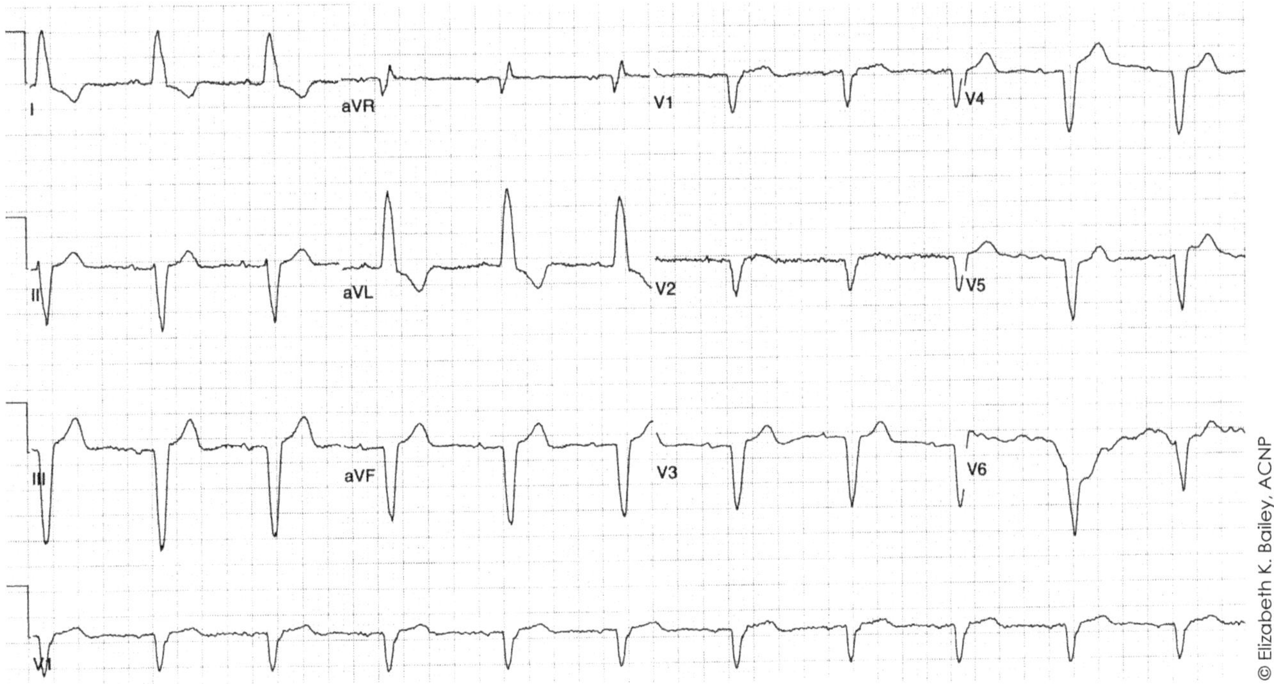

FIGURE 8.8 Abnormal 12-lead ECG in an 87-year-old White female patient. The ECG shows normal sinus rhythm with left axis deviation and LBBB.

LBBB most often occurs in patients with underlying heart disease and may be associated with progressive conducting system disease. However, LBBB can also be seen in asymptomatic patients with a structurally normal heart. The presence of LBBB complicates the diagnosis of myocardial ischemia/infarction and interferes with the interpretation of exercise testing. In patients with significant left ventricular dysfunction, LBBB results in left ventricular **dyssynchrony** and may contribute to heart failure. The electrocardiographic changes in LBBB can cause diagnostic problems in a variety of clinical conditions:

- left ventricular hypertrophy—diagnosis of left ventricular hypertrophy can be established only by echocardiography in an individual with LBBB because the two disorders produce similar ECG changes
- myocardial ischemia—LBBB masks the ability to identify ischemia during exercise because of the associated ST and T wave abnormalities acute myocardial infarction—LBBB complicates and often prevents the electrocardiographic diagnosis of acute myocardial infarction

Hemiblocks

Hemiblocks, also called fascicular blocks, are more complicated than what we have seen to this point. Recall that the LBB is not a single pathway but actually a trifascicular structure involving posterior, anterior, and septal fascicles (Fig. 8.1). The bundle of His divides at the juncture of the fibrous and muscular boundaries of the interventricular septum into the right and left bundle branches. The main left bundle branch penetrates the membranous portion of the interventricular septum under the aortic ring and then divides into several fairly discrete branches. Large individual variability is present in the size and distribution of the left fascicles. Most individuals present with two main fascicles of the left bundle branch. The left anterior fascicle crosses the left ventricular outflow tract and terminates in the Purkinje system of the anterolateral wall of the left ventricle. The left posterior fascicle fans out inferiorly and posteriorly into Purkinje fibers. About 65% of hearts have a left septal fascicle (variously called the left middle or left median fascicle) that serves the interventricular septum.

Anatomically variable, it arises from the common left bundle or from the anterior, posterior, or both fascicles and has many interconnections. In the normal heart, the three fascicles of the left bundle are simultaneously depolarized.

Blocks in the RBB have been discussed. Blocks in the LBB are more complicated because of the distinct anatomy involved, that is, occurring at any single point (or in multiple points) in either of the three divisions. A block in any one of these fascicles is called a hemiblock, and unlike right or left bundle blocks, which widen the QRS complex, hemiblocks do not markedly widen the QRS complex.

Left septal hemiblock is a hemiblock occurring only in the septal fascicle. It mainly affects the direction, but not the duration, of the QRS complex because the conduction disturbance primarily involves the early phase of activation. Myocardial activation may be affected in two ways by a conduction disturbance in the left septal fascicle: (1) apparent gain of anterior forces or (2) apparent loss of anterior forces. With a gain in anterior depolarization forces, there is an early precordial transition/counterclockwise rotation with prominent R waves in the right precordial leads like those that occur in posterior myocardial infarction. The loss of anterior forces is thought to be related to a functional loss or hyperkalemia-induced dysfunction in the left septal fascicle. The result is a transient development of q waves in leads V_1 and V_2, which normally have a positive initial deflection owing to septal depolarization. Similar changes occur with permanent left septal fascicular block and are indistinguishable from septal fibrosis or infarction. The major clinical implication of LSFB, then, is that the ECG mimics the changes induced by a septal or posterior myocardial infarction.

Left anterior hemiblock, if isolated, involves a mean QRS axis $\geq -45°$ (S wave in lead aV_F is $\geq$ the R wave in lead I) and a QRS width of < 0.12 s (Fig. 8.9). There are qR complexes in the inferior leads and rS complexes in the high lateral leads.

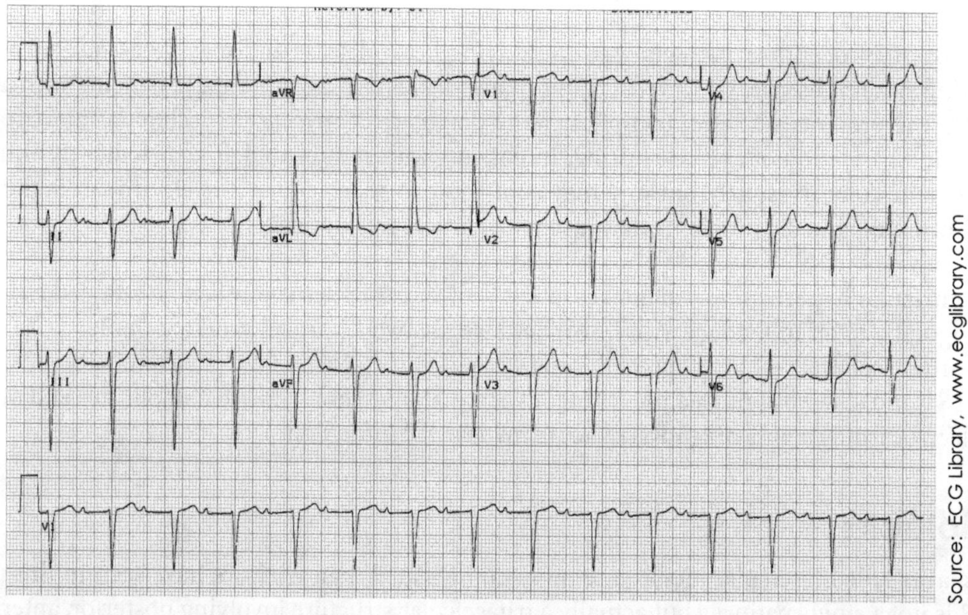

FIGURE 8.9 Left anterior hemiblock: QRS axis $\geq -45°$, initial R wave in inferior leads, absence of any other cause of LAD. First-degree heart block is also present. Interestingly, in the presence of left anterior hemiblock the diagnostic criteria of LVH are changed. In this case, an S wave in lead III deeper than 15 mm is predictive of LVH.

Left posterior hemiblock, if isolated, involves a finding of a mean QRS axis $\geq +120°$ with a QRS width of < 0.12 s (Fig. 8.10). There are rS complexes in the inferior leads and qR complexes in the high lateral leads. However, isolated left posterior hemiblock is very rare. The condition most often occurs with RBBB. The proper interpretation of left posterior hemiblock, however, is made after the usual causes of RAD (right ventricular hypertrophy, emphysema, lateral wall MI, pulmonary embolism) are excluded.

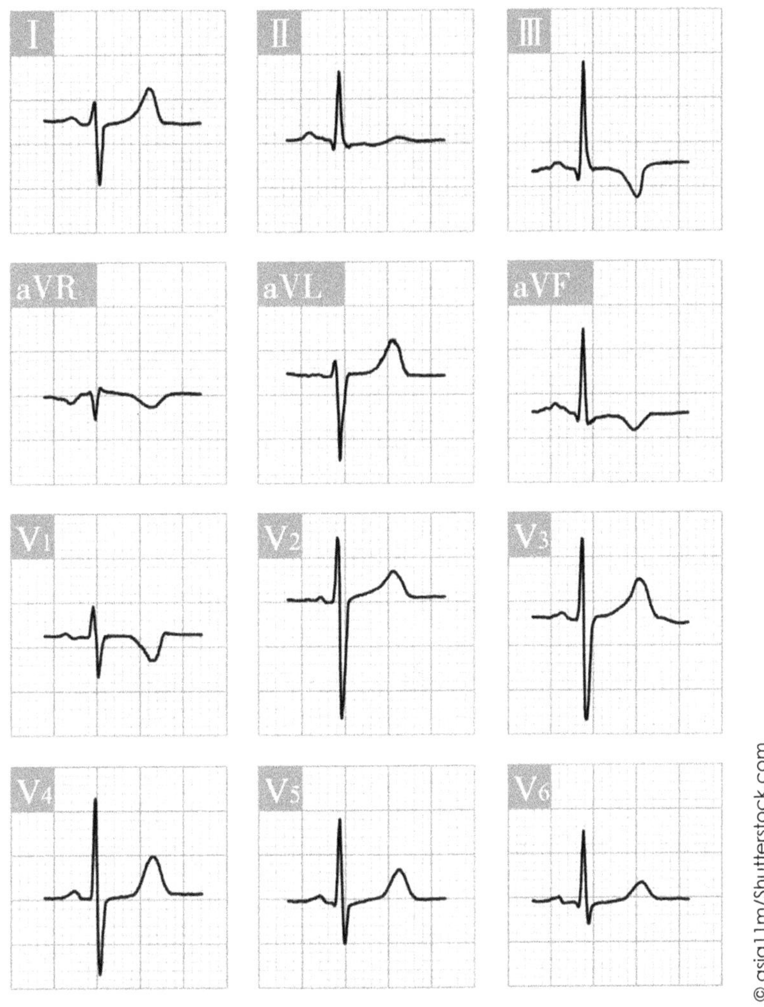

FIGURE 8.10 Left posterior hemiblock—QRS duration modestly prolonged at 102 ms, RAD, qR complexes in the inferior leads and rS complexes in the high lateral leads.

Bifascicular and Trifascicular Blocks

A bifascicular block combines a RBBB with either a left anterior hemiblock (common) or a left posterior hemiblock (less common) (Fig. 8.11). Bifascicular blocks put patients at risk of complete heart block (third-degree AV block). Although many patients have chronic bifascicular block for years and do not develop concerning symptoms, we should be mindful of the fact that patients with syncope and bifascicular block may be experiencing transient episodes of third-degree AV block or even asystole (third-degree AV block with no escape rhythm). Bifascicular blocks make ventricular conduction dependent on the single remaining fascicle.

Blockage of just the left anterior fascicle produces left anterior hemiblock with left axis deviation. Blockage of just the left posterior fascicle produces left posterior hemiblock with right axis deviation. It is also possible that in individuals with a septal portion of the LBB there can be a left septal fascicle block producing left septal hemiblock. This is a more recent finding. Historically, the LBB was thought to be only bifascicular. Therefore, terminology was adopted for the combination of LBBB with both left anterior and left posterior blockage—a trifascicular block. If indeed a septal branch is anatomically present in individuals, the existence of a quadfascicular block is a possibility. These are very rare occurrences, however. Chapter 13 introduces AV heart blocks, blocks that occur in the AV junction before the bundle of His bifurcates into right and left bundle branches.

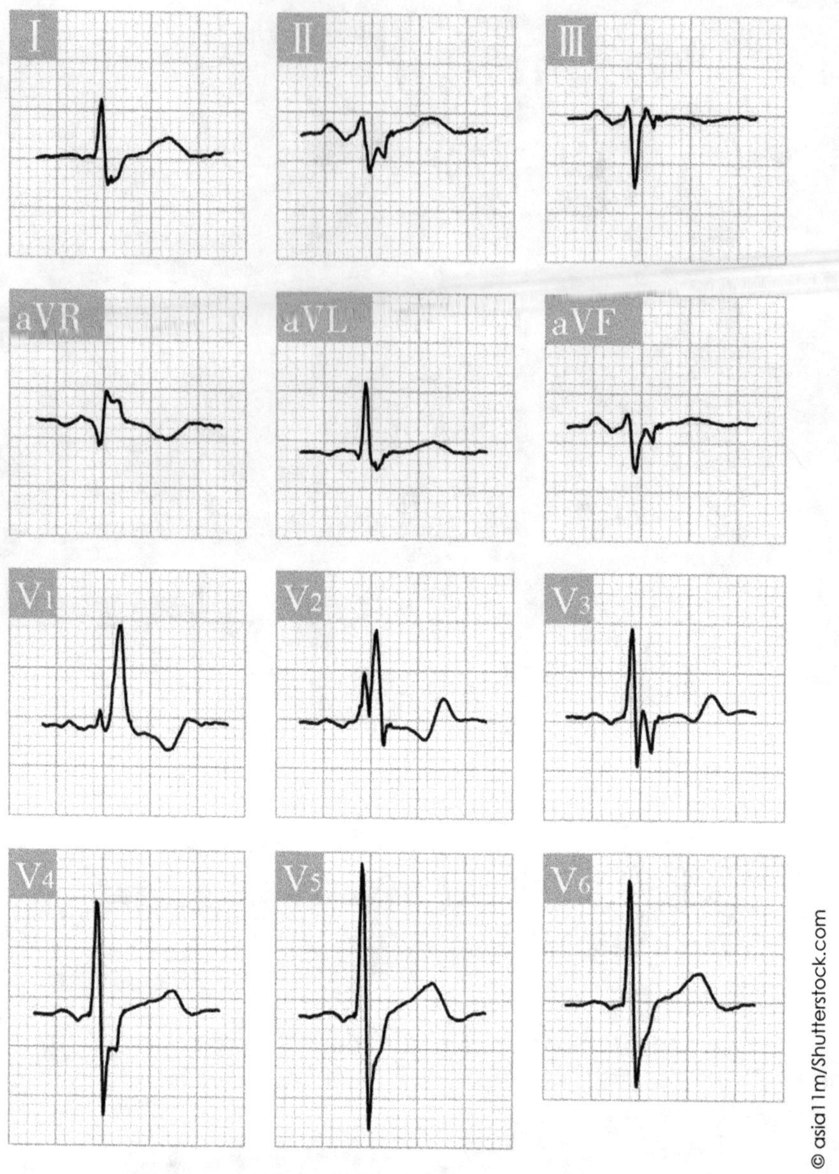

FIGURE 8.11 Complete RBBB with left anterior hemiblock. There is an rsR' complex in lead V_1 and V_2, LAD, and rS complexes in the inferior leads and qR complex in the high lateral lead aVL.

Chapter Questions

1. Practice your knowledge of ventricular activation by drawing the usual shape of the QRS complex from memory and how this shape is changed with either RBBB or LBBB.
2. Which BBB is more clinically significant? Why?

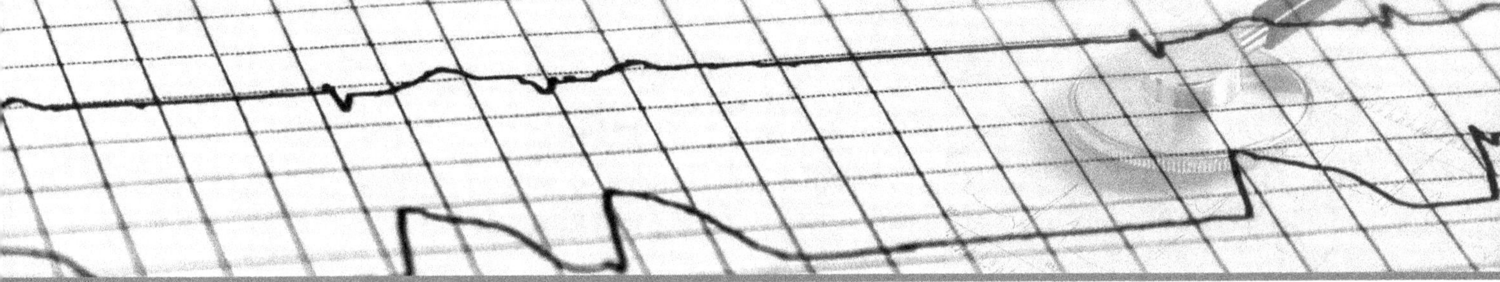

CHAPTER 9

Myocardial Ischemia and Infarction

Ischemia denotes diminished volume of perfusion, whereas infarction is the cellular response to lack of perfusion.

CONTENT OUTLINE

- Myocardial Ischemia
- Myocardial Infarction
  - Left ventricular infarction
  - Right ventricular infarction
  - Subendocardial infarction
- Special Considerations
  - Myocardial infarction with bundle branch block
  - Ventricular aneurysm
- Case Study

The heart is the systolic pump for the pulmonary and systemic circuits but receives its own blood supply during diastole through the coronary circulation. The coronary circulation opens via the proximal aorta into right and left main coronary arteries (Fig. 9.1). The left coronary artery (LCA) has two main branches: the left anterior descending artery (LAD) and the left circumflex artery (LCX). The right coronary artery (RCA) supplies the right ventricle and the inferior region of the heart. The LAD supplies the anterior side of the left ventricle and the interventricular septum. The LCX encircles the heart to supply the lateral and posterior side of the left ventricle.

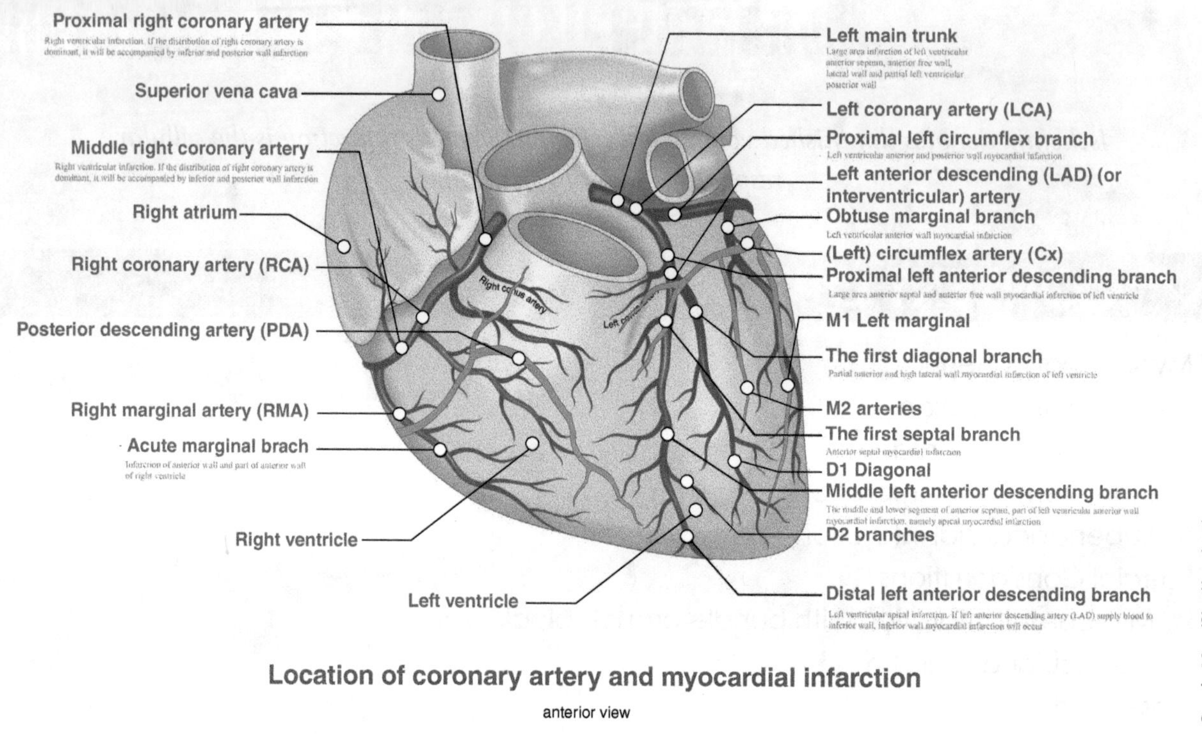

FIGURE 9.1 The coronary tree.

Heart dominance is described by which coronary artery branch gives rise to the posterior descending artery (PDA), which supplies the inferior wall. Heart dominance is characterized as left, right, or codominant. The PDA supplies the posterior third of the interventricular septum, including the posterior and inferior wall of the left ventricle. The PDA most commonly originates from the RCA (right dominant), LCX (left dominant), or both (codominant). It is estimated that approximately 70% to 80% of the population is right-heart dominant, 5% to 10% are left-heart dominant; and about 10% to 20% are codominant, with the PDA supplied by both the LCX and the RCA. Cardiac dominance plays an important role in coronary artery bypass graft surgery, where precise knowledge of a patient's coronary anatomy is needed to identify which vessels are best suited to the distal anastomosis of the venous graft.

Myocardial Ischemia

An inadequate blood supply to the heart muscle results in myocardial ischemia. Myocardial ischemia and infarction result in ECG changes that can usually be approximated to the offending artery. Knowing the location allows for timely and targeted therapy to provide better clinical outcomes.

Extending the period of acute myocardial ischemia for more than 20 minutes leads to cardiomyocyte death, beginning in the **subendocardium** and extending across the extent of the myocardial wall toward the pericardium. During acute myocardial ischemia, the lack of oxygen switches cell metabolism to anaerobic respiration with lactate accumulation, ATP depletion, Na^+ and Ca^{2+} overload, and inhibition of myocardial contractile function. This extended lack of blood supply results in a myocardial infarction (MI), the death of the affected region of the heart muscle.

Myocardial ischemia is usually attributable to severe narrowing of a coronary artery. Figure 9.2 depicts a simplified schema of lesion diversity in human coronary atherosclerosis, showing two morphological extremes of coronary atherosclerotic plaques. Stenotic lesions tend to have smaller lipid cores (more fibrosis and calcified), thick fibrous caps, and less compensatory enlargement. The ischemia they produce is typically managed by combined medical therapy and revascularization to relieve symptoms. Nonstenotic lesions outnumber stenotic plaques and tend to have large lipid cores and thin, fibrous caps susceptible to rupture and thrombosis. They often undergo substantial compensatory enlargement that leads to underestimation of lesion size by angiography. Nonstenotic plaques may cause no symptoms for many years but when disrupted can provoke episodes of unstable angina or MI. Management of nonstenotic lesions includes lifestyle modification and pharmacotherapy in high-risk individuals.

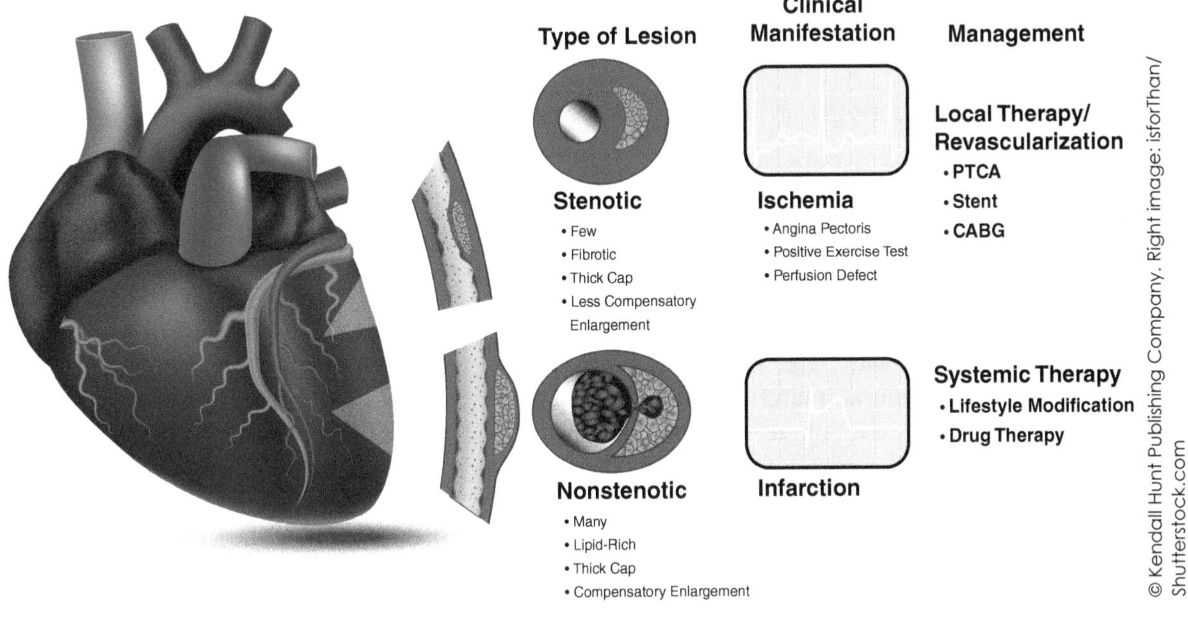

FIGURE 9.2 Atherosclerosis is the process of laying down fatty deposits in the lumen of arteries. The enlarged segments of the schematic show longitudinal section (left) and cross section (right). Many coronary atherosclerotic lesions may lie between these two extremes, produce mixed clinical manifestations, and require multipronged management. Because both types of lesions usually coexist in given high-risk individuals, optimum management often requires both revascularization and systemic therapy. PTCA (percutaneous transluminal coronary angioplasty), CABG (coronary artery bypass graft).

Myocardial ischemia produces diverse ECG changes owing to the various ways ischemia can manifest in the myocardium. As shown in Figure 9.3, ischemia may be persistent, producing infarction, or transient, producing anginal attacks. The extent of the ischemia is also important. Worse-case scenarios involve ischemic attacks across the entirety of the myocardial wall, leading to a transmural infarct. Notice in Figure 9.3 the top two scenarios are limited to ischemic episodes localized to the subendocardium, whereas the bottom two involve ischemia across (trans) the myocardial wall. Further, the top scenarios, whether noninfarction or infarction, involve ST depression as the principal ECG change, and the bottom scenarios involve ST elevations.

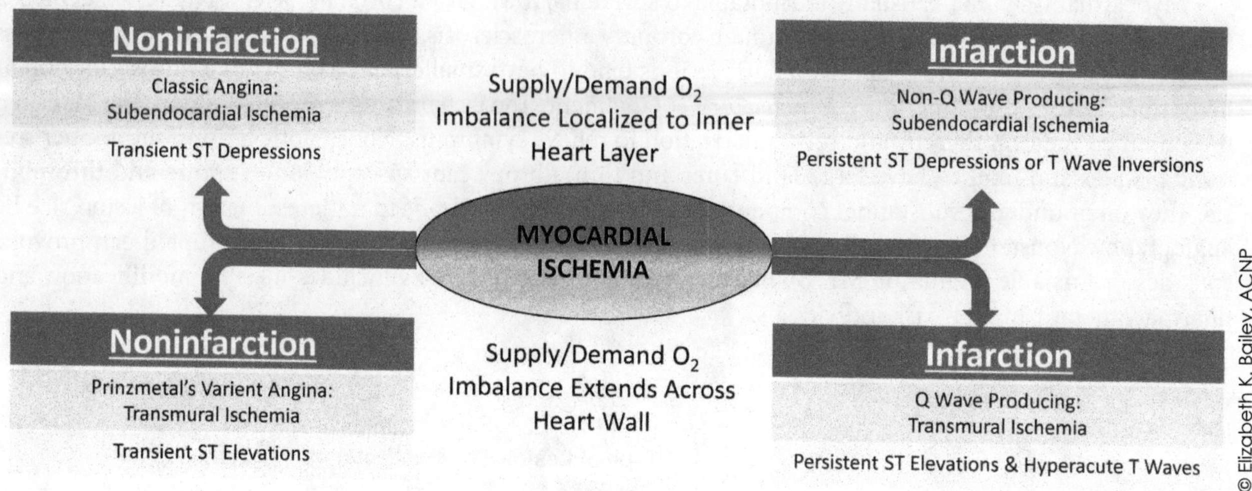

FIGURE 9.3 Myocardial ischemic paradigm for infarctional and noninfarctional ischemia with principal ECG changes.

When transient, an ischemic attack results in angina pectoris (either the classic variety, top left panel of Fig. 9.3) or variant "atypical" angina (bottom left panel of Fig. 9.3). In the case of Prinzmetal's variant angina, the chest pain is associated with ST elevations (Fig. 9.4) that resolve back to the baseline without later Q wave formation typical of transmural infarction. The classic symptoms of angina pectoris include substernal chest pressure and dull pain. The pain often radiates to the neck, jaw, or left shoulder (Fig. 3.1). This pain is usually brought on by the exertion of exercise or various other forms of physical activity as a result of an imbalance between the heart's demand for oxygen and its supply. Ischemia producing angina pectoris may be reversed with rest or with medication such as nitroglycerin, which acts as a vasodilator to allow increased blood flow to the affected area of the heart.

Given that exercise can precipitate subendocardial ischemia, an exercise stress test is often used as part of the workup for someone with worrisome or unexplained angina pectoris. In its classic form, an exercise stress test includes recording the ECG while the patient is walking on a treadmill. A positive stress test results when the patient develops angina and/or when ST segment changes are diagnosed. It must be remembered that a negative stress test does not always rule out coronary artery disease. A negative stress test in the presence of coronary artery disease is classed as a false negative test (See Chapter 4).

If the aforementioned ischemia involves only the inner portion of the cardiac chamber, it is referred to as subendocardial ischemia. This area of the heart is vulnerable to ischemia because it is the most distant from the blood supply of the coronary arteries. The classic ECG change of subendocardial ischemia is ST-segment depression (Fig. 9.4). If blood flow is not restored, subendocardial ischemia can progress into the outer layer of the heart, the epicardium, a condition known as transmural ischemia. Myocardial ischemia, whether sub-endocardial or transmural, can deteriorate into **necrosis** of the affected area of heart muscle, which is more commonly known as MI. Case Study 9.1 presents a patient who has had an ischemic episode entering an exercise program.

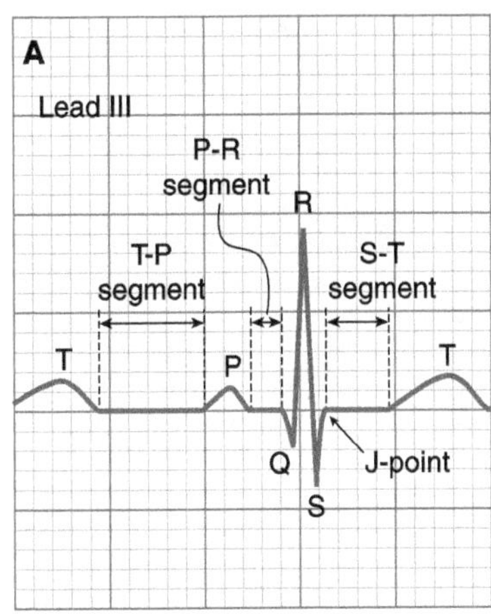

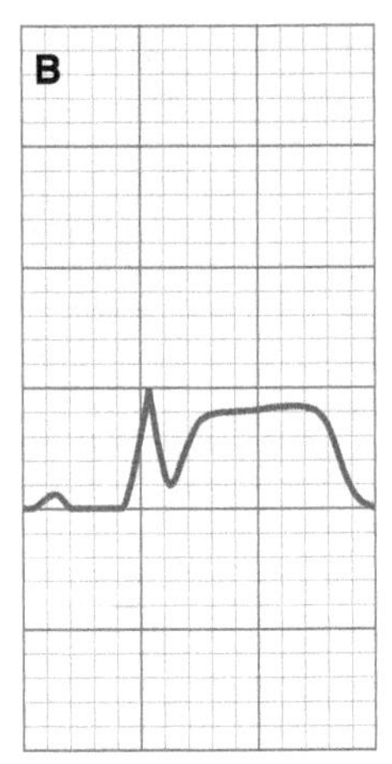

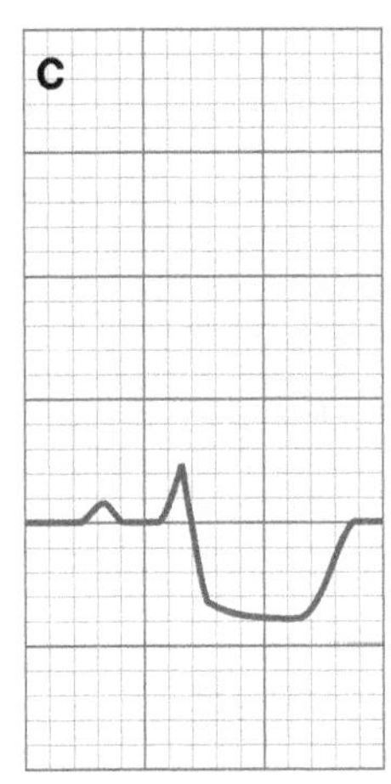

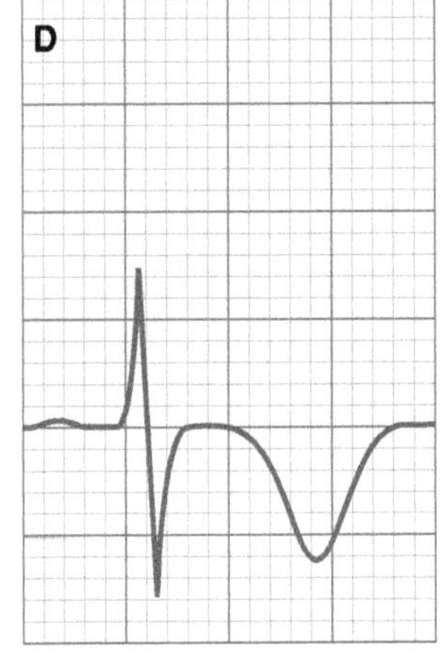

ST-Segment Deviation

A Normal ECG complex, the TP or PR is used to define the isoelectric line. ST-segment is measured at 60–80 ms after the J point

B ST- elevation—the ST-segment is abnormally raised at a measurement of 60–80 ms after the J point

C ST- depression—the ST-segment is abnormally depressed 60–80 ms after the J point

D T-wave inversion describes a T wave of regular morphology but negative polarity. It is often referred to as "flipped" i.e. below the isoelectric line

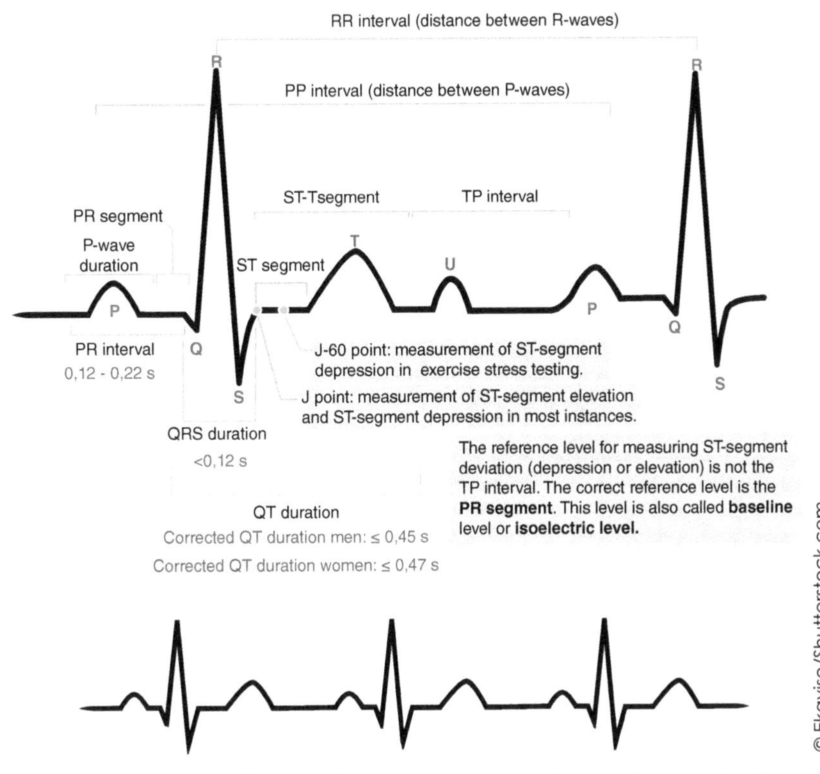

FIGURE 9.4 **A–D** shows the normal ECG waveform versus waveforms demonstrating ST segment elevation and depression with subsequent T wave morphological changes. Recall that in the normal ECG waveform, identification of the isoelectric line is important. **E** shows important durations on the electrocardiogram over two cardiac cycles. The PR segment and the ST segment are normally isoelectric. Deviations from the isoelectric line (**B–D**) of the ST segment has important implications.

CASE STUDY 9.1: MYOCARDIAL ISCHEMIA WITH ECG CHANGES

John is a 51-year-old male who was recently admitted to the hospital with chest pain while walking up three flights of stairs. Past medical history includes peptic ulcer disease, for which he takes medication. The patient is 30 pounds overweight and has a sedentary lifestyle. Family history is positive for heart disease—his father died of a myocardial infarction (MI) at the age of 60. Medical workup in the hospital included examination of cardiac enzymes, a resting ECG, determination of blood cholesterol levels, and a cardiac catheterization. Based on the cardiac enzymes, the patient did not have an MI. Total blood cholesterol levels were 250 mg·dL^{-1}. Results of the cardiac catheterization showed an 80% blockage in the left anterior descending coronary artery. Subsequently, the patient underwent the percutaneous transluminal coronary angioplasty (PTCA) procedure to open the narrowed coronary artery. The patient was discharged from the hospital in 3 days and was referred to an outpatient cardiac rehabilitation program. The patient is now on medication to reduce cholesterol levels and anticoagulant therapy to prevent the formation of blood clots.

Description

The development of coronary atherosclerosis begins with a small, local accumulation of lipids and fibrous tissue. This local accumulation progressively increases in size over time, resulting in narrowing of the lumen of the coronary arteries. Symptoms of cardiac ischemia usually appear when the cross-sectional area of the artery is reduced by 75%. Often these fatty lesions are accompanied by hemorrhage, development of clots, and calcification. Ischemia occurs when the O_2 demand of the heart tissue is greater than the ability of the circulation to deliver O_2 to the myocardium. Often revascularization of these occluded arteries is done via coronary artery bypass grafting; the PTCA procedure is also often performed. The use of electrocardiography is one way to assess cardiac ischemia, especially during exercise. Ischemia on the ECG is evidenced by ST-segment depression and T wave inversion as shown in the following figure.

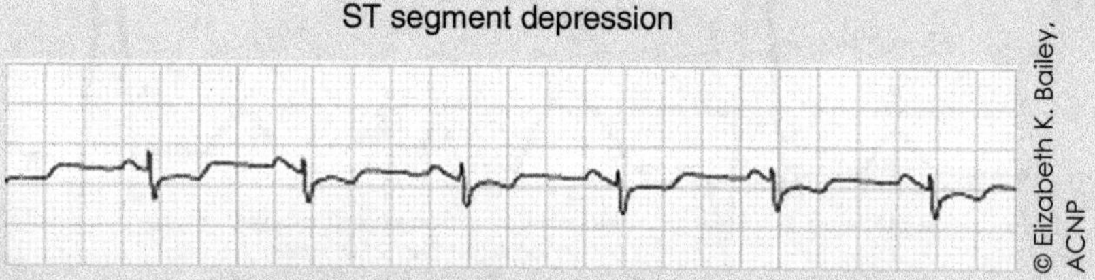

Intervention

The overall goal for this patient is to engage in lifestyle changes designed to slow the rate of further atherosclerotic development. These lifestyle changes include the following:

- Proper diet to decrease cholesterol levels
- Engage in regular aerobic exercise
- Reduction in body weight
- Education about his disease process

The multidisciplinary approach to treating this patient includes the physician, dietitian, physical therapist and/or exercise physiologist, and nurse. The exercise physiologist develops an exercise prescription and goals to improve physical work capacity. Improved exercise capacity results in decreased heart rate and a reduction in myocardial O_2 demands at rest and with activity. Because restenosis of coronary arteries following PTCA does occur, it would be important to monitor John's ECG during exercise sessions at the beginning of his cardiopulmonary rehabilitation program. He should be educated regarding the signs and symptoms of angina.

Myocardial Infarction

As with ischemia, MI can be classified as subendocardial or transmural. As we have seen, there are clinical and ECG differences between these two types. Most of our discussion on MI deals with transmural infarctions resulting from full-thickness necrosis of an area of the heart. Additionally, this chapter centers on transmural infarcts of the left ventricle and only briefly includes discussions of right ventricle transmural infarcts and subendocardial infarctions.

Left Ventricular Infarcts

Given that transmural infarcts involve the full thickness of the ventricular wall, there are both depolarization and repolarization ECG changes. As you recall, depolarization changes are manifest in the QRS complex, and repolarization changes are localized to the ST-T complex.

Acutely, transmural infarction is usually first seen in the ST-T complex by causing ST segment elevation (STEMI) and peaked T waves. An example is shown in Figure 9.5. The shape of the STEMI can be variable, but it is often dome shaped, explaining why it is nicknamed a "tombstone" wave. If not fatal, the ST-T changes will begin to evolve after a variable period of time. The leads showing STEMI will return to baseline, and the peaked T waves will often become inverted.

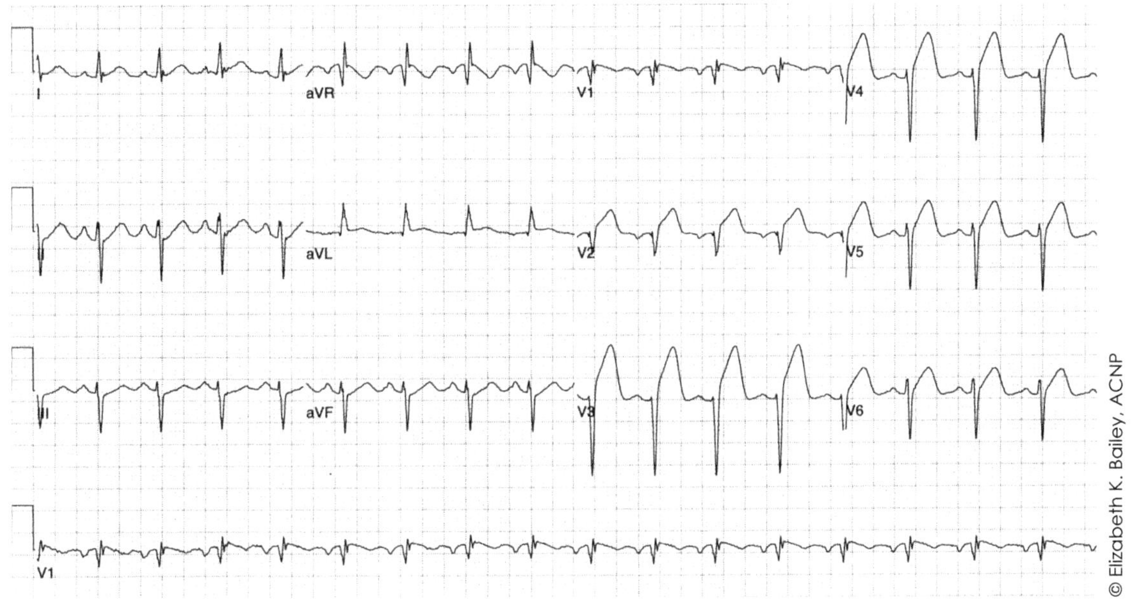

FIGURE 9.5 ECG demonstrates acute transmural MI (STEMI). In this case, the MI is localized to the anteroseptal walls with ST elevations extending across the precordium ($V_{1\text{-}6}$) to include lateral wall involvement.

After the acute ST-T complex changes, QRS complex changes usually occur within the first couple of days. The classic finding is the development of new Q waves in the affected leads. Recall that a Q wave is the first negative (downward) deflection of the QRS complex. This is the result of electrical activity being directed away from the ECG lead in which the Q wave appears. Following a transmural infarct, necrosis of an area of myocardium leads to loss of electrical activity through that area and thus a loss of a positive electrical charge on the ECG. In addition to the new Q wave, there is sometimes the development of a QS complex.

It is important to note that transmural infarctions are localized to an anatomical area of the heart. ST-T segment changes and the development of Q waves localize the pathology to certain coronary arteries. This location is based on the abnormalities seen in particular ECG leads. The following are a few examples:

- Septal MI is most likely affected via the proximal LAD, manifesting in ECG changes in leads V_1 & V_2 (Fig. 9.6). Significant Q waves signify an MI of indeterminant age.

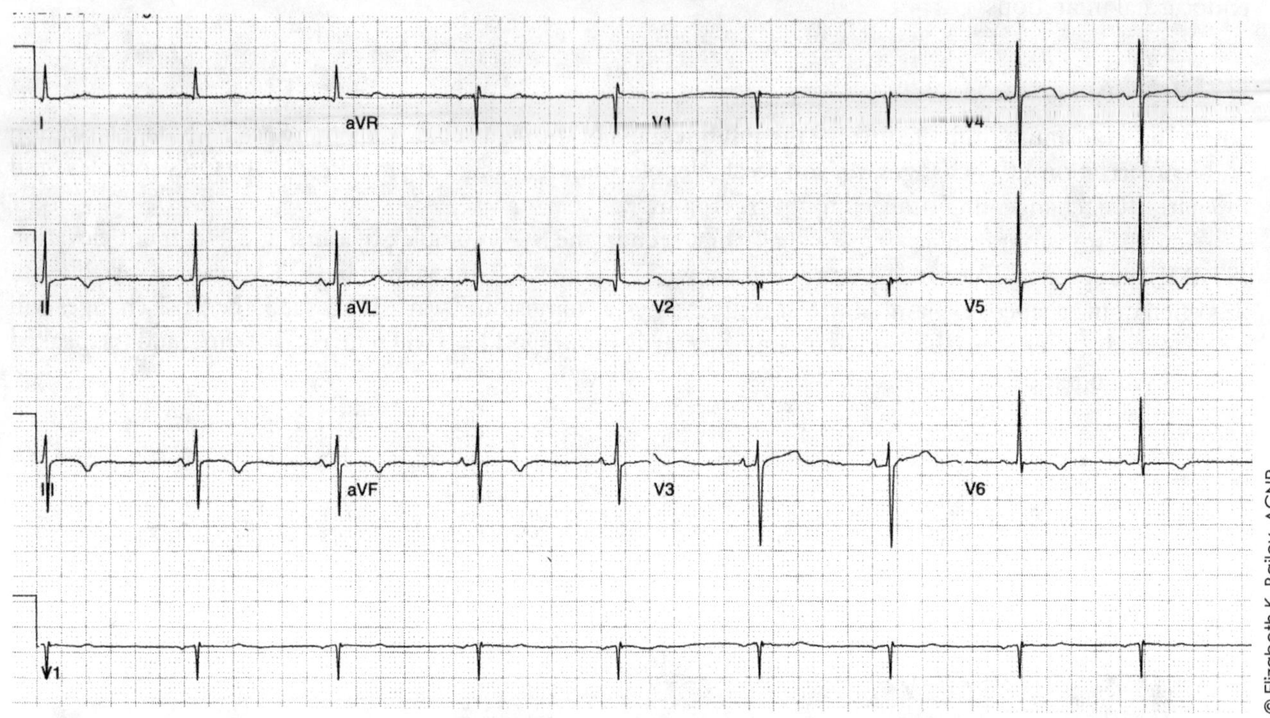

FIGURE 9.6 Old septal MI (age is indeterminant). Note the significant Q waves in leads V_1 and V_2.

- Acute anterolateral wall MI involving the anterior wall of the left ventricle is caused by atherosclerotic blockages in the territory of the distal LAD. The ECG changes of an anterior MI are best seen in the anterior chest leads V_3–V_4 (Fig. 9.7), whereas the high lateral involvement is seen in I and aVL. Reciprocal changes (ST depressions) are seen in the inferior leads.

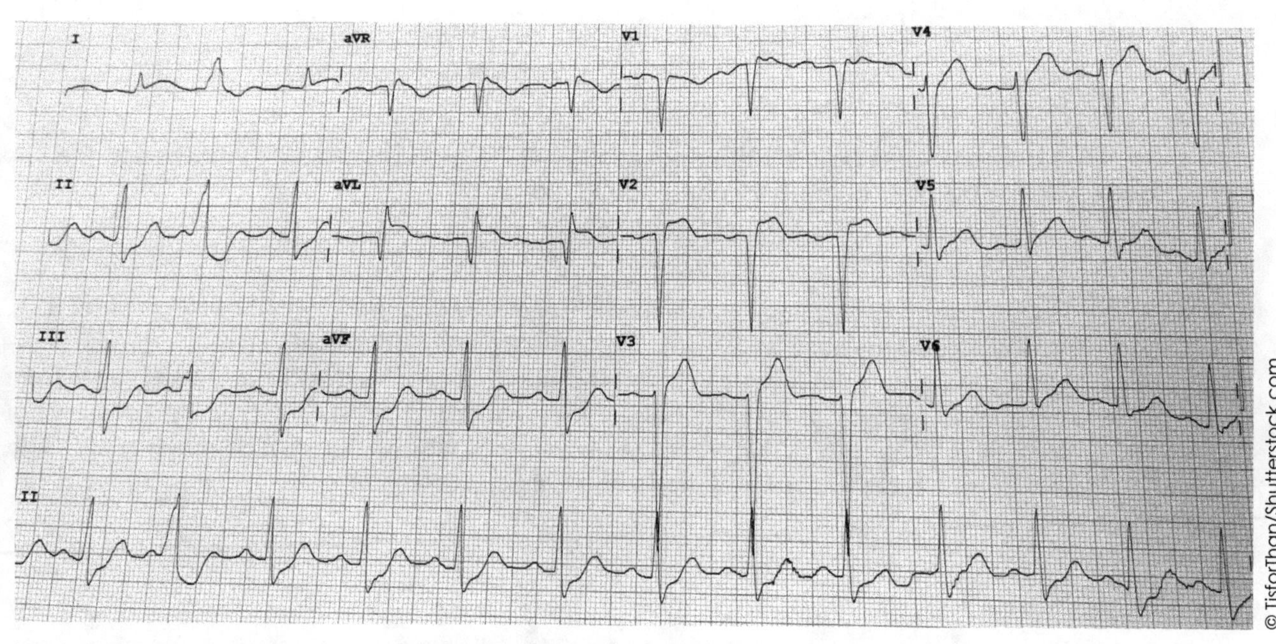

FIGURE 9.7 Acute transmural anterolateral wall MI.

- Old inferior wall MI (**A**) is caused by the involvement of the RCA, with ECG changes best seen in leads II, III, and aVF. The same leads are involved in an acute transmural inferior wall MI, with the exception that an acute infarct involves the injury current of ST elevation (**B**) (Fig. 9.8).

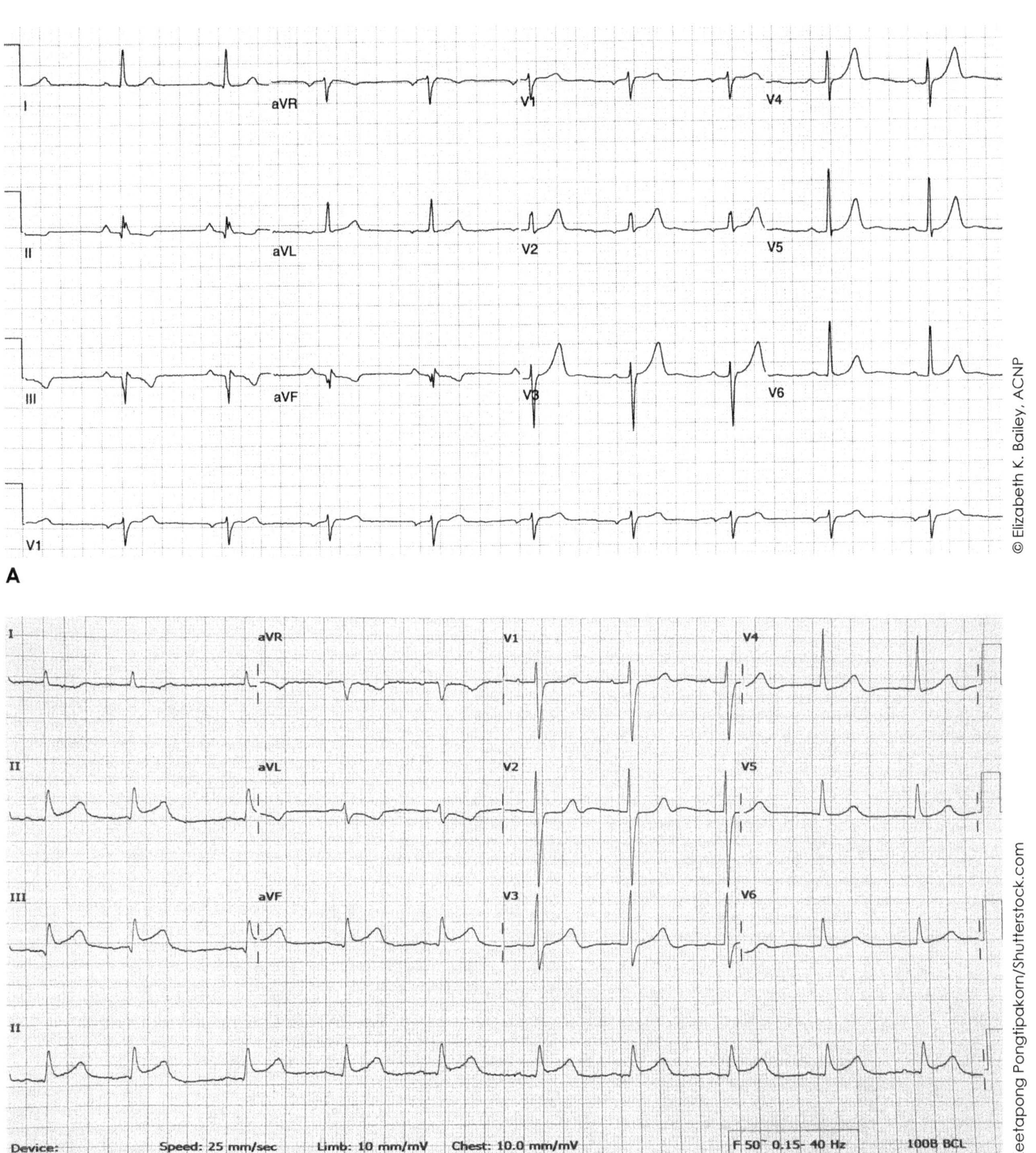

FIGURE 9.8 Old inferior wall MI showing significant Q waves in the inferior leads (**A**) and acute inferior wall MI showing ST elevations in leads II, III, and aVF (**B**).

- MI involving the lateral wall of the left ventricle is also caused by LCX involvement (Fig. 9.9).

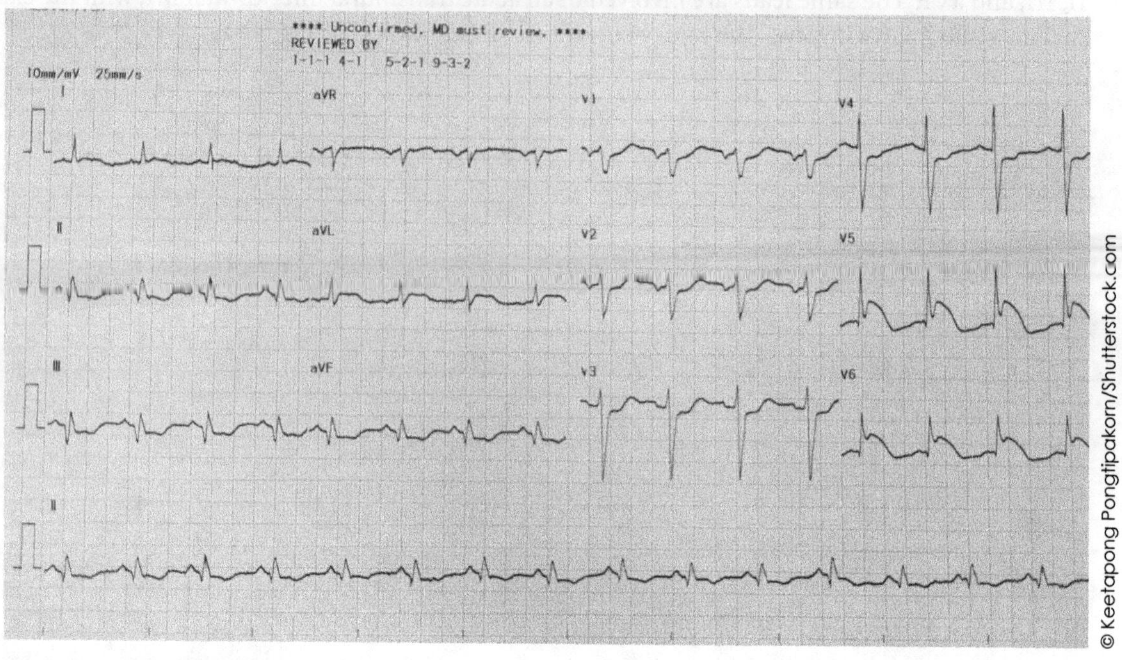

FIGURE 9.9 Acute lateral wall transmural MI (ST elevations in leads I, aVL, and $V_{5\text{-}6}$). The 12-lead ECG also shows an old inferior wall MI of indeterminant age (significant Q waves in leads II, III, and aVF).

Also, an infarction may involve more than one area of the heart. For example, an anteroseptal wall MI would show ECG changes in both the septal leads (V_1 & V_2) and in the anterior leads (V_3 & V_4).

Right Ventricular Infarcts

Most of what we have learned thus far about MI has focused on left ventricular infarcts. Right ventricular (RV) infarcts seldom occur as isolated events. Often, they occur in conjunction with inferior MI of the left ventricle. RV infarcts are confirmed with right sided precordial ECG leads (Fig. 9.10). The primary effects of RV ischemia and infarction result from decreased RV contractility. This leads to a reduction in blood flow from the venous system to the lungs and to the left heart. This produces an increased right heart pressure, increased pulmonary artery systolic pressure, and decreased left ventricular preload. As a result, symptoms include peripheral edema, especially distention of the jugular vein, hypoxemia, and hypotension. If severe enough, RV infarcts can cause cardiogenic shock. Case Study 9.2 details this situation. Additionally, as the RV dilates, the motion and function of the interventricular septum are altered. If the right ventricle dilates secondary to overload or if the septal myocardium is jeopardized by simultaneous left ventricular ischemia, symptoms of hypotension and cardiac failure can become pronounced. If the septum shifts leftward during diastole, it may impede left ventricular filling, decreasing cardiac output and resulting in a loss of **biventricular interdependence.**

Subendocardial Infarcts

As you recall, subendocardial ischemia results in transient ST segment depression. As subendocardial ischemia gives way to subendocardial infarction, the ST segment depression persists and inverted T waves can develop. Also, because subendocardial infarctions generally affect repolarization rather than depolarization, Q waves typically do not appear in subendocardial infarcts.

Subendocardial ischemia produces ST segment depression on the ECG (Fig. 9.11A). The ST depression is reversible if ischemia is transient but persists if ischemia is severe enough to produce infarction. T wave inversion with or without ST segment depression is sometimes seen but not STEMI or Q wave formation. Subendocardial infarction is also called non-ST-elevation myocardial infarction (NSTEMI).

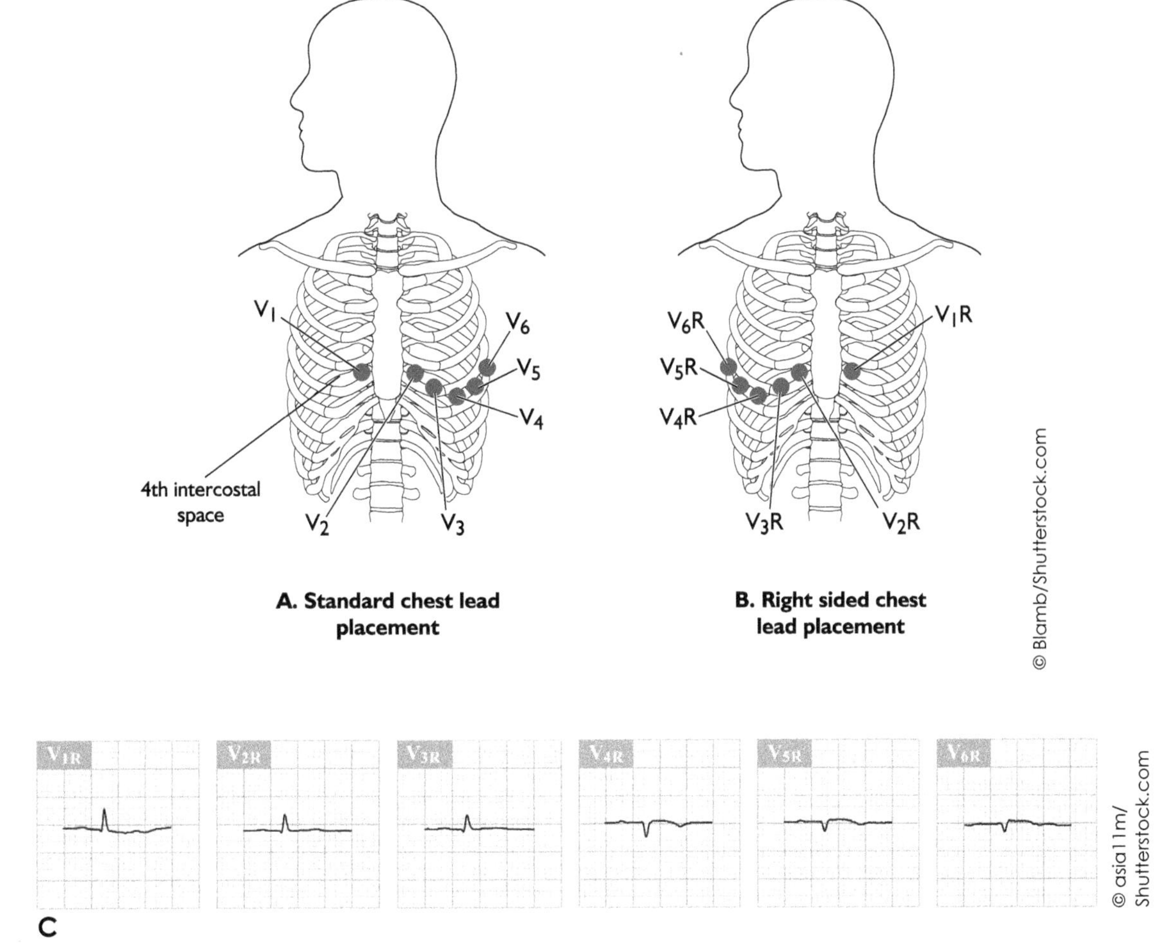

FIGURE 9.10 **A & B** show the lead placements for the left chest and right chest. **C** shows the ECG for a right ventricular MI.

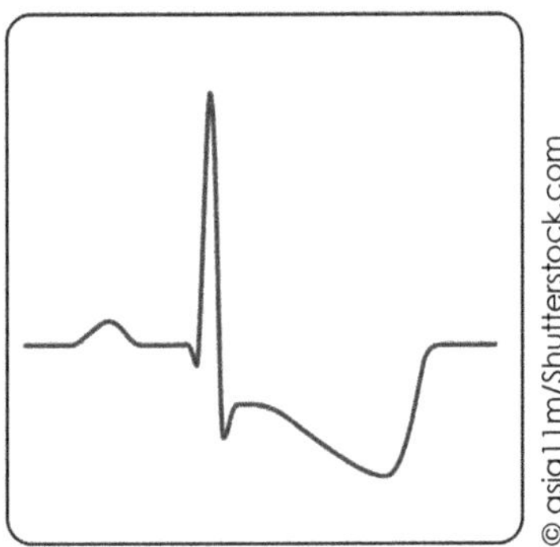

FIGURE 9.11 ST depression in subendocardial ischemia.

ST segment depression seen in subendocardial ischemia or infarction can manifest differing morphologies. The most common pattern is horizontal or down-sloping depression. Generally, up-sloping ST depression is less specific for ischemia. In exercise stress tests, horizontal or down-sloping depression of 1 mm or more (Fig. 9.12A–C) or up-sloping depression of the same magnitude 80 ms beyond the J point (Fig. 9.12D) is considered a positive sign of ischemia. Up-sloping depression of less than 1 mm at 80 ms beyond the J point (Fig. 9.12E) is considered J point depression, not ST segment depression.

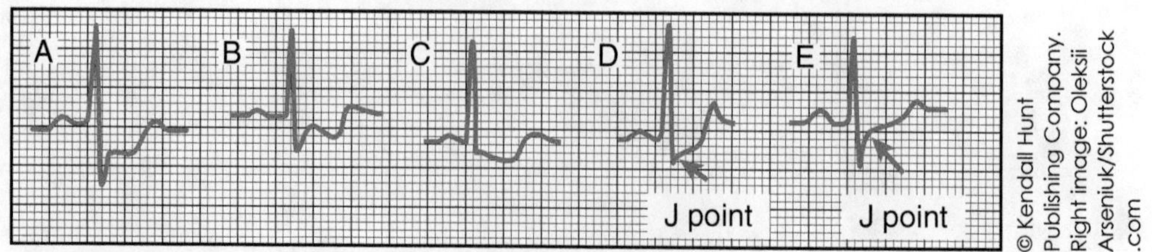

FIGURE 9.12 Five different patterns of ST segment depression.

Special Considerations

Thus far, we have discussed classic examples of MIs and their associated ECG changes. There are some special circumstances that warrant discussion.

Myocardial Infarction with Right Bundle Branch Block (RBBB)

Diagnosing an acute MI in the setting of RBBB is not as difficult as with a left bundle branch block. Recall that RBBB typically affects the second half of ventricular depolarization. Thus, the classic ECG changes of RBBB include a wide QRS complex (> 0.12 seconds), an rSR' in V_1–V_2, and a wide S wave in V_6. In contrast, MIs affect the first half of ventricular depolarization, thereby producing abnormal Q waves. In an acute inferior MI with RBBB, ST elevation is noted in II, III, & aVF (Fig. 9.13).

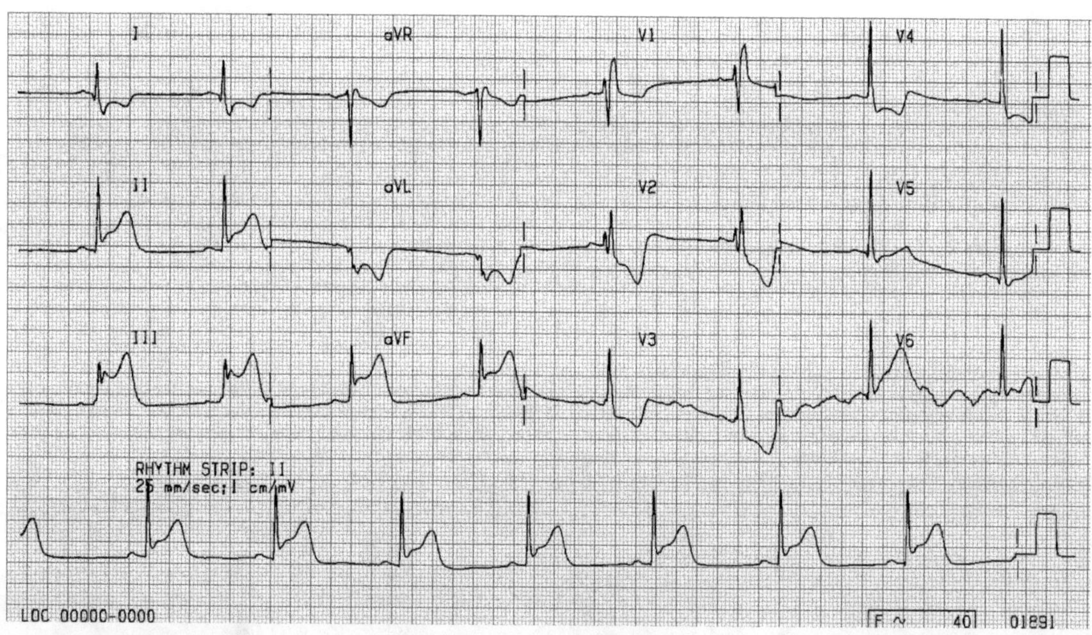

FIGURE 9.13 Acute transmural inferior wall MI in a 55-year-old man with 4 hours of "crushing" chest pain. Note the reciprocal ST depression in the anterior leads and the presence of RBBB.
Source: https://ecglibrary.com/infmi.php

Myocardial Infarction with Left Bundle Branch Block (LBBB)

Diagnosing an acute MI in the setting of LBBB can be more difficult owing to LBBB interrupting the entire depolarization cycle of the ventricles. LBBB also causes ST-T changes thereby making STEMI more difficult

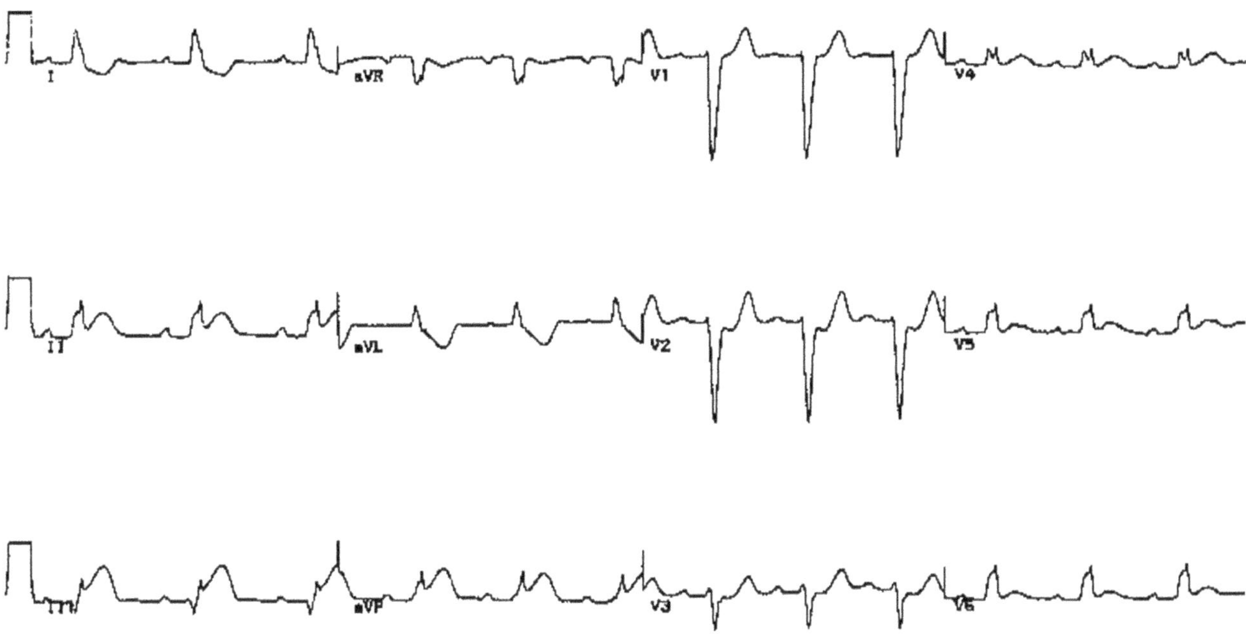

FIGURE 9.14 Acute inferior wall transmural MI in the presence of LBBB.
Source: https://ecglibrary.com/lbbbimi.html

to ascertain. Hints of an acute MI in the setting of LBBB include ST segment changes that are in the same direction as the primary direction of the QRS complex, deep negative T waves in leads with predominately negative QRS complexes (V_1–V_3), and ST segment elevation (STEMI) in leads with prominent R waves (Fig. 9.14). The occurrence of LBBB is known to mask ECG changes indicative of anterior wall MI because of the changes it causes in the ST-T complex of the precordial leads. However, the ECG changes of inferior wall infarction that affects the limb leads are usually unaffected by the intraventricular conduction abnormality caused by LBBB.

There is a system available to clinicians to increase the specificity of diagnosing MI in the presence of LBBB. The Sgarbossa criteria work on a scale of 0 to 5. A minimal score of 3 is required for a specificity of 90%. Three criteria are included in Sgarbossa's classification system, with a score of ≥3 points producing a 98% probability of STEMI.

- Rule 1: ST elevation ≥ 1 mm in a lead with positive QRS complex (concordant)—5 points
- Rule 2: ST depression ≥ 1 mm in lead V_1, V_2, or V_3—3 points
- Rule 3: ST elevation ≥ 5 mm in a lead with negative QRS complex (discordant)—2 points

These original criteria had a low sensitivity (20%) and a high specificity (98%). However, the original criteria have recently been updated, resulting in an improved sensitivity (91%) for a slightly lower specificity (90%). The newer criteria change Rule 3 of Sgarbossa's original criteria as follows: *ST elevation at the J-point, relative to QRS onset, is at least 1 mm AND has an amplitude at least 25% of the preceding S-wave (an ST/S ratio of 0.20 is also very high and almost as specific as a 0.25 ratio).* This change increases the sensitivity from 52% to 91% at the expense of reducing specificity from 98% to 90%. Figure 9.15 details these issues using the ECG.

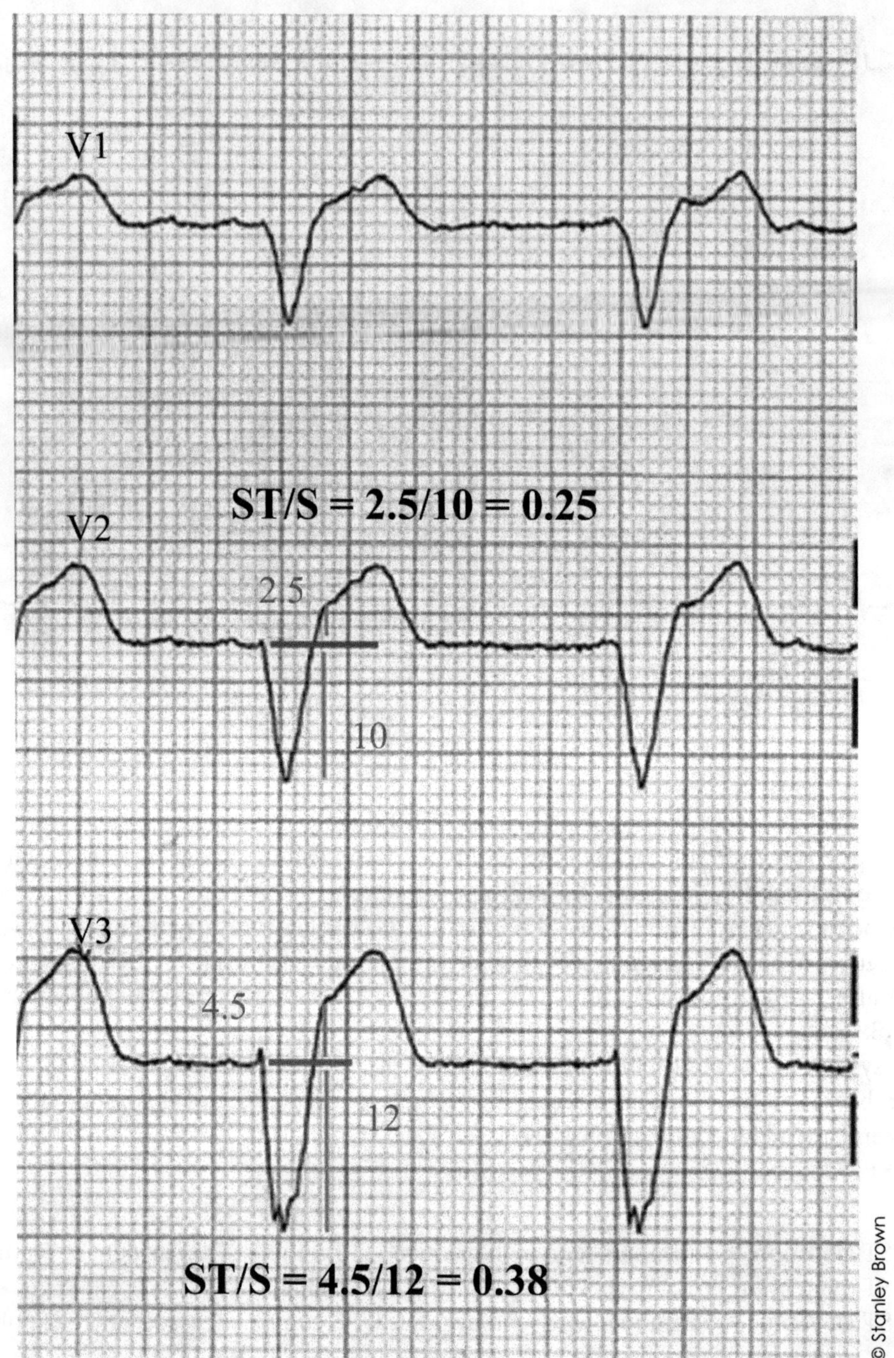

FIGURE 9.15 Demonstration of the Sgarbossa criteria.

Ventricular Aneurysm

A ventricular aneurysm is one of the complications of a large, usually anterior, MI. If an infarct occurs in a large enough area of myocardium, an aneurysm, or a weakened area of the wall of the heart, can occur. This area of myocardium will move paradoxically during systole as compared to the unaffected area. A ventricular aneurysm can result in heart failure, arrhythmias, embolic strokes, and, rarely, free wall rupture of the ventricle. As mentioned earlier, the ST elevation in an acute STEMI usually resolves over a few days. If a ventricular aneurysm develops, ST elevation will persist for a longer period (Fig. 9.16).

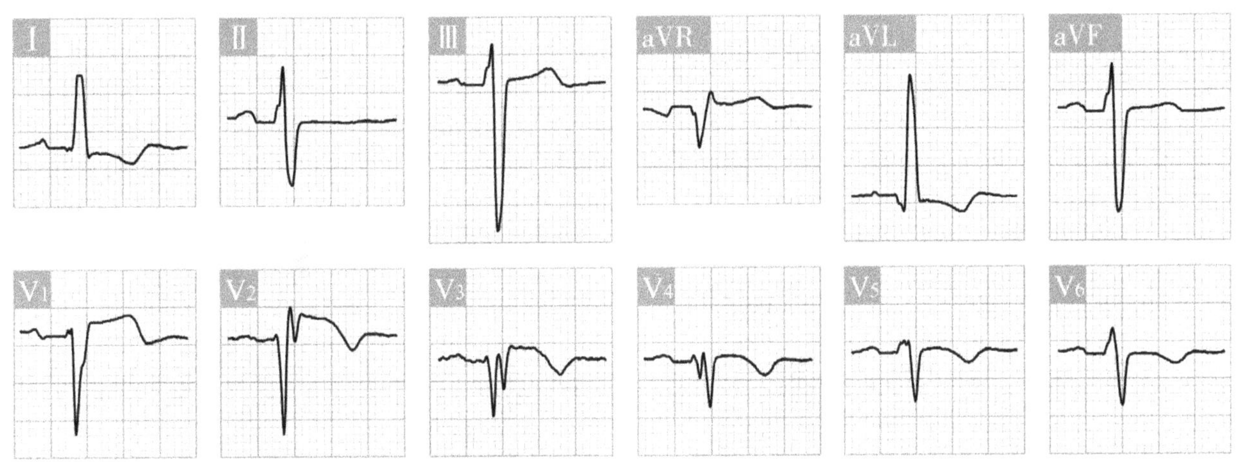

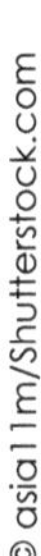

FIGURE 9.16 The patient, female, 57 years old, suffered an MI one year ago. Follow-up ECG with persistent ST-segment elevation indicates the formation of a ventricular aneurysm.

CASE STUDY 9.2

Mr. Smith is a 77-year-old man who is currently admitted to the hospital for a urinary tract infection. He has a past medical history of poorly controlled hypertension and diabetes. On hospital day two, he suddenly develops chest pain. He describes the pain as severe and squeezing in nature. It is associated with dyspnea and nausea. He appears to be in distress. He is **diaphoretic**, and his breathing is labored.

On physical exam, his blood pressure is 110/60 mmHg with a heart rate of 95 beats per minute. His O_2 saturation on room air is 95%. His physical exam reveals jugular venous distention (Fig. A). Auscultation of his chest reveals clear lung sounds and no heart murmurs. His chest X-ray is unremarkable (Fig. B). His ECG shows ST elevation in leads II, III, and aVF (Fig. C). The internal medicine resident on call accurately diagnoses him with an acute inferior myocardial infarction (MI) and begins appropriate acute coronary syndrome management. Additionally, the resident believes that the patient has acute congestive heart failure (given the distended neck veins) and administers intravenous furosemide as a diuretic. Following this, the patient's condition suddenly deteriorates. He becomes more lethargic, and his blood pressure drops to 80/60 mmHg with a heart rate of 125 beats per minute. The cardiology fellow arrives at bedside and quickly reviews the chart, including the ECG. He immediately places right-sided chest leads and repeats the ECG (Fig. D). With the new results, he orders a one-liter saline bolus. The patient's hemodynamics quickly improve, and his mental status returns to normal. As the patient is being taken to cardiac catheterization lab, the cardiology fellow explains to the medicine resident what has just happened.

Discussion

Mr. Smith was correctly diagnosed with an acute inferior MI, but the concomitant right ventricular (RV) infarct was initially missed. Remember, the RV pumps blood to the lungs. If the RV becomes dysfunctional, blood volume backs up into the central venous circulation, resulting in distended neck veins, and, if severe enough, hypotension and cardiogenic shock attributable to right heart failure. Therefore, it is imperative to evaluate a patient with an inferior left ventricular infarct who presents with distended neck veins and hypotension for an RV infarct.

ECG changes of RV infarction are often more difficult to discern because they require special placement of right-sided anterior leads. The reason it is important to diagnose RV infarct has to do with therapy. It is almost counterintuitive, but the treatment of cardiogenic shock in the setting of an RV infarction is to administer aggressive IV fluid therapy.

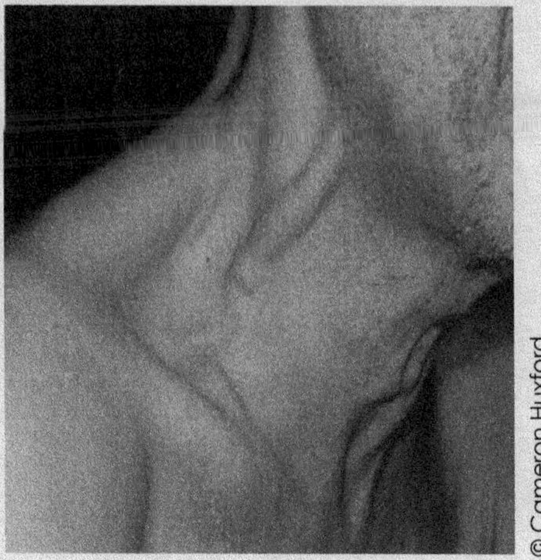

© Cameron Huxford

FIGURE A. Jugular vein distention.

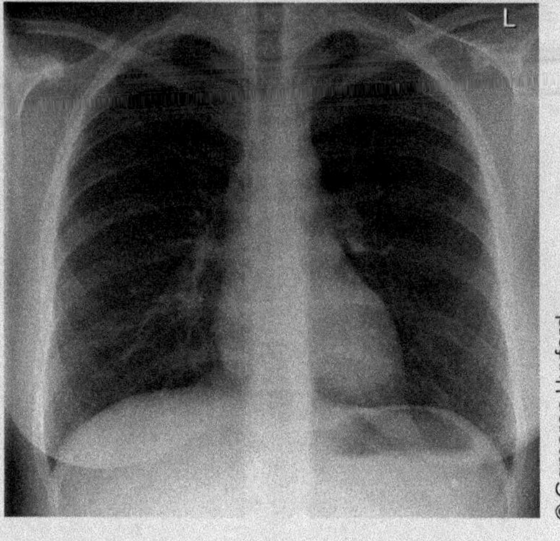

© Cameron Huxford

FIGURE B. The patient presented with a normal chest X-Ray.

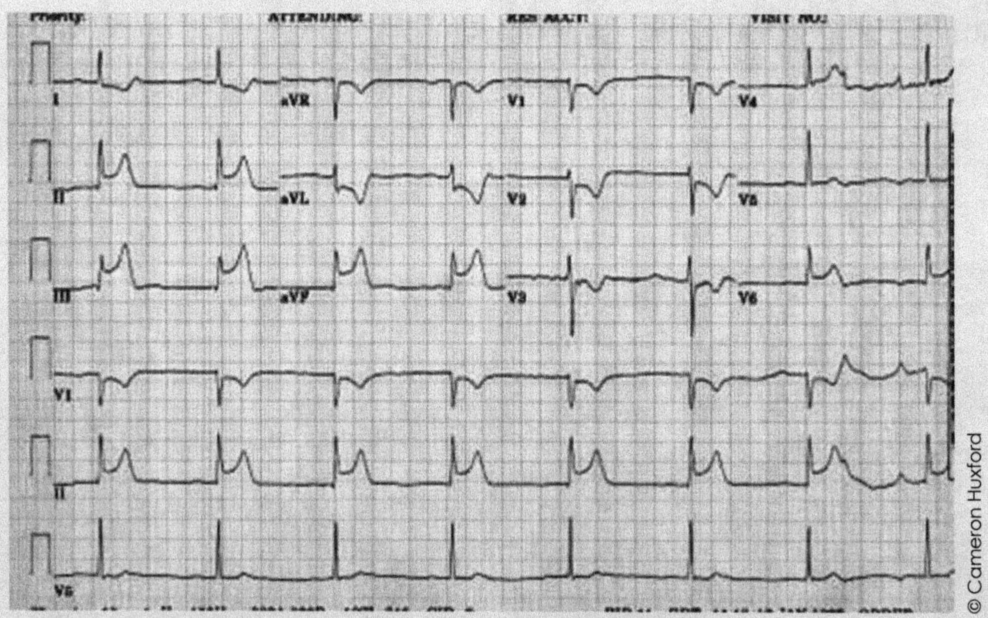

© Cameron Huxford

FIGURE C. Acute inferior STEMI as seen in leads II, III, and aVF.

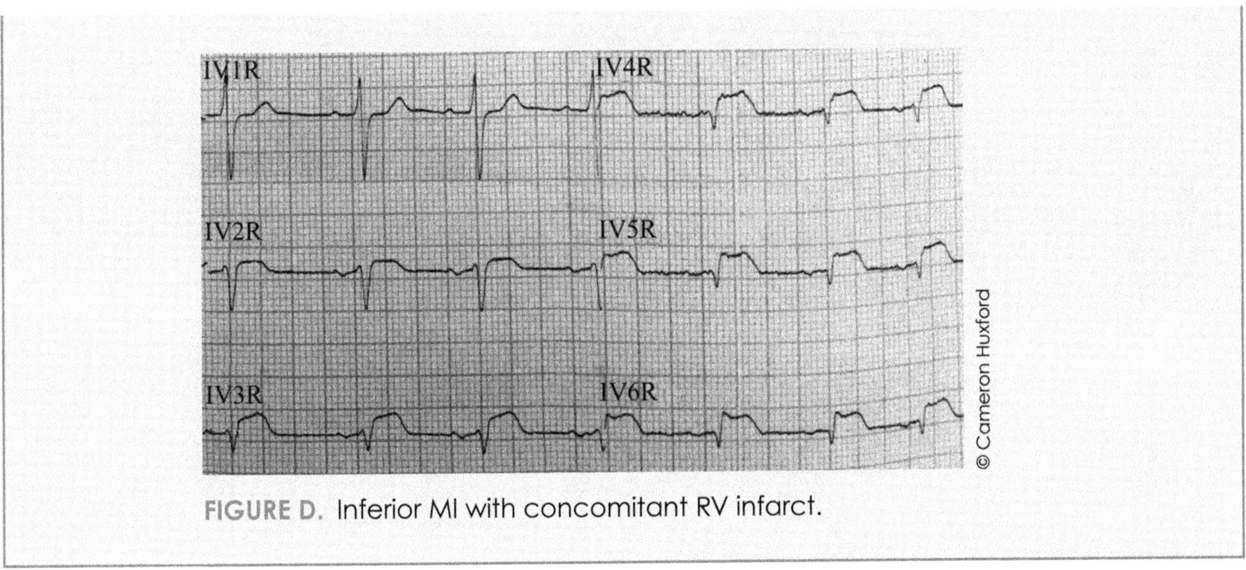

FIGURE D. Inferior MI with concomitant RV infarct.

Chapter Questions

1. Describe the difference between classic angina and acute MI.
2. In acute transmural MI, what are reciprocal ECG changes?

PART THREE

CARDIAC RHYTHM BASICS

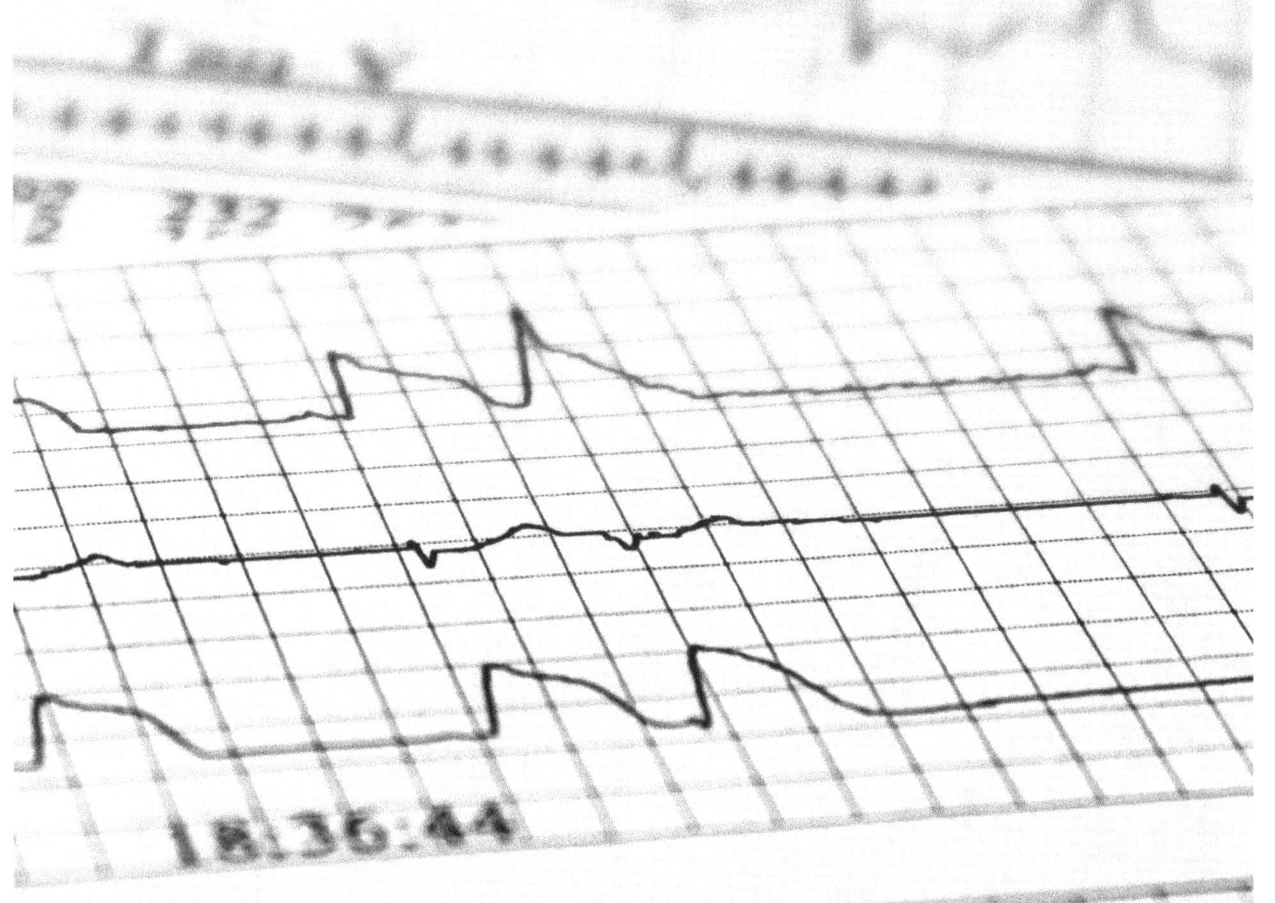

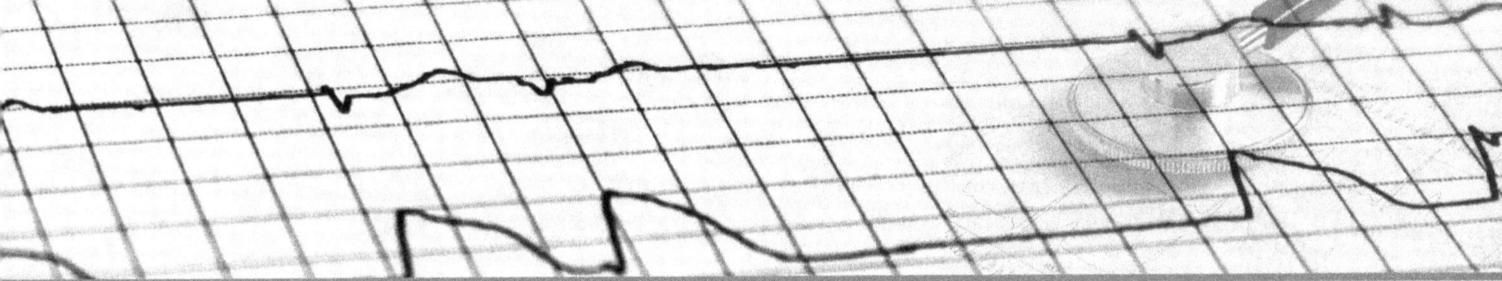

CHAPTER 10

Sinus and Escape Rhythms

In this final section of the text, rhythm origination is introduced with discussions of deviations from normal sinus pacing of the heart.

CONTENT OUTLINE

- Evaluating Cardiac Rhythms
- Normal Sinus Rhythm
- Sinus Bradycardia
- Sinus Tachycardia
- Sinus Arrhythmia
    - Sinus Pause and Exit Block
- Chapter Questions

Disturbances of cardiac rhythm can be divided into those of *supraventricular* origin and those of *ventricular* origin. This convenient division follows the normal cardiac electrical activation pathway:

Sinus Node ⟶ Atria ⟶ AV Junction ⟶ Ventricles

Arrythmias can originate from each of these four locales, but the prefix *supra* specifically refers to arrythmias that originate in the atria or atrioventricular (AV) junction, that is, coming from above the ventricles, versus those that are of ventricular origin, that is, starting within the ventricles themselves.

Arrythmias can be dangerous, but which origination locale is more dangerous? Consider the following. Supraventricular arrythmias usually produce normal QRS complexes unless a normal sinus activation pattern is aberrantly conducted through the ventricles that can appear to be of ventricular origin when it is not. On the other hand, arrythmias originating from either ventricle produce a bizarre QRS complex (and an amorphous T wave) with a prolonged QRS interval. There is always the possibility that abnormal conductions through the ventricles are occurring with supraventricular rhythm disturbances. For example, supraventricular tachycardia (SVT; covered in Chapter 12) could coincide with a temporary intraventricular block. The resultant fast rhythm with wide, bizarre QRS complexes would make it hard to distinguish between SVT and ventricular tachycardia (VT; covered in Chapter 11). As will be discussed in their respective chapters, SVT is far less worrisome clinically than is VT.

Evaluating Cardiac Rhythms

Interpreting/diagnosing arrhythmias can be done at a glance, but often it is only with painstaking study that a final accurate finding is made. For this reason, it is best to be systematic in approaching the interpretation of cardiac rhythm disturbances. Refer to Box 10.1 for a simplified approach.

BOX 10.1: SEVEN STEP APPROACH TO ECG RHYTHM ANALYSIS

The Lead II rhythm strip is the best location to confirm an arrhythmia but needs to be confirmed by checking other leads.

Step 1. Pattern of QRS complexes

- Is the rhythm strip regular or irregular?
- If irregular, is the pattern regularly irregular or irregularly irregular?

Step 2. Rate

- Is the rhythm strip tachycardic or bradycardic?
- Or is the rate normal (60–100 beats per minute)?

Step 3. QRS complex morphology

- If narrow, then look for the origin being sinus, atrial, or junctional.
- If wide, then look for the origin being ventricular or supraventricular (with aberrant conduction).

Step 4. P waves

- If absent, then look for sinus arrest or atrial fibrillation.
- If present, then the morphology and PR interval suggest sinus, atrial, junctional, or retrograde from the ventricles.

Step 5. Relationship between P waves and QRS complexes

- If there is AV dissociation, it will be difficult to distinguish from isorhythmic dissociation.
- If there is complete AV dissociation, then atrial and ventricular activity is always independent.
- If there is incomplete AV dissociation, then there is intermittent capture of the signal.

Step 6. Onset and termination

- Abrupt: reentrant process
- Gradual: increased automaticity

Step 7. Response to vagal maneuvers

- Sinus tachycardia, ectopic atrial tachyarrhythmia: gradual slowing during the vagal maneuver but resumes on cessation
- Atrioventricular nodal reentry tachycardia (AVNRT) or atrioventricular reentrant tachycardia (AVRT): abrupt termination or no response
- Atrial fibrillation and atrial flutter: gradual slowing during the maneuver
- VT: no response

A basic definition is a good starting point. Rhythm refers to the pattern of ECG complexes that occur over time. Usually, rhythm strips lasting longer than 3 seconds are the easiest to evaluate. Second, ECG leads with large P waves (Lead II and V_1) are best for rhythm interpretation, with the rhythm judged either regular or irregular. Irregular rhythms can be either **regularly irregular** or **irregularly irregular** (completely irregular). An irregularly irregular rhythm is defined as a pulse in which the heart beats are spaced irregularly with no discernible pattern. Conversely, a regularly irregular rhythm is a patterned (consistent) irregularity. Both examples are discussed in Chapter 12. Third, for all rhythms look for and evaluate the P waves in the underlying rhythm first and then evaluate the presence, or absence, and appearance of P waves occurring in association with additional or dropped beats. Make a note that P waves may "hide" in preceding QRS complexes or T waves or may not be seen well in all leads and may be aberrant in their appearance. The following questions are relevant.

- *Does a P wave precede every QRS complex?*
- *Does a QRS complex follow every P wave?*
- *Do the P waves have a normal configuration and the same configuration with each cardiac cycle?*
- *Is the PR interval normal, short, or prolonged?*

Within this evaluative exercise in rhythm recognition, an important step is to look at the QRS complexes:

- Evaluate the underlying QRS rhythm first. Then evaluate other QRS complexes that appear to be expressing a different, secondary rhythm.
- Look for any P waves found to be in association with the QRS complexes in question.
- Look for aberrancy in the appearance of the QRS (QRS duration $\geq$ 0.12 seconds) and then compare the appearance and duration of any additional complexes with the complexes of the underlying rhythm.

Normal Sinus Rhythm

Before we can proceed with a full discussion of ventricular and supraventricular rhythm disturbances in the next two chapters, there is another origination locale of cardiac arrhythmias, the sinus node. In sinus rhythms, there is a normal impulse formation at the sinoatrial (SA) node that spreads from there to the AV node. This spread through the atria produces a normal P wave, which is the hallmark of all sinus rhythms.

The normal cardiac rhythm is called normal sinus rhythm (NSR) because it begins, as we have seen, with an impulse from the SA node and conducts through normal pathways to the AV node and junction and, finally, to the ventricles. NSR has the following characteristics (Fig. 10.1):

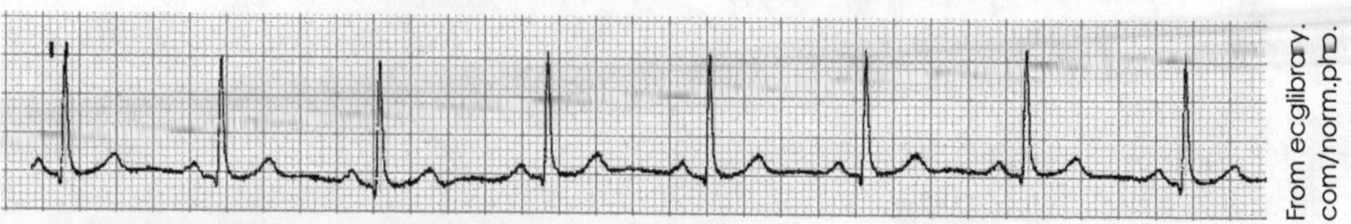

From ecglibrary.com/norm.php.

FIGURE 10.1 Normal sinus rhythm (71 beats per minute). Lead I is shown.

- Regular rhythm (with slight respiration variation).
- Rate is between 60 and 100 beats per minute.
- Normal P waves of consistent morphology precede every QRS complex (1:1 P to QRS ratio) and are positive in lead II and negative in lead aVR.
- All waves are of normal size and morphology.
- All intervals are of normal length.

Sinus Bradycardia

Sinus bradycardia is a sinus rhythm with a heart rate of less than 60 beats per minute (Fig. 10.2). Sinus bradycardia may occur with the following conditions:

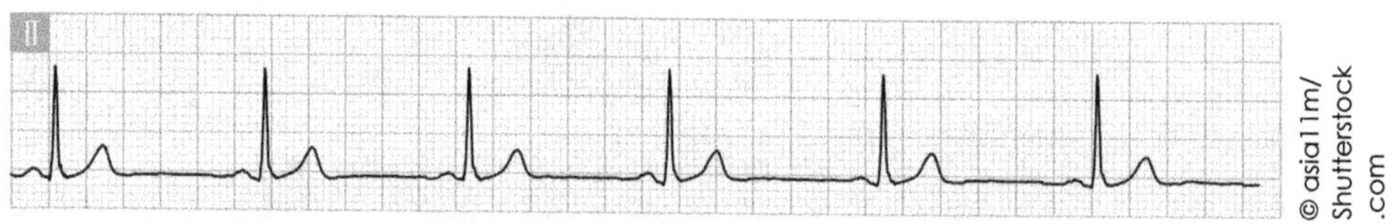

© asia11m/ Shutterstock .com

FIGURE 10.2 Sinus bradycardia (53 beats per minute).

- Normal variant such as in individuals who are aerobically trained
- Drugs that increase vagal tone (digitalis) or decrease sympathetic tone (beta blockers)
- Hypothyroidism
- Increased intracranial pressure
- Inferior myocardial infarction
- Hyperkalemia
- Sick sinus syndrome
- Sleep apnea syndrome

If sinus bradycardia is moderate, no symptoms are usually apparent. Very slow rates may produce light-headedness and syncope owing to reduced cardiac output. If symptomatic (hypotension, chest pain, heart failure, altered mental status), therapy is directed primarily at correction of the underlying cause.

Sinus Tachycardia

Sinus tachycardia is a sinus rhythm with a heart rate of more than 100 beats per minute, usually between 100 and 180 beats per minute (Fig. 10.3). In general, sinus tachycardia occurs with any condition that produces an increase in sympathetic tone or a decrease in vagal tone. The following conditions are commonly associated with sinus tachycardia:

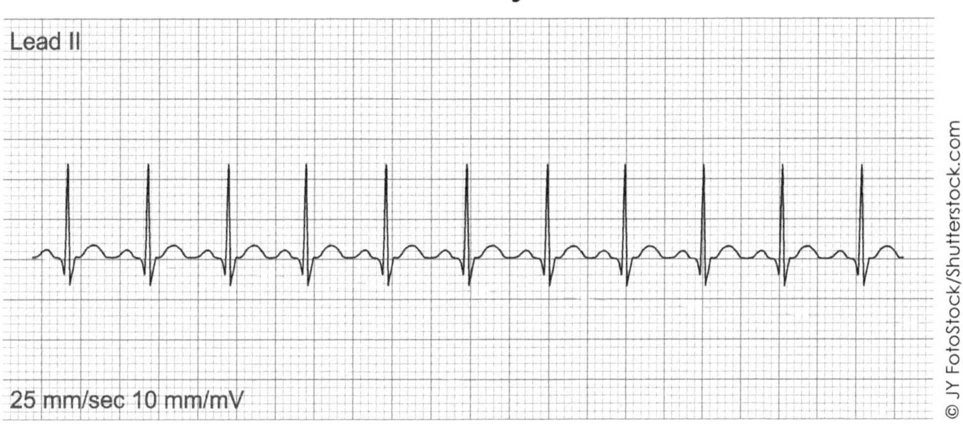

FIGURE 10.3 Sinus tachycardia shown in lead II (150 beats per minute).

- Fever
- Shock
- Eating
- Infection
- Congestive heart failure
- Hypoxia
- Anxiety, excitement, pain
- Physical exertion
- Drugs that increase sympathetic tone or block vagal tone
- Acute myocardial infarction
- Pulmonary embolism
- Hypovolemia
- Anemia
- Hyperthyroidism
- Bleeding, vomiting, diarrhea, or dehydration resulting in intravascular volume loss.

Treatment associated with a pathologic condition is directed at correction of the underlying cause. Slower tachycardias usually do not produce symptoms, but faster tachycardias can produce symptoms associated with reduced cardiac output owing to a reduced filling time.

Sinus Arrhythmia

Sinus arrhythmia is an irregularity in rhythm in which the impulse is initiated by the SA node but the rhythm is not perfectly maintained; the impulses formed by the SA node are formed irregularly. There is an accentuated beat-to-beat variation caused most commonly by the respiratory cycle (Fig. 10.4). Sinus arrhythmia is a normal variation of sinus rhythm and usually occurs when respirations are exaggerated, such as in recovery from exercise or owing to obstructive lung conditions. If sinus arrhythmia is not associated with respirations, the underlying cause needs to be determined.

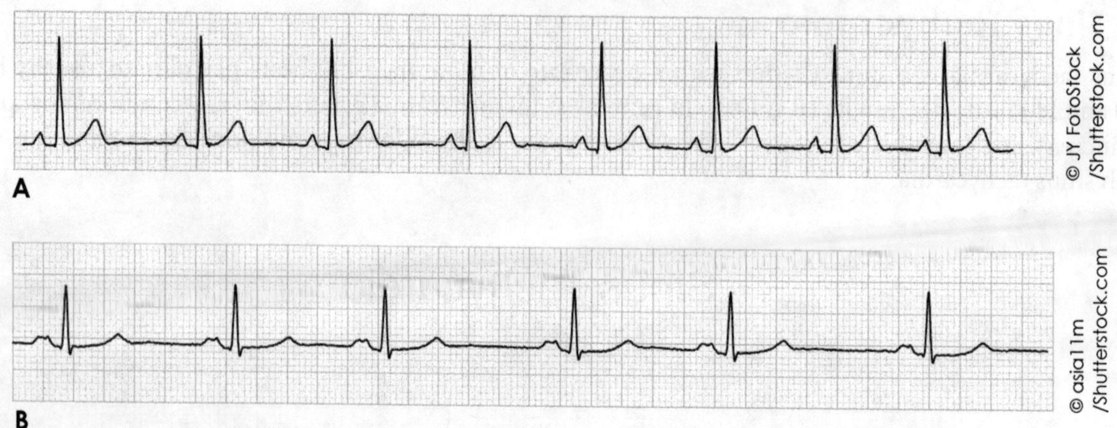

FIGURE 10.4 Strip **A** shows sinus arrhythmia caused by the respiratory cycle (heart rate increases with inspiration and decreases with expiration). Strip **B** shows nonrespiratory sinus arrhythmia.

Sinus Pause/Arrest and Sinoatrial Exit Block

The SA node represents the joined activity of pacemaker cells (P cells) and transitional cells (T cells). Pacemaker cells generate impulses, and transitional cells propagate these electrical impulses from the SA node to the right atrium. SA nodal dysfunction typically results from either an abnormality in impulse generation by P cells or an abnormality in conduction across T cells. This dysfunction can produce symptoms or may be entirely asymptomatic. The etiology of sinus pause and exit block is varied: (1) hyperkalemia, (2) excessive vagal tone, (3) ischemic, inflammatory, or infiltrative or fibrotic disease of the SA node, (4) sleep apnea, (5) digitalis toxicity and other drugs.

Sinus pause and arrest occur when there is a transient absence of P waves on the ECG, with sinus pause lasting less than two seconds and sinus arrest lasting two seconds or longer. The cause is an alteration in the discharge of P cells and often allows escape beats or rhythms to occur. However, lower pacemakers may be lethargic or absent in SA node dysfunction. A pause of two seconds or somewhat longer can occur in the normal heart in the absence of disease. Longer episodes of sinus arrest can produce dizziness and syncope. Sinus pause/arrest can be associated with escape beats arising out of the atria, AV node, or ventricles (Fig. 10.5). They occur intermittently with no P wave or QRS complex appearing where they should be. The appearance on the ECG is an area that lacks electrical activity from the end of one T wave until the eventual appearance of the next P wave. These escapes can also originate from the sinus node.

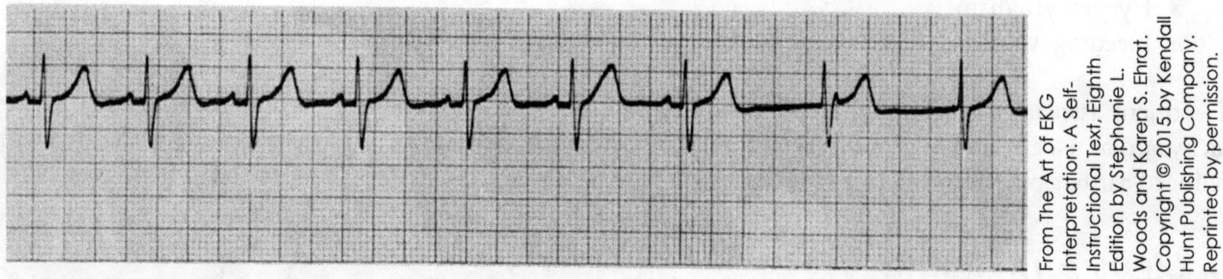

FIGURE 10.5 Reading from left to right, there is normal sinus rhythm present of about 88 beats per minute, followed by a pause after complex 7. This is followed by a junctional escape beat (8th and 9th complex). The sinus mechanism has failed owing to the lack of an upright P wave before the QRS complexes for the last two beats on the strip, demonstrating that the AV junctional pacemaker is now generating the rhythm at a rate of about 68 beats per minute.

Interference with the delivery of impulses from the SA node to atrial tissue describes the process of SA node exit block. When this happens, P waves are absent on the ECG. Following the convention for AV nodal block (discussed in Chapter 13), SA nodal exit block can be classified as first, second, or third degree with the following specifics:

- Input is from the SA nodal pacemaker (SA node electrical activity is not visible on the ECG but is merely inferred from the P waves of atrial activation—the relationship between impulse generation and transmission must be inferred from the P waves alone).
- Exit block involves T cells, and the type of exit block in perinodal tissue is inferred from P waves.
- P wave abnormalities reflect the type of exit block present.
- Only second-degree SA block (types I and II) can be diagnosed from the 12-lead ECG.

As mentioned earlier, the scheme for SA nodal exit block is analogous to AV blocks discussed in Chapter 13:

- *First-degree SA exit block*—conduction time between the sinus node impulse and atrial tissue depolarization increases. Sinus node depolarization produces no waveform on the surface ECG; therefore, first-degree SA exit block cannot be recognized on the surface ECG. Thus, first-degree SA exit block cannot be diagnosed without performing an electrophysiologic study.
- *Type 1 second-degree SA exit block*—progressive shortening of the P-P interval before a P-QRS-T complex is dropped. The shortening of the P-P interval is helpful in distinguishing this condition from sinus pause.
- *Type 2 second-degree SA exit block*—the P-P interval surrounding the dropped complexes is twice (or a multiple of) the baseline P-P interval, distinguishing this type of SA exit block from sinus pause.
- *Third-degree SA exit block*—characterized by asystole or junctional rhythm on the ECG. Diagnosis on surface ECG is often difficult or impossible and often requires invasive electrophysiologic study.

In SA node exit block, the diagnostic approach and treatment are similar to sinus pause. The duration of the pause with SA node exit block is a direct multiple of the R-R interval of the underlying rhythm. In sinus pause and arrest, the duration of the pause is not a direct multiple of the R-R interval of the underlying rhythm.

Chapter Questions

1. Analyze this tracing using the seven steps of rhythm analysis and give an interpretation.

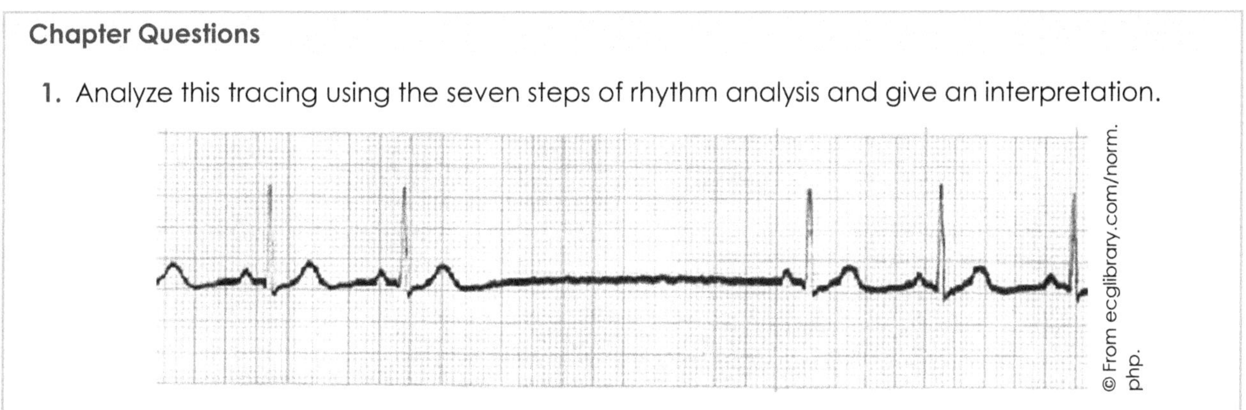

© From ecglibrary.com/norm.php.

2. After reading Chapter 13, distinguish between SA nodal block and AV nodal block.

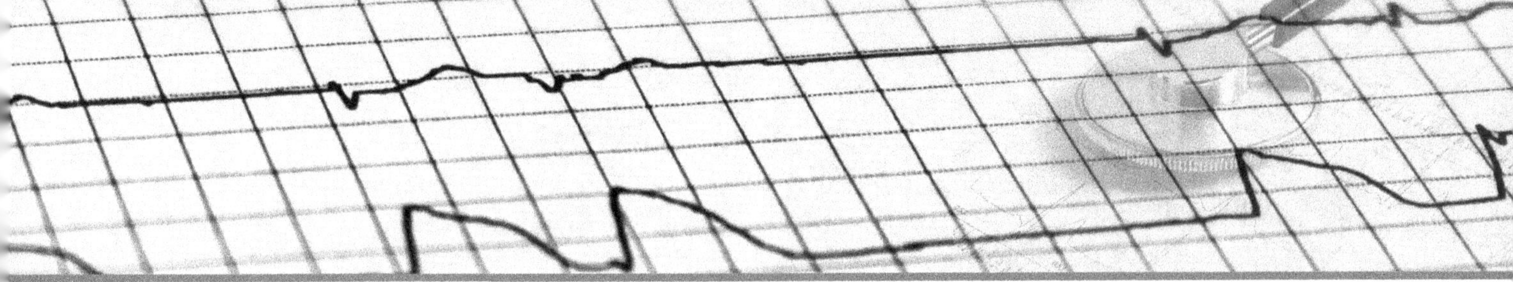

CHAPTER 11

Ventricular Arrhythmias

Ventricular arrhythmias are abnormal heart rhythms that originate in the lower chambers of the heart. They are often benign but may also be life threatening, prompting exercise personnel to regard them with care and sometimes urgency.

CONTENT OUTLINE

- Appearance
- Effects
- Premature Ventricular Complexes
  - Appearance
  - Patterns and Origination
- Ventricular Escape Beats, Idioventricular Rhythm (IVR), and Accelerated Idioventricular Rhythm (AIVR)
- Ventricular Tachycardias
- Torsades de Pointes (TdP)
- Ventricular Fibrillation (VF)
- Chapter Questions

This chapter and the next examine **ectopic** activity in the heart. **Ventricular arrhythmias** arise from ectopic activity originating in the ventricles below the bundle of His. The ventricles may initiate an electrical impulse when higher areas (sinoatrial [SA] node, atria, or atrioventricular [AV] junction) are unable to or when enhanced automaticity of the ventricles overrides activation from above. When the ventricles initiate an impulse, depolarization throughout the ventricles is very unorganized and chaotic because the flow of the impulse throughout the ventricles proceeds very differently than normal. Although some ventricular dysrhythmias are benign, many may become life threatening and are therefore of great clinical concern.

Although it would be more logical from the standpoint of the order of progression of the heart's normal electrical activation to cover atrial and junctional arrhythmias first, this text presents ventricular arrhythmias, followed by atrial and junctional arrhythmias. The reason for this is primarily for ease of student learning. Ventricular complexes are much simpler to recognize than are either atrial or junctional complexes. Therefore, once the characteristics of ventricular complexes are mastered, the student may then turn to the more challenging topic of how atrial and junctional complexes differentiate from the normal activation pattern.

Appearance

Cardiac impulses of ventricular origin display several common features on the ECG, as seen in Figure 11.1. These include lack of a P wave, wide, bizarre-looking QRS complexes, and an inverted T wave.

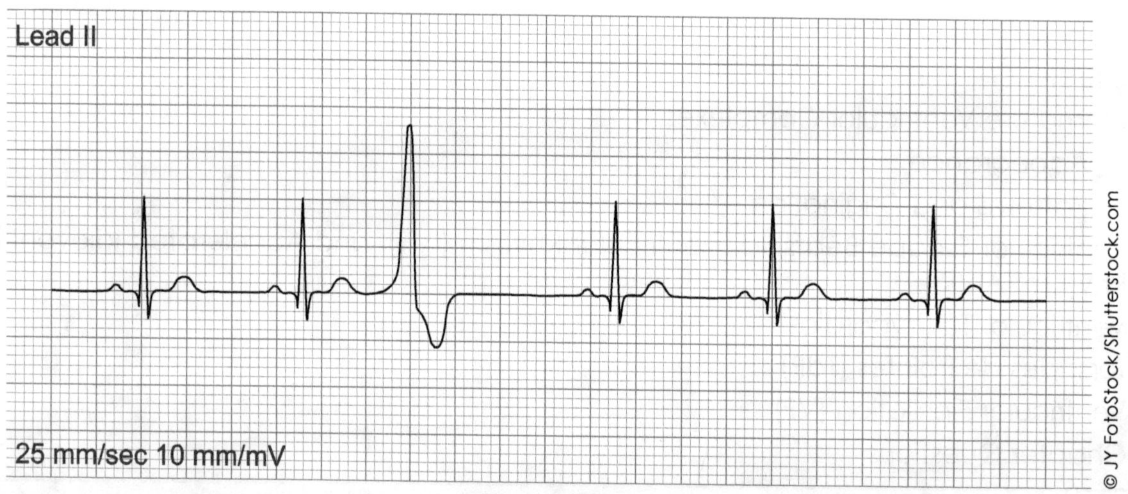

FIGURE 11.1 Premature ventricular complexes have the following characteristics: no P wave, wide QRS, very short down-sloping ST segment, inverted T wave, occurs early, contains a compensatory pause.

When the impulse initiates within the ventricles, the ventricles depolarize first. Most typically, the impulse does not travel back up through the AV node to the atria. If it does travel to the atria, the P wave is buried within the abnormal QRS complex and not observed. There is a small chance of observing a P wave after the QRS complex, during the ST segment, but ST segments are usually very short to nonexistent in ventricular complexes, because there is little to no time between the end of depolarization and the beginning of repolarization. If a P wave appears to occur before a ventricular complex, then either the P wave occurred independently of the QRS complex, as occurs in third degree AV block (see Chapter 13), or the impulse originated above the ventricles and was conducted aberrantly through the ventricles.

The QRS complex of ventricular complexes is wide (>0.12 s) because in such cases depolarization depends wholly on the slow wavelike spread of the impulse from myocyte to myocyte, instead of through the faster His/Purkinje system. The ST segment is usually very short to nonexistent and is either elevated if the QRS complex is negative or depressed if the QRS complex is positive. The T wave is inverted (in the opposite direction from that of the QRS complex). Thus, if the QRS complex is positive, the T wave will be negative, and if the QRS complex is negative the T wave will be positive.

Effects

Ventricular complexes result in several effects on the body. First, the loss of atrial kick reduces the end-diastolic volume (EDV) of each heartbeat and thus decreases stroke volume (SV) and the resultant cardiac output ($\dot{Q}$) to some degree. If a ventricular rhythm exists, the rate of discharge of ventricular impulses is usually in the range of 20 to 40 beats per minute. This rate is so slow that $\dot{Q}$ will be too low to adequately meet the body's demand for blood flow. If there is a ventricular tachycardia (VT) present, ventricular filling time is reduced, again resulting in reductions in $\dot{Q}$. Thus, almost all symptoms attributable to ventricular dysrhythmias are a result of decreased $\dot{Q}$, which can be significant enough to result in death.

Premature Ventricular Complexes

As indicated in the first word of their title, **premature ventricular complexes** (PVC) are ectopic complexes that occur early. They occur earlier than the next expected sinus complex and nearly always interrupt the sinus rhythm. Although there are many causes of PVCs, the causes can generally be grouped into one of four types: sympathomimetic changes (those causes that stimulate the sympathetic nervous system), hypoxic factors, heart disease, and electrolyte imbalances. PVCs can even occur from time to time in healthy hearts. When PVCs occur in isolation and infrequently, they are usually of no significant consequence. As the frequency of PVCs increases, however, so does their clinical significance.

Appearance

In addition to the three characteristics of ventricular complexes noted earlier in this chapter (no P wave, wide QRS, and inverted T wave), PVCs have two additional characteristics, both of which are related to the rhythm. PVCs appear early and are followed by a compensatory pause. Regarding the early appearance, the distance from the sinus beat prior to the appearance of a PVC is shorter than the normal RR interval. When a compensatory pause is present, the next sinus beat after the PVC appears when expected. To measure a compensatory pause, the distance from the sinus beat before the PVC to the sinus beat after the PVC is equal to two normal RR intervals. In Figure 11.1, the normal RR interval is approximately 22.5 small boxes, whereas the distance from the pre-PVC sinus to the post-PVC sinus complex is 45 small boxes.

$$45 \div 22.5 = 2.0$$

The reason for the compensatory pause is that the PVC prevents one normal sinus impulse from depolarizing the ventricles because they are refractory during the PVC. The following sinus beat can proceed normally because the ventricles are no longer refractory by the time it arrives. PVCs can occur in different patterns and arise either from one location or multiple locations within the ventricles (**multifocal PVC**).

Patterns and Origination

PVCs may originate from one or more locations (foci) within the ventricles. When PVCs arise from only one location, they all look the same and are referred to as either **monomorphic** or **unifocal** (Fig. 11.2). Note that these PVCs will all look the same within the same lead, but they will look different in different leads, just as QRS complexes normally look somewhat different in different leads, because each lead presents a view of the heart from a different angle. When PVCs arise from two or more sites within the ventricles, they are called **polymorphic** or multifocal (Fig. 11.3). Multifocal PVCs are of greater concern than unifocal PVCs because they indicate that the ventricular myocardium is agitated in more than one locale.

Certain patterns of PVCs have been assigned specific names. When two unifocal PVCs occur consecutively, it is called a ventricular **couplet** or a couplet of PVCs (Fig. 11.2). When a run of three or more PVCs occurs in a row at a rate of at least 100 beats per minute, it is known as **ventricular tachycardia.** Anywhere from 3 consecutive unifocal PVCs to a run of 30 seconds of consecutive PVCs is known as **nonsustained ventricular tachycardia** (NSVT) (Fig. 11.4). A run of PVCs lasting greater than 30 seconds is called **sustained ventricular**

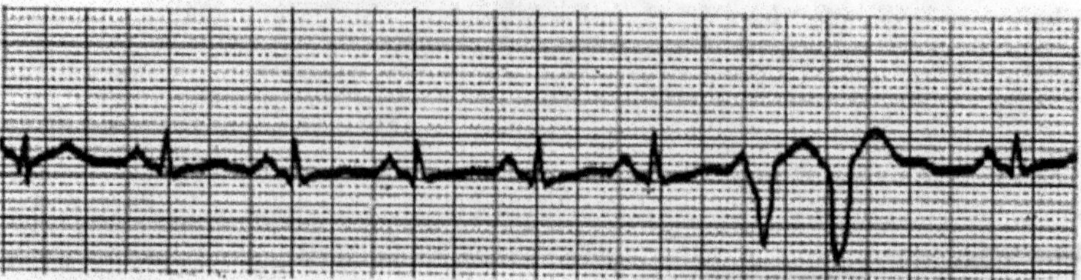

FIGURE 11.2 Ventricular couplet (couplet of PVCs). Two unifocal PVCs occurring in in consecutive cardiac cycles. The PVCs look the same within the same lead.

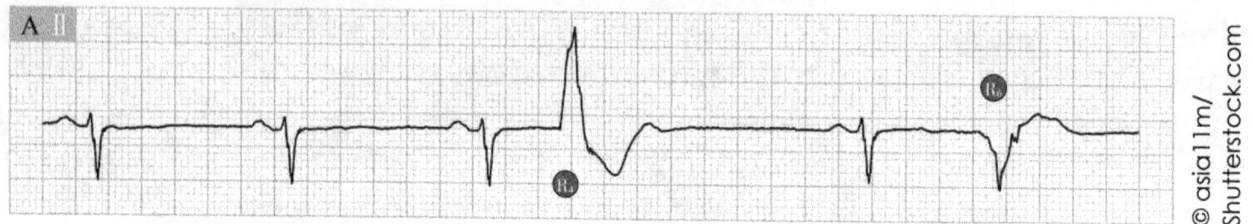

FIGURE 11.3 Multifocal PVCs. The two PVCs have different appearances within the same lead because they arise from different locations (foci) within the ventricles.

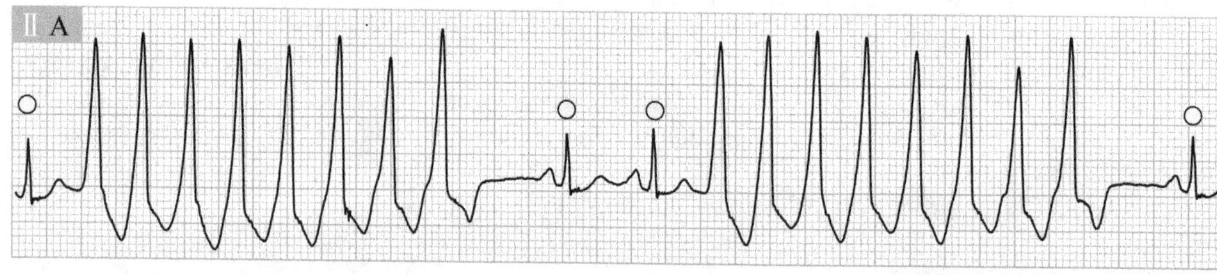

A

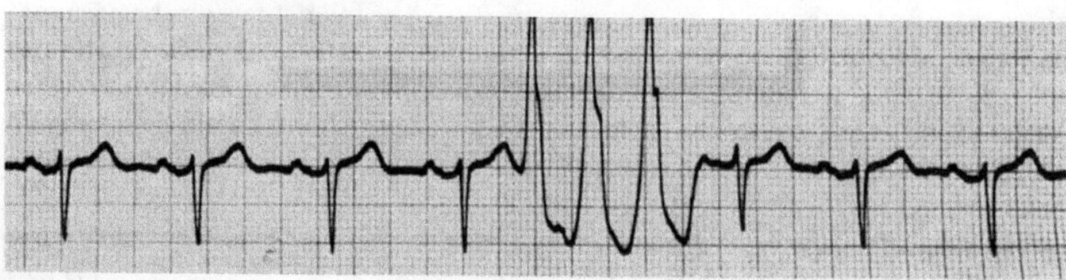

B

FIGURE 11.4 Nonsustained ventricular tachycardia (NSVT). **A** shows two runs of NSVT (8 PVCs each) with two sinus beats in between the two runs of NSVT. **B** shows a salvo or burst of NSVT (in this case consisting of three consecutive PVCs).

tachycardia (SVT) (Fig. 11.5). Usually, SVT occurs in the presence of coronary artery disease (CAD). When there are three consecutive PVCs, it is called a "salvo" or "burst" of NSVT (Fig. 11.4b). When unifocal PVCs are present every other beat, it is known as ventricular **bigeminy** or bigeminal PVCs (Fig. 11.6). When PVCs are present every third beat, it is known as ventricular **trigeminy** or trigeminal PVCs (Fig. 11.7). When PVCs are present every fourth beat, it is known as ventricular **quadrigeminy** or quadrigeminal PVCs (Fig. 11.8). Remember that the more frequent the PVCs, the greater is the cause for concern. Thus, ventricular bigeminy is generally more concerning than trigeminy and trigeminy more so than quadrigeminy.

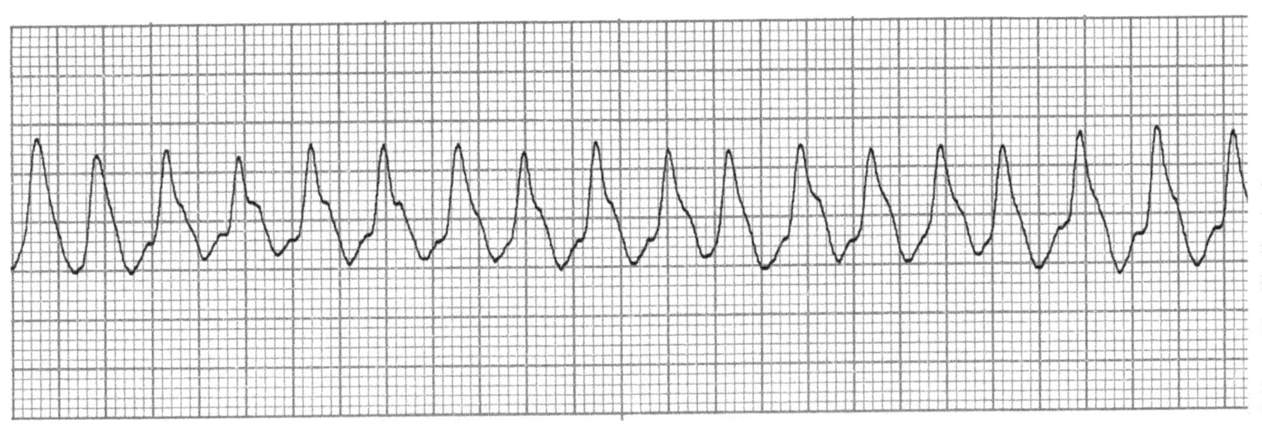

FIGURE 11.5 Sustained ventricular tachycardia (SVT).

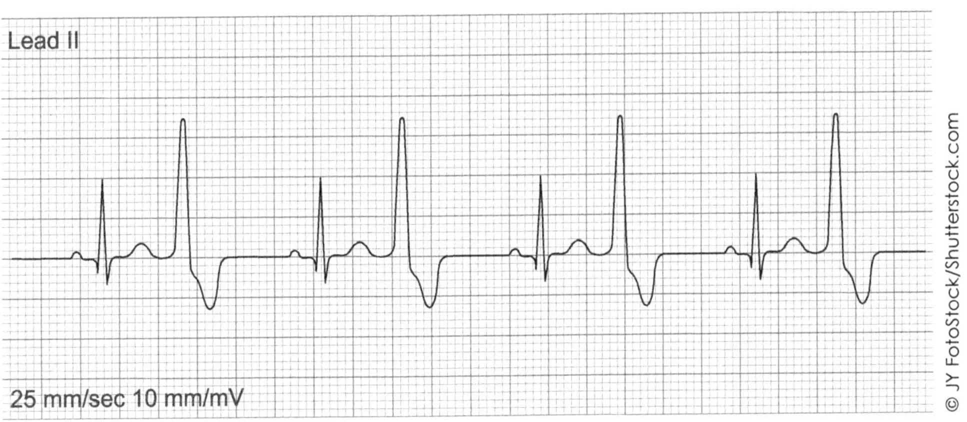

FIGURE 11.6 Ventricular bigeminy (bigeminal PVCs). PVCs occurring every other beat.

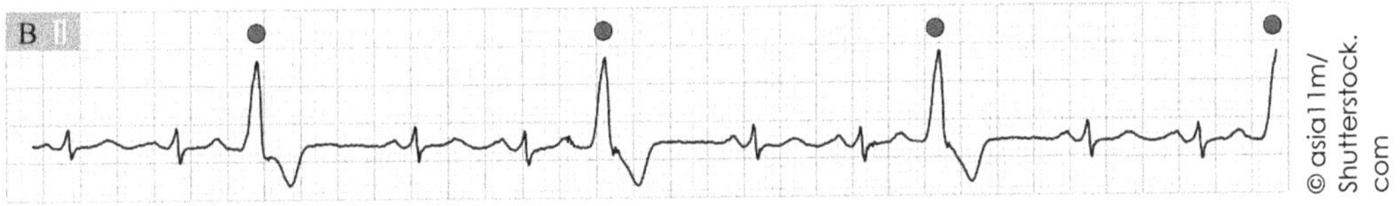

FIGURE 11.7 Ventricular trigeminy (trigeminal PVCs). PVCs occurring every third beat.

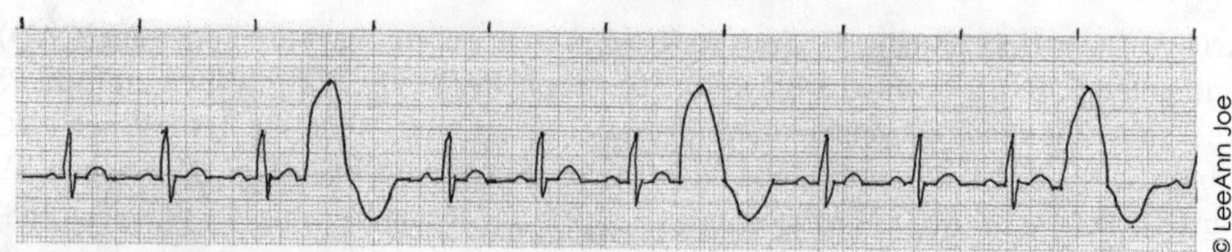

FIGURE 11.8 Ventricular quadrigeminy (Quadrigeminal PVCs). PVCs occurring every fourth beat.

Sometimes, a PVC occurs without interrupting the normal cardiac cycle. This is known as an **interpolated PVC** (Fig. 11.9) and appears as a PVC squeezed between two regular complexes. It does not have a compensatory pause because it does not interrupt the normal cardiac cycle. The distance between the pre-PVC sinus beat and the post-PVC sinus beat is one RR interval. Interpolated PVCs are more likely to occur when there is a slower sinus rate.

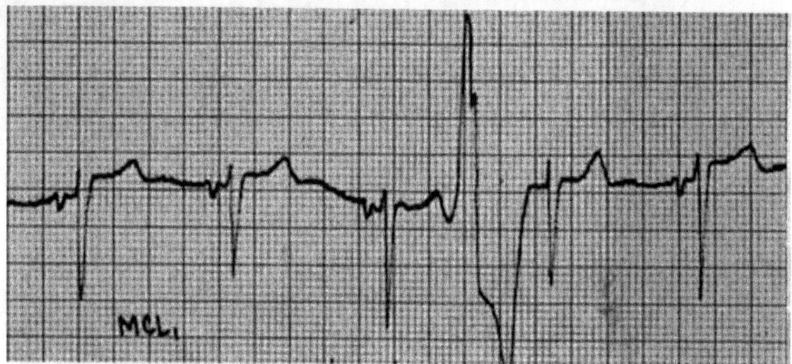

FIGURE 11.9 Interpolated PVC. The PVC does not interrupt normal sinus rhythm. Distance from pre-PVC sinus to post-PVC sinus beat is 1 RR interval.

When a PVC appears on the T wave of the previous sinus beat, it is known as **R on T phenomenon** (Fig. 11.10). This ventricular ectopic beat occurs while the ventricles are in the relative refractory period before they have completely repolarized. An R on T is a very unstable occurrence and is highly susceptible to progress to life-threatening dysrhythmias such as ventricular fibrillation (VF).

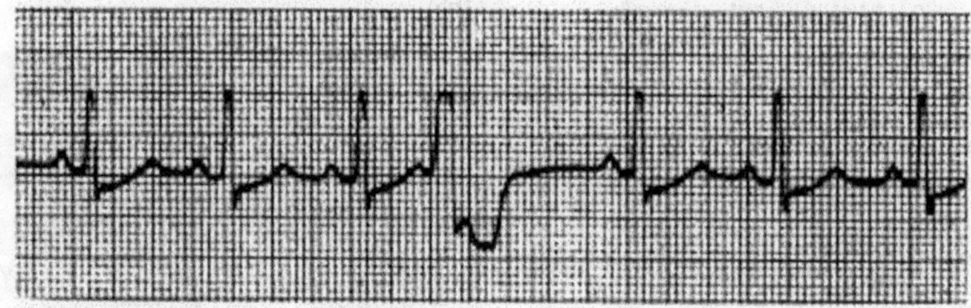

FIGURE 11.10 R on T phenomenon. The PVC occurs during the T wave of the previous sinus beat.

Treatment for PVCs can vary widely. Asymptomatic patients usually don't require treatment. Treatment is usually directed at identifying and correcting the underlying cause. Pharmacologic management with antiarrhythmic drugs may be used, or if a single focus can be mapped during an electrophysiologic study, **catheter ablation** may be performed to rid the individual of the irritable focus.

Ventricular Escape Beats, Idioventricular Rhythm (IVR), and Accelerated Idioventricular Rhythm (AIVR)

Ventricular escape beats sometimes occur after a period of no higher electrical activity, as in sinus arrest. When electrical activity fails to reach the ventricles from a higher center for a period of time, the ventricles will spontaneously generate their own impulse in an effort to avoid cardiac arrest. It may be that one or two ventricular escape beats occur, and then the sinus node or other higher pacemaker is able to resume activity. If not, then ventricular depolarizations will continue producing a ventricular rhythm, usually resulting in what is known as an **idioventricular rhythm (IVR)** (Fig. 11.11).

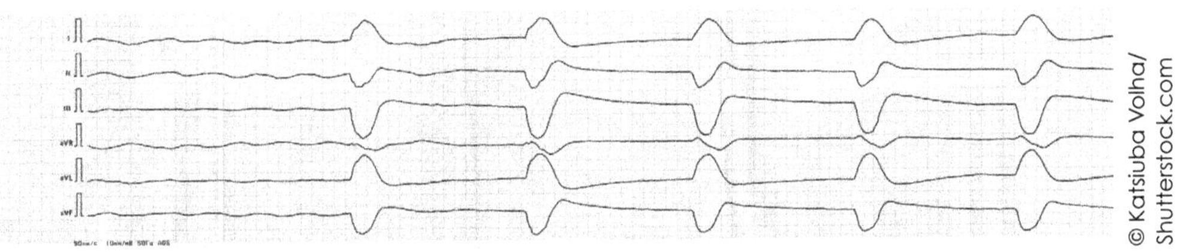

© Katsiuba Volha/ Shutterstock.com

FIGURE 11.11 Idioventricular rhythm (IVR). Ventricular rhythm with a heart rate of less than 40 beats per minute (most commonly between 20 and 40 beats per minute). Here, the heart rate is approximately 19 beats per minute.

If one or two ventricular escape beats occur before a higher pacemaker resumes activity, what will be observed is the normal underlying rhythm, followed by an area of lack of electrical activity (isoelectric area), then one or more ventricular beats, and, finally, the underlying rhythm picks back up (Fig. 11.12).

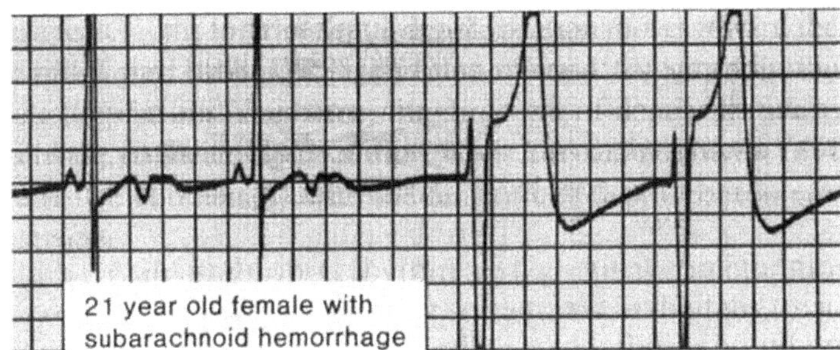

FIGURE 11.12 Ventricular escape beats. Following a long pause, as occurs with sinus arrest, the ventricles may generate a beat to cause contraction of the ventricle and to prevent cardiac arrest.

IVR occurs when higher pacemakers fail or there is a block in the conductive system between the atria and the ventricles. In these cases, a ventricular pacemaker takes over to maintain some amount of cardiac output and preserve life. In IVR, the rate is usually between 20 and 40 beats per minute, because that is the intrinsic rate of ventricular pacemaker cells. IVR may be the final rhythm observed before going into cardiac arrest as well as the first organized rhythm noted following defibrillation. IVR may be referred to as an **agonal rhythm** if the heart rate is less than 10 beats per minute, as may occur in the final stages prior to death. An agonal rhythm does not produce significant cardiac output.

The causes of IVR include cardiac diseases such as myocardial ischemia and MI, certain drugs, increased vagal tone, and metabolic acidosis. As with most other conditions in this chapter, symptoms associated with IVR are attributable to decreased $\dot{Q}$. With IVR, the reduced $\dot{Q}$ is highly significant. Treatment will focus on maintaining the airway, breathing, and circulation and treating any underlying causative conditions.

An IVR on the ECG appears as a ventricular rhythm with a regular rhythm rate of 20 to 40 beats per minute (Fig. 11.12). However, as the heart dies, it may become irregular. P waves are typically absent but may be present with no predictable relationship to the QRS complex as occurs in third degree AV block (see Chapter 13).

Accelerated idioventricular rhythm (AIVR) is very similar in appearance to IVR (Fig. 11.13). It is a ventricular rhythm where the rhythm is regular and the rate is between 40 and 100 beats per minute, which is in excess of the inherent rate of the ventricles. AIVR can have the same causes as IVR, but it is also a very common occurrence following an acute MI, especially after the administration of thrombolytic medications. Thus, it is commonly referred to as a **reperfusion dysrhythmia.**

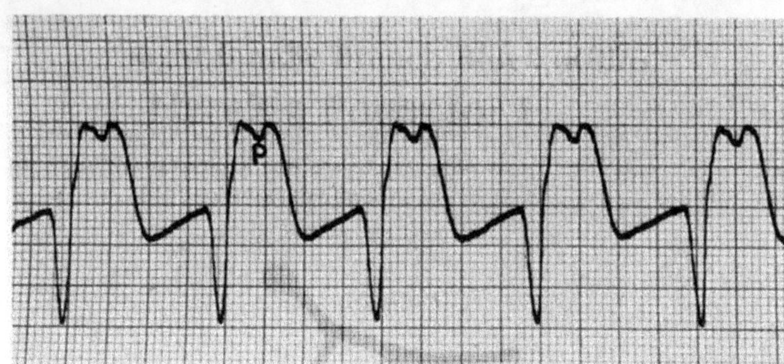

FIGURE 11.13 Accelerated idioventricular rhythm (AIVR). Ventricular rhythm with a heart rate between 40 and 100 beats per minute. Here, the heart rate is approximately 75 beats per minute.

Because the rate is faster in AIVR, often few to no symptoms are noted. If symptoms do occur, most likely in slower AIVRs, symptoms are again attributable to low $\dot{Q}$. Thus, treatment will be aimed at increasing $\dot{Q}$, primarily through pharmacologic means.

Ventricular Tachycardias

VTs include any ventricular rhythms where the rate is greater than 100 beats per minute. Usually, VT occurs with myocardial ischemia or other cardiac disease, but there are other causes too, such as the use of certain drugs or electrolyte imbalances. NSVT and SVT (refer to Fig. 11.4–11.15), discussed earlier in this chapter, are VTs, but VT also includes Torsades de Pointes (TdP). All VTs should be considered clinically significant. Even when a pulse is produced by a VT, it should be closely monitored because it could easily degrade into a life-threatening cardiac arrest. Between the loss of atrial kick and the decreased ventricular filling time due to the fast rate, $\dot{Q}$ is reduced. Thus, symptoms will be those of reduced $\dot{Q}$, and treatment will be aimed at maintaining $\dot{Q}$ and treating underlying causes. Slower VTs, however, may not produce any symptoms. If a VT is pulseless, it should be treated like VF.

Torsades de Pointes (TdP)

Torsades de Pointes (TdP) is a form of polymorphic VT. In French, it literally means twisting around the points. TdP has a very characteristic look to it in that the QRS complexes alternate in shape and height and width and appear to cycle from taller to shorter complexes in a repeating pattern (Fig. 11.14). They appear to twist themselves around the isoelectric axis, similar to the look of a towel being wrung out.

TdP is associated with long QT syndrome, a condition in which there are long QT intervals present on the ECG. Most commonly, long QT syndrome occurs owing to either certain drugs or electrolyte imbalances but

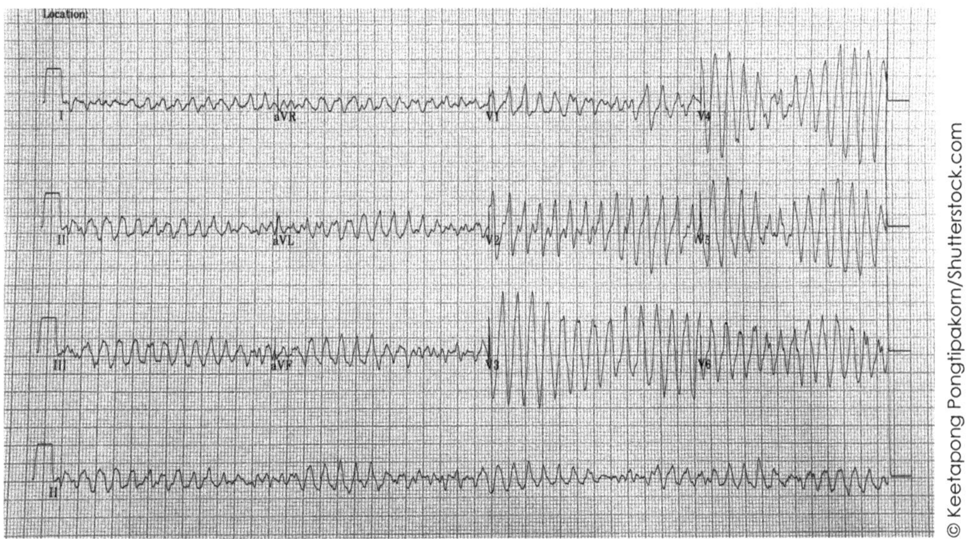

FIGURE 11.14 Torsades de Pointes. A form of polymorphic ventricular tachycardia in which the QRS complexes are of varying shapes, widths, and heights and appear to twist around the isoelectric axis.

can also be an inherited condition. Symptoms associated with TdP vary widely with the rate and duration of TdP. Treatment will usually begin with an initial unsynchronized shock. Standard antidysrhythmic drugs can often worsen the condition. Any drugs causing the condition should be stopped and electrolyte imbalances treated. If TdP is pulseless, it should be treated as VF.

Ventricular Fibrillation (VF)

VF is caused by very fast and chaotic firing of multiple sites in the ventricles. It appears as a wavy, chaotic line without clearly discernible complexes (Fig. 11.15). The ventricular impulses typically fire at a rate somewhere between 300 and 500 times per minute. The depolarizations are so chaotic that the ventricles essentially quiver and do not contract as a unit to produce any $\dot{Q}$ and thus blood pressure. Individuals in VF are pulseless, and it is the most common initial form of cardiac arrest. Most commonly, VF is associated with significant cardiac conditions but can also occur because of the use of certain drugs or as the result of noncardiac sources like electrical shock, acid–base imbalances, and electrolyte imbalances. Because it is pulseless, immediate treatment is necessary to prevent death. Immediate treatment includes prompt CPR, followed by defibrillation as soon as it becomes available.

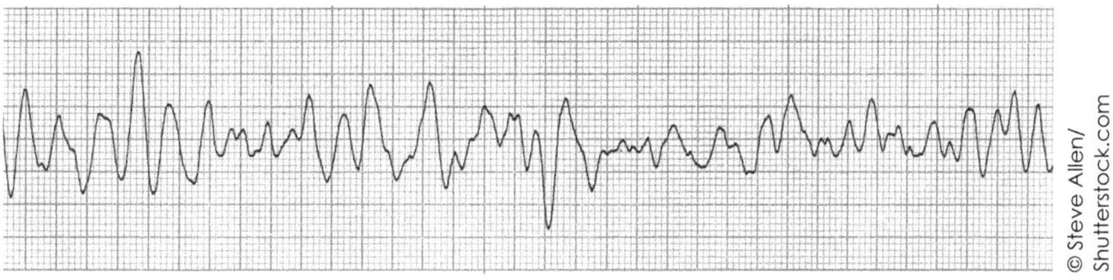

FIGURE 11.15 Ventricular fibrillation (VF). Chaotic firing of impulses from multiple sites within the ventricles. Creates an erratic wavy line with no clearly discernible waves.

Chapter Questions

1. Explain why ventricular ectopic complexes do not contain P waves.
2. Explain why isolated PVCs are of little concern but those that occur more frequently are more worrisome.

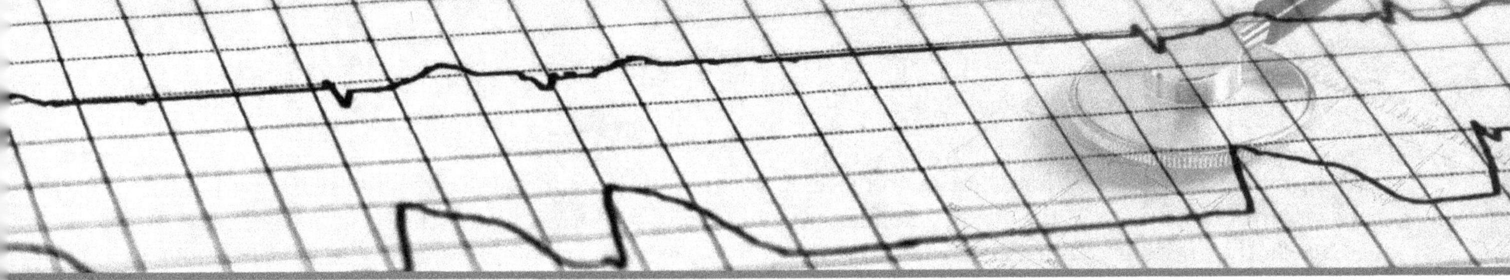

CHAPTER 12

Supraventricular Arrhythmias

Supraventricular arrhythmias can cause uncomfortable symptoms that interfere with patients' ability to exercise. An understanding of these arrhythmias is essential for the clinical exercise physiologist to provide proper therapy when treating cardiac patients.

CONTENT OUTLINE

- Premature Atrial Complexes
- Wandering Atrial Pacemaker
- Premature Junctional Complexes
- Supraventricular Tachycardias
  - Atrial Tachycardia
  - Multifocal Atrial Tachycardia
  - Atrioventricular (AV) Nodal Reentrant Tachycardia (AVNRT)
  - Atrioventricular Reciprocating Tachycardia (AVRT)
  - Atrial Flutter
  - Atrial Fibrillation
- Chapter Questions

Supraventricular arrhythmias arise from ectopic activity originating above the ventricles, particularly either in the atria or at the atrioventricular (AV) junction. In contrast to ventricular ectopic activity, discussed in the previous chapter, atrial and junctional ectopic activity exhibit more subtle changes in the ECG and are relatively harder to identify. Atrial dysrhythmias tend to be more benign than ventricular dysrhythmias, but some may still produce life-threatening complications.

Premature Atrial Complexes

Premature atrial complexes (PAC) (Fig. 12.1) originate within the atria, but the shape of the P wave produced may or may not be noticeably different from the sinus P wave. If the origination of atrial ectopic activity is in proximity to the sinoatrial (SA) node, the wave of depolarization will proceed in a similar fashion to that which was created by the SA node, and the P' wave (ectopic waves are denoted with the prime symbol) appearance may be indistinguishable from that of P waves originating in the SA node. However, all atrial ectopic activity (P' waves) distal to the SA node is likely to be different in shape and/or size from the sinus P wave. Additionally, the P'RI may be different in length from the sinus PRI. The P'RI will most often be shorter, but it could be longer if the origination point is far in the left atrium. If origination is very close to the AV node, the P' wave may be inverted, and there will be a very short P'RI.

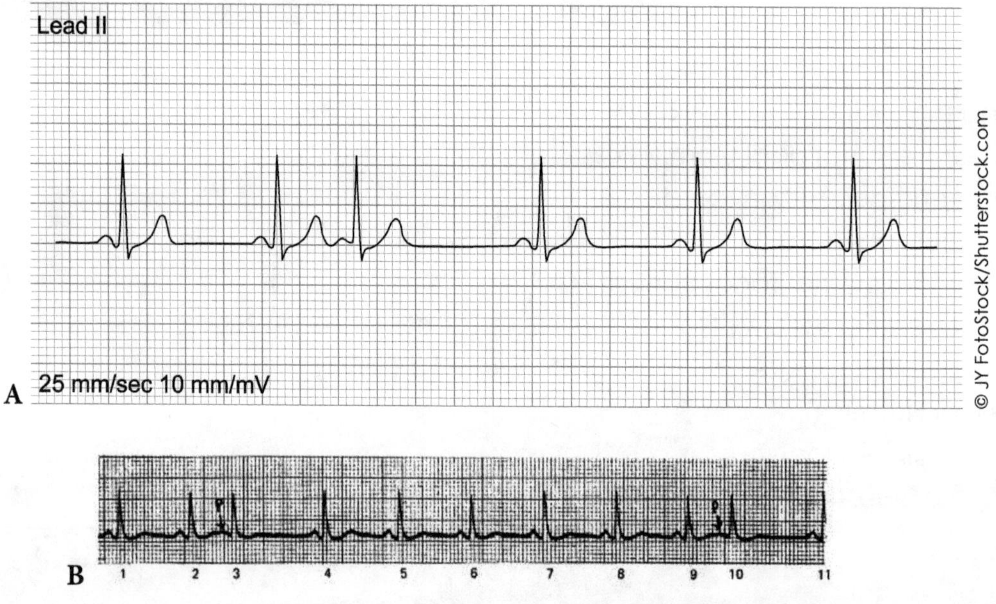

FIGURE 12.1 Premature Atrial Complex. **A** – The PAC appears early, has a P' wave that is different in shape from the sinus P wave, has a short PRI, and a noncompensatory pause. **B** – There are two PACs, at complexes 3 and 10 in this rhythm strip. Note that both PACs are identical because they both arose from the same focus within the atria (unifocal PACs).

Once the wave of depolarization from the ectopic atrial focus reaches the AV node, the signal usually proceeds normally throughout the rest of the conductive system. Thus, the QRS complex, ST segment, and T wave should all appear normal if no other types of arrhythmias are present. The two exceptions to this rule are a blocked PAC and a PAC with aberrant conduction.

A **blocked PAC** (nonconducted PAC) occurs when the wave of depolarization created by the atrial focus reaches the AV node while it is refractory from the preceding sinus depolarization (preceding cardiac cycle), preventing conduction to the ventricles. The appearance of a blocked PAC on the ECG is a premature P' wave that is not followed by a QRS complex (Fig. 12.2). Blocked PACs can sometimes be confused with either sinus pause/block/arrest or second-degree AV blocks. In the case of sinus block/pause/arrest, there is not a premature P' wave following a T wave, but rather the area that lacks electrical activity immediately follows the T wave. Blocked PACs can be distinguished from AV blocks because the P' wave appears early. In the case of second-degree AV blocks, the P waves appear on time.

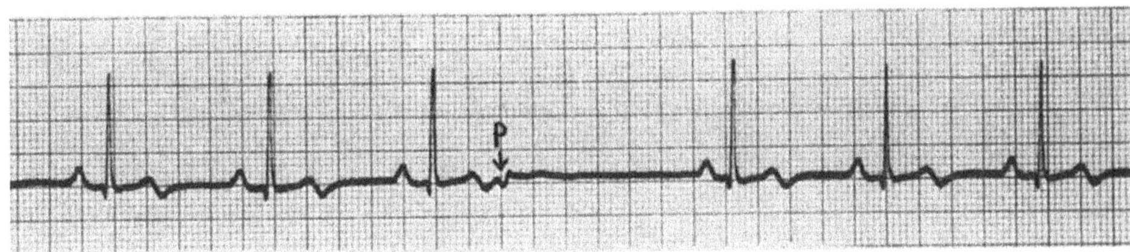

FIGURE 12.2 Blocked PAC (Nonconducted PAC). A P' wave appears early, during the downstroke of the previous sinus T wave, without being followed by ventricular depolarization. Note that there is also a noncompensatory pause present. Blocked PACs usually happen when the electrical impulse reaches the ventricles while they are refractory.

A **PAC with aberrant conduction** (PAC with aberrancy) occurs when the impulse that reaches the AV node does not conduct through the ventricles normally (Fig. 12.3). This sometimes occurs if one of the bundle branches or fascicles of the left bundle branch is still refractory when the impulse reaches the ventricles. When this happens, the impulse doesn't spread throughout the ventricles normally and instead spreads through with either a bundle branch block or fascicular block pattern. The PAC with aberrancy looks very much like a premature ventricular complex (PVC) but is preceded by the P' wave. Thus, the presence of the P' wave is the characteristic distinguishing it from a PVC.

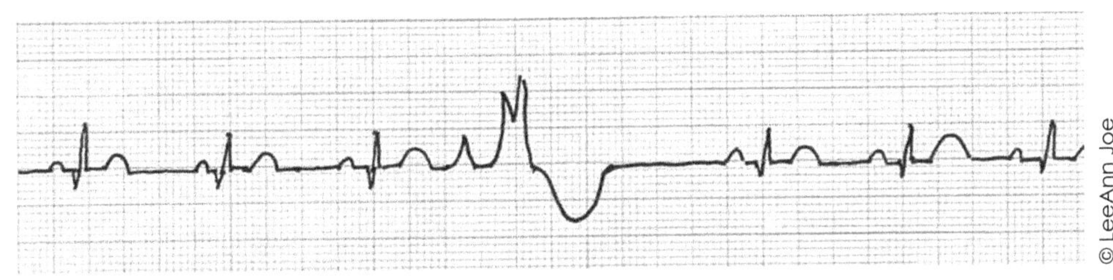

FIGURE 12.3 Aberrant PAC (PAC with aberrancy). P' wave of PAC is significantly different in shape from sinus P waves. The electrical signal reaches the ventricles in such a way that it does not proceed normally through the His-Purkinje system but rather in a wavelike fashion similar to the conduction that happens with PVCs. The resultant QRS appears to depict a PVC, but these beats are actually of atrial origin owing to the presence of the P' wave.

As with PVCs, PACs appear early. If they appear early enough, they can sometimes be buried within the T wave of the preceding complex. If a P wave is buried within a T wave, that T wave usually has a higher amplitude than other T waves, but not always. However, PACs do not exhibit a compensatory pause noted with PVCs. Thus, PACs are said to have noncompensatory pauses. In this case, the RR interval from the pre-PAC sinus complex to the post-PAC sinus complex is not equal to two RR intervals, but instead is one plus a part of an RR interval, as the PAC resets the sinus node timing, allowing it to fire earlier than its next scheduled discharge.

PACs may appear in nearly all the same patterns that we saw in Chapter 11 for PVCs. There may be **atrial couplets** (Fig. 12.4), runs of **nonsustained atrial tachycardia** (including "salvos" or "bursts" of nonsustained atrial tachycardia) or **sustained atrial tachycardia** (Fig. 12.5), and **atrial bigeminy, atrial trigeminy,** and **atrial quadrigeminy** (Fig. 12.6). PACs may be either unifocal or multifocal. The presence of multifocal PACs (Fig. 12.7) can be detected by the presence of P' waves of differing shapes and/or sizes.

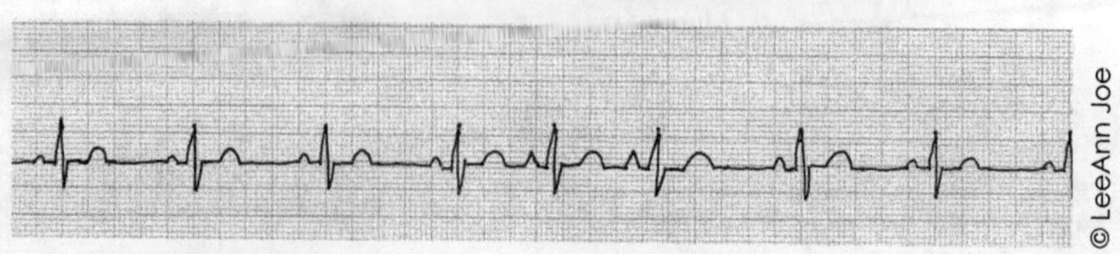

FIGURE 12.4 Atrial couplet (couplet of PACs). Two unifocal PACs in a row (the 5th and 6th complexes) are known as an atrial couplet.

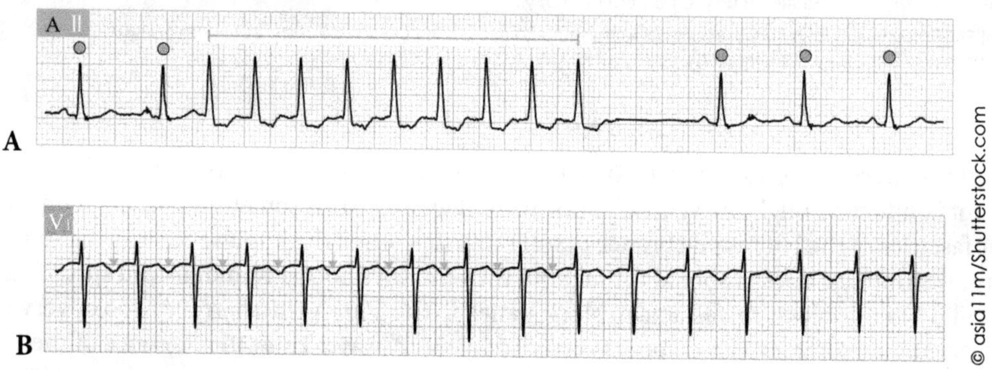

FIGURE 12.5 **A**, nonsustained atrial tachycardia. **B**, sustained atrial tachycardia. It is difficult to distinguish atrial tachycardia from sinus tachycardia if no sinus P waves are present to compare the P' wave to, as seen here.

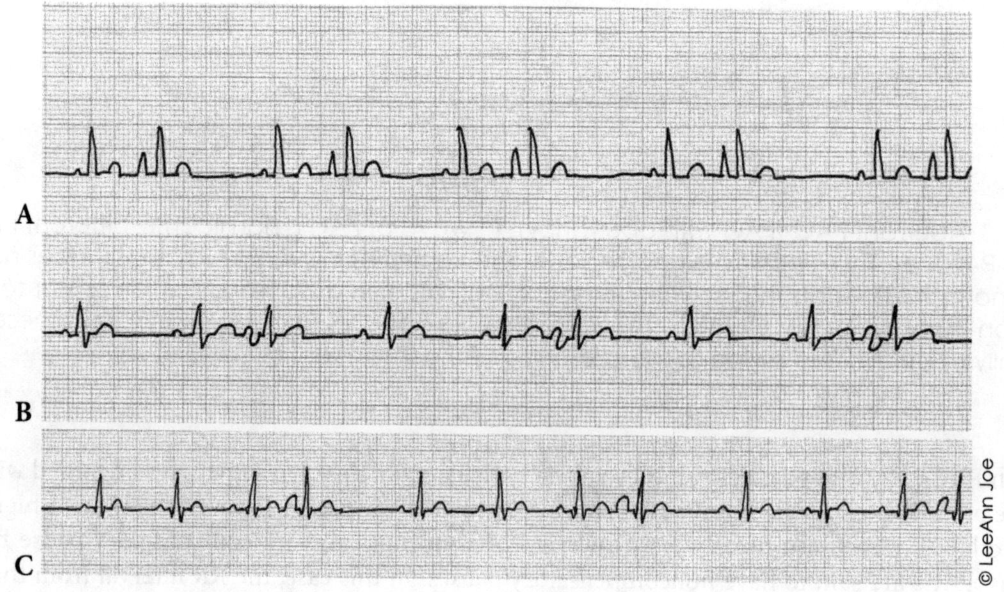

FIGURE 12.6 **A**, atrial bigeminy (PACs present every other complex). Note the different shape of P and P' waves. **B**, atrial trigeminy (PACs present every third complex). C, atrial quadrigeminy (PACs present every fourth complex).

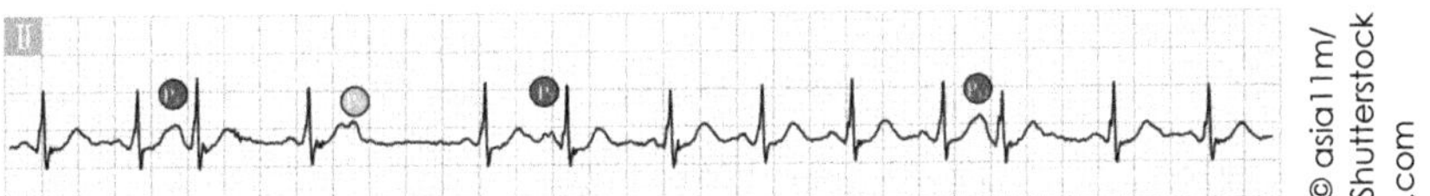

FIGURE 12.7 Multifocal PACs are from different foci and have different P' waves within the same lead. P'RIs and how early the PAC appears are likely to be different from each other.

Most PACs are asymptomatic and are often found incidentally. They do appear more commonly at night or during other periods of deep relaxation when the SA node slows down. Symptoms, if present, are usually associated with "feeling" a skipped beat or extra beat or palpitations owing to the early beat that has occurred. If PACs occur frequently, they should be monitored, because they can lead to more serious dysrhythmias or may be signs of the presence of other serious conditions.

Wandering Atrial Pacemaker

Wandering atrial pacemaker (WAP) is a rhythm in which there are multiple ectopic atrial sites firing from beat to beat. In appearance, if at least three different P wave morphologies appear (SA node and at least two ectopic sites), WAP is likely present (Fig. 12.8). WAP occurs most commonly when there is increased parasympathetic stimulation to the heart. It is commonly seen in children, well-conditioned adults, and the elderly. The condition is usually asymptomatic. WAP is usually transient, disappearing when vagal stimulation decreases in the individual. In addition to P waves of varying morphology, there are usually slight variations in PRIs and in the regularity of the rhythm.

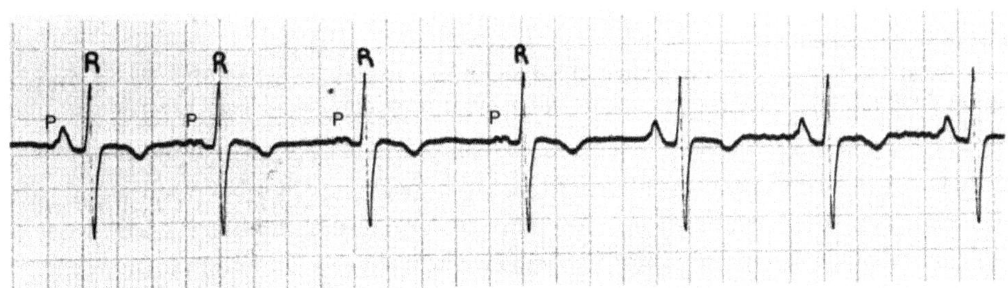

FIGURE 12.8 Wandering Atrial Pacemaker. At least three different P wave morphologies are present, and heart rate is less than 100 beats per minute.

Premature Junctional Complexes

Premature junctional complexes (PJC) (Fig. 12.9) include complexes originating in or between the AV node and/or the AV bundle (bundle of His). Because the impulse originates somewhere between the atria and ventricles, these complexes are referred to as junctional complexes and have a more varied appearance than those seen with either PACs or PVCs. If the impulse travels to the atria before going to the ventricles, a P wave will appear before the QRS complex, and it will typically be inverted, because it proceeds primarily in the opposite direction throughout the atria compared to the SA node as the origination point. If both the atria and ventricles depolarize at the same time, a P wave may not appear owing to the more

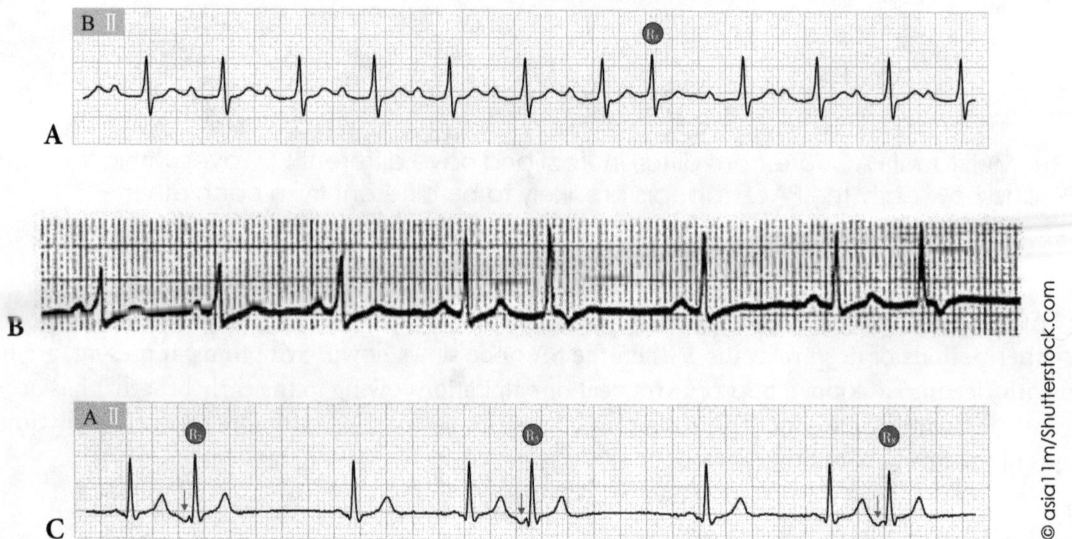

FIGURE 12.9 PJCs. **A**, arrows indicate PJC. This PJC is unifocal and does not have a P' wave (absent P' wave). **B**, arrow indicates PJC. This PJC has a P' wave after the QRS complex. This is known as a retrograde PJC. In this case, the ventricles depolarized before the atria. **C**, arrow indicates PJC. The P wave in this PJC is inverted.

dominant ventricular depolarization. Also, the impulse may fail to travel from the junctional origination point up through the atria, which would also result in the lack of a P wave. Additionally, if the ventricles depolarize before the atria, a **retrograde P wave** may appear. In this case, the P wave would appear after the QRS complex, most commonly within the ST segment. It could potentially also be fused or partially fused with the T wave, but this is uncommon. Thus, the three appearances of P waves in junctional complexes are inverted, absent, or retrograde. Even when the P wave is retrograde, it is also very likely to be inverted.

PRIs are very short or nonexistent in PJCs. Often, the P wave has barely ended when the QRS complex starts. The QRS complex is most commonly normal, as ventricular depolarization most often proceeds normally. However, it can sometimes be long, especially when there is an origination point closer to the AV junction. In these cases, it may range from fairly normal in shape but a little long in duration to ventricular conduction that has a more PVC-like appearance. The ST segment and T wave are normal unless the ventricular conduction is more aberrant. In those few cases, the ST and T appearance will again mimic that of a PVC. Of course, as with all premature complexes, PJCs appear early. Finally, PJCs can't be said to always have a compensatory or noncompensatory pause. The presence of either is possible with PJCs.

If junctional complexes take over the entire rhythm of the heart, they are named according to their rate. A junctional rhythm is said to exist if the rate is between 40 and 60 beats per minute, because that is the inherent pace of the AV node. If the rhythm is less than 40 beats per minute, a slow or **bradycardic junctional rhythm** exists. An **accelerated junctional rhythm** occurs if the HR is between 60 and 100 beats per minute, and it is called **junctional tachycardia** (Fig. 12.10) if the HR is greater than 100 beats per minute.

As with PACs, most PJCs are primarily asymptomatic and are often found incidentally. They do appear more commonly at night or during other periods of deep relaxation when the SA node slows down. Recall that the AV node is the second highest order pacemaker after the SA node. Causes of PJCs are the same as those for PACs plus failure of the SA node. If symptoms are experienced, it is usually associated with loss of $\dot{Q}$ because there may be the loss of the atrial kick. If PJCs occur frequently, they should be monitored, because they can lead to more serious dysrhythmias or may be signs of other serious conditions present.

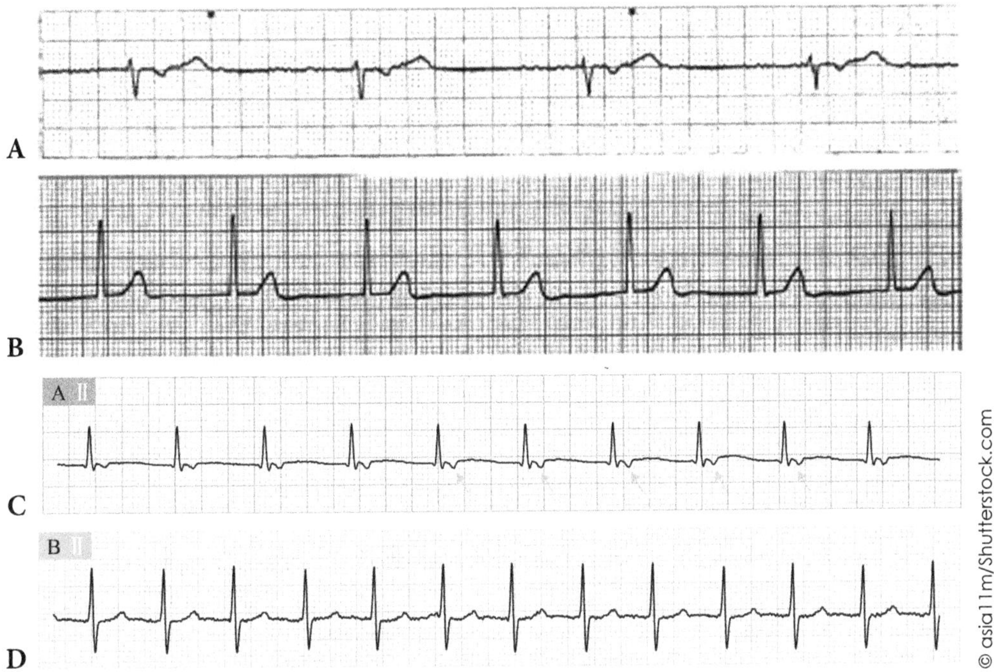

FIGURE 12.10 **A.** Bradycardic junctional rhythm with a heart rate below 40 beats per minute. HR is approximately 33 beats per minute in this 12-lead ECG. P' waves are absent in this example. **B.** Junctional rhythm with a heart rate between 40 and 60 beats per minute. HR is approximately 50 beats per minute in this rhythm strip. The P' waves are inverted in this example. **C.** Accelerated junctional rhythm with a heart rate greater than 60 but less than 100 beats per minute. HR is approximately 83 in this rhythm strip. The P' waves are retrograde in this example. **D.** Junctional tachycardia with a heart rate greater than 100 beats per minute. HR is approximately 115 beats per minute. P' waves are absent in this example.

Supraventricular Tachycardias

Supraventricular tachycardias are tachycardias whose origination point is above the ventricles. Some people consider sinus tachycardia (covered in Chapter10) as a supraventricular tachycardia too because it does originate above the ventricles. However, we are defining supraventricular tachycardia as originating not only above the ventricles but also outside of the SA node. This text abbreviates these as PSVT for two reasons. One, most of these conditions are **paroxysmal** in nature (the P part of the abbreviation—PSVT). Two, the P is also added to help distinguish the abbreviation from that of sustained ventricular tachycardia (SVT), covered in Chapter 11. Thus, our definition of PSVTs includes the following conditions: **atrial tachycardia**, **multifocal atrial tachycardia** (MAT), AV nodal reentrant tachycardia (AVNRT), **AV reciprocating tachycardia** (AVRT), junctional tachycardia (discussed earlier under PJCs), **atrial flutter**, and **atrial fibrillation** (AF or A fib).

Atrial Tachycardia

Atrial tachycardias are unifocal, fast atrial rhythms of greater than 100 beats per minute (Fig. 12.5), but most commonly they are between 150 and 250 beats per minute. Both the onset and the termination of atrial tachycardias tend to be sudden and are therefore usually referred to as paroxysmal atrial tachycardias. Unless the onset of atrial tachycardia is witnessed, it may be difficult to distinguish atrial tachycardia from sinus tachycardia. As with all other atrial complexes, P' waves may differ in appearance from the sinus P wave, and the P'RI may be different (most commonly shorter) than the PRI. Sometimes, the rate is so fast that the P' gets buried in the T of the preceding complex.

In some instances, the AV junction is unable to conduct all the atrial impulses to the ventricles. In these cases, atria tachycardia with block (see chapter 13 for a discussion of heart blocks) occurs, and more than one P' wave will be seen preceding each QRS complex. Most commonly, a two to one block (2 P' waves before each QRS) occurs, but the block can occur in different intervals or irregularly.

Causes of atrial tachycardia are varied and include various cardiac diseases, electrolyte imbalances, and the use of certain drugs. A few of the most common causes, however, are digitalis toxicity, Wolff–Parkinson–White syndrome, and various congenital heart anomalies. As with all tachycardias, there is decreased ventricular filling time, which if severe reduces stroke volume and cardiac output, resulting in a reduction in blood pressure. Thus, most symptoms are attributable to loss of blood pressure.

Multifocal Atrial Tachycardia

In appearance, MAT looks like WAP but with a fast rate (>100 beats per minute) (Fig. 12.11). However, unlike WAP, MAT is almost always caused by a pathological condition. MAT is commonly associated with chronic cardiac and pulmonary disorders, but it can also occur with the use of certain drugs. Again, signs and symptoms will primarily be those associated with low cardiac output. Treatment should be aimed at correcting the underlying condition.

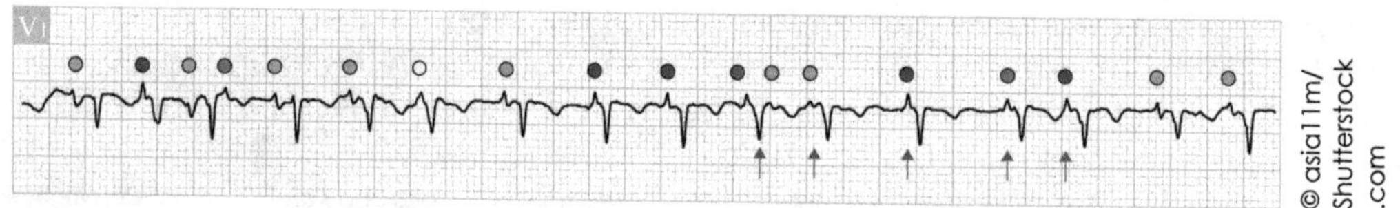

FIGURE 12.11 Multifocal Atrial Tachycardia. Similar in appearance to WAP but with a fast rate. Arrows indicate P' waves of differing shapes.

Atrioventricular (AV) Nodal Reentrant Tachycardia (AVNRT)

A reentrant mechanism is responsible for AVNRT. In the normal heart, there is only one pathway present between the atria and the ventricles. When a reentrant mechanism (reentrant circuit) is present, there is at least one additional, congenital pathway present in the individual between the atria and the ventricles. Specifically, in AVNRT, there are two separate pathways present within the AV node, and these are commonly known as the slow and fast pathways. The fast pathway is the normal tract, whereas the slow pathway is the accessory pathway. The fast pathway has a long refractory period, whereas the slow pathway has a shorter refractory period. Figure 12.12 depicts both pathways and what happens most of the time in the individual. As the impulse starts down both pathways, it reaches the end of the fast pathway first, which transfers the signal to the His-Purkinje system to depolarize the ventricles, and the refractory wake of the fast pathway terminates the signal traveling down the slow pathway. Thus, most of the time, the individual's ECG appears normal, barring the presence of other conditions. However, if the timing of the pathways is affected, as happens when there is a premature ectopic complex (especially a PAC) generated, the signal can proceed down the slow pathway first and loop around the fast pathway without a signal simultaneously coming down the fast pathway. In this case, there is no canceling effect and a looping of the electrical impulse results. Each time the signal loops, a signal is sent to the ventricles, which creates ventricular depolarization and the fast rate, as seen in Figure 12.13. The signal loops around until an event occurs to interrupt the looping, such as another premature complex. Most commonly, PACs are the cause of both the initiation and termination of runs of AVNRT. The appearance of AVNRT

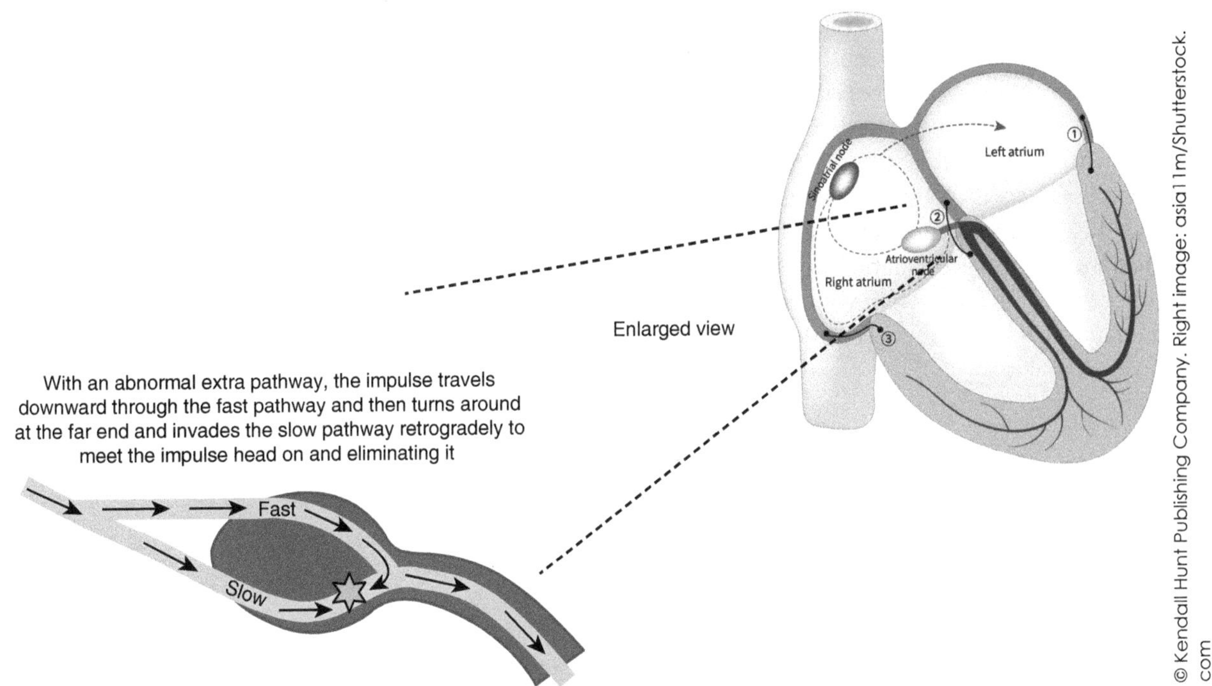

FIGURE 12.12 Accessory pathway and normal pathway present within AV node in AVNRT. The fast pathway is the normal pathway through the AV node, whereas the slow pathway is the accessory pathway. Normally, the impulse proceeds down the fast pathway first, transferring the signal to the ventricles and then proceeds up the slow pathway. The impulse heading down the slow pathway meets the impulse heading upward, which is then eliminated.

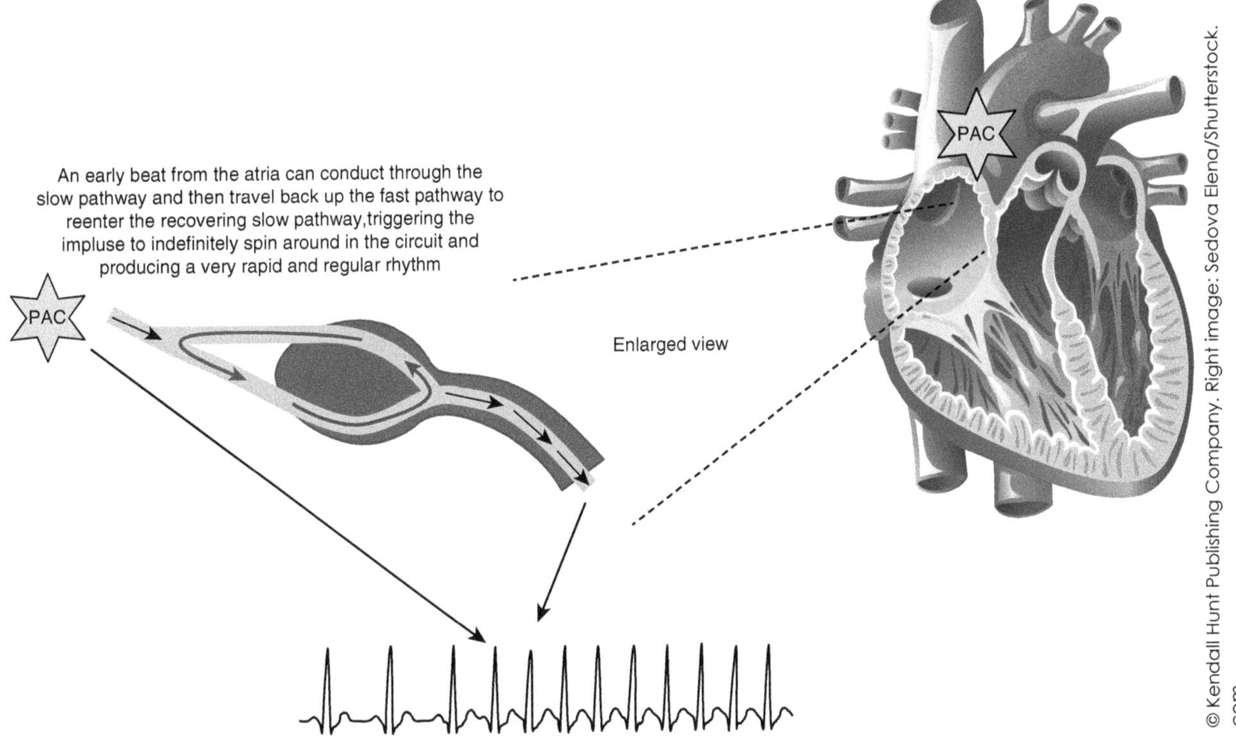

FIGURE 12.13 Accessory pathway and normal pathway present within AV node in AVNRT. The fast pathway is the normal pathway through the AV node, whereas the slow pathway is the accessory pathway. When the timing down the pathways is disrupted, as may happen when a PAC fires, the impulse proceeds down the slow pathway first, transferring the signal to the ventricles, and can loop around the fast pathway, triggering the reentry circuit, producing the AVNRT pattern on the ECG.

commonly exhibits the following characteristics, as seen in Figure 12.14: a HR of greater than 100 beats per minute (most typically between 140 and 240 beats per minute), a regular or slightly irregular rhythm, normal width QRS complexes, P waves either not visible (they are usually lost in the QRS or T) or appearing as pseudo r' or s' waves, and ST segment depression.

As with most supraventricular tachycardias, AVNRT is most typically paroxysmal in nature. The patient usually presents with a history of paroxysmal palpitations, which may produce symptoms such as light-headedness/dizziness, shortness of breath, chest pain or pressure, activity intolerance, fatigue, and anxiety. Owing to the nature of the presentation, AVNRT is, at times, misdiagnosed as anxiety disorder or panic attacks. Most commonly, AVNRT is seen in younger women. Several different treatments may be used to manage the condition including vagal maneuvers, adenosine, or catheter ablation.

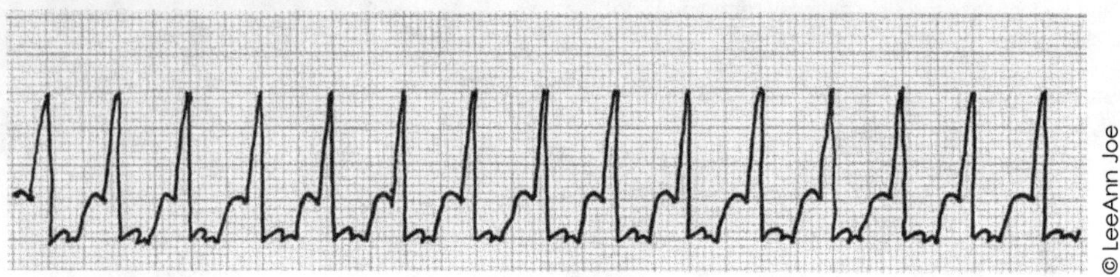

FIGURE 12.14 The characteristics of AVNRT are a regular or slightly irregular (regular here) rhythm (rate greater than 100 beats per minute (approximately 188 beats per minute here), either P' waves are not visible or appear as pseudo r' or s' waves (pseudo s' here), and, most notably, ST segment depression.

Atrioventricular Reciprocating Tachycardia (AVRT)

The name of this condition, atrioventricular reciprocating (or reentrant) tachycardia (AVRT) (a.k.a. macroreentrant tachycardia), is obviously very similar to and can easily be confused with the previous condition. It may help the student to focus on the difference in the abbreviations of AVNRT versus AVRT. AVRT is less common than AVNRT, but there is also a reentrant circuit present, as the name suggests, in the individual with AVRT. However, the accessory circuit present in AVRT is not the same circuit present in AVNRT. In fact, episodes of AVRT may be caused by one of several different types of accessory pathways.

Episodes of AVRT are produced by accessory tracts that are involved in preexcitation syndromes, the most common and best understood of which is Wolffe-Parkinson-White (WPW) Syndrome. In WPW, the accessory pathway fibers form the Bundle of Kent. This pathway may occur either between the left atrium and the left ventricle, known as type A pre-excitation, or between the right atrium and the right ventricle, known as type B preexcitation. In type A preexcitation, a positive R wave is noted in V_1, whereas in type B, a negative R wave is seen in V_1. In preexcitation, the signal from the atria travels faster from the atria to the ventricles than it does through the AV node, as accessory tracts do not have the conduction delay present in the AV node. Thus, the ventricles are stimulated early, from which comes the preexcitation part of the name. On the ECG, the preexcitation pattern produces a short PRI and a delta wave. A delta wave is an early, slurred takeoff of the QRS complex (Fig. 12.15), which occurs as the transfer of the signal to the ventricles initially arises via wavelike myocyte to myocyte transfer but then normalizes as it encounters the His-Purkinje system. The PRIs are short because of not only the faster ventricular activation through the accessory pathway but also the slurred takeoff of the QRS complex. Not all preexcitation syndromes produce a delta wave, however, such as Lown–Ganong–Levine (LGL) Syndrome. The main characteristic of LGL on the ECG is a shortened PRI.

Tachycardias may sometimes occur owing to a looping that results, similarly to what was noted in the discussion of AVNRTs. The initiation and termination of runs of the AVRT are usually premature complexes (particularly PACs), just as with AVNRTs. With AVRTs, the signal most often goes through the accessory pathway first and then loops back through the AV node, with each loop sending a signal to depolarize the ventricles, creating the tachycardia. In some instances, the looping occurs in the opposite direction, that is, it goes through the AV node first and then loops back through the accessory pathway. When the signal heads through

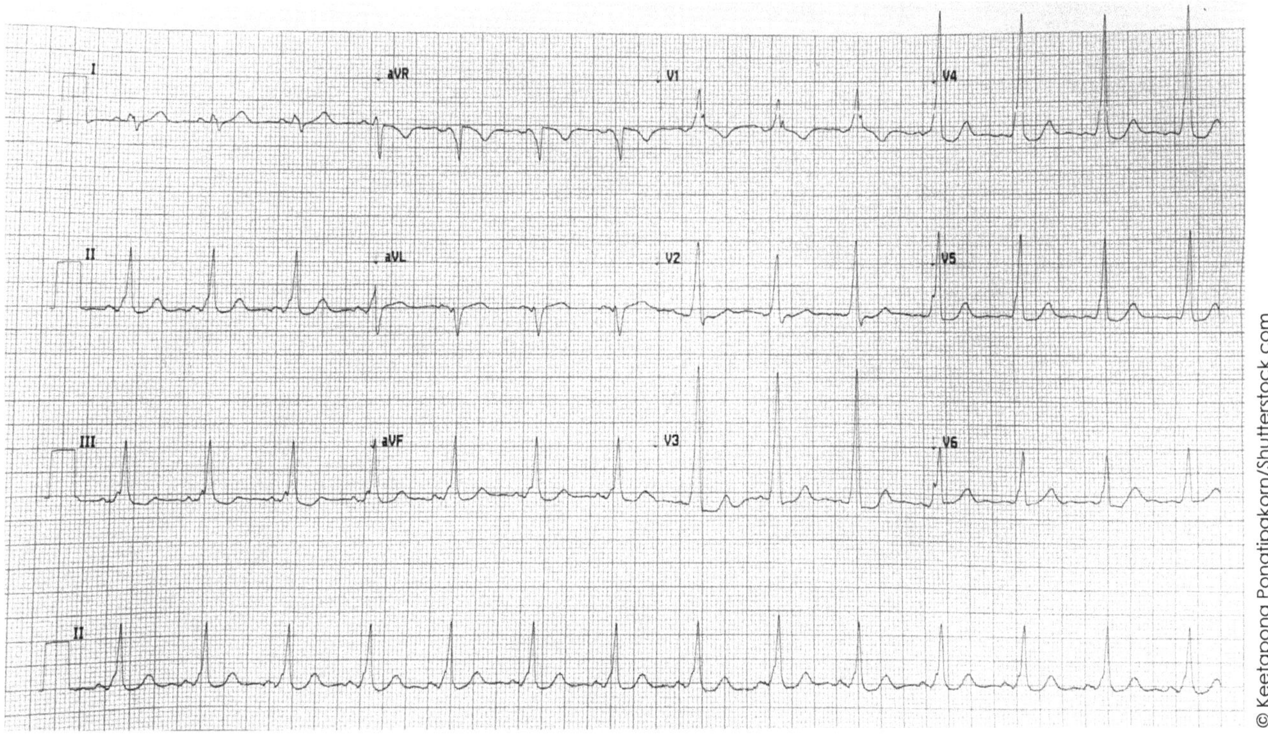

FIGURE 12.15 Wolfe–Parkinson–White preexcitation syndrome. Note the early takeoff of the QRS complex known as a delta wave, which are marked by arrows.

the accessory pathway first and then loops back through the AV node, it is known as an antidromic AVRT (Fig. 12.16B). When the signal heads through the AV node first and then loops back through the accessory pathway, it is called an orthodromic AVRT (Fig. 12.16A). AVRT characteristics on the ECG include a fast heart rate (usually 200–300 beats per minute), P waves are often either buried in QRS or retrograde, normal length QRS complex, QRS alternans (QRS complex varies in height from complex to complex), ST segment depression, and T wave inversion. During an episode of AVRT, symptoms are very similar to those described in regard to AVNRT. Treatment may involve synchronized cardioversion, medications, and catheter ablation.

Atrial Flutter

Atrial flutter (AFL) is a unifocal atrial tachycardia in which the rate is typically between 250 and 350 beats per minute. It is characterized by the presence of **flutter waves** (F waves) (Fig. 12.17). Flutter waves give the baseline a characteristic appearance similar to waves on the ocean or teeth on a saw. Owing to the slower conduction through the AV node, not all atrial depolarizations make their way to the ventricles. Thus, there is some degree of block (see chapter 13 for a discussion of blocks) that happens, most commonly a 2:1 block (atria fire twice for each time the ventricles fire). The ventricular rate tends to be fast but not nearly as fast as the atrial rate (half as fast if there is a 2:1 block). When the atria fire this rapidly, atrial contraction is not efficient, causing blood pooling in the atria. Blood that is more stagnant tends to clot. That clot can subsequently be pumped out of the heart, becoming an **embolus**, and lodge in a vessel elsewhere in the body, most commonly in a brain artery, resulting in a stroke. AFL can be asymptomatic or can include symptoms common to many heart conditions such as shortness of breath, light-headedness, pressure or tightness in the chest, heart palpitations, and fatigue. AFL is primarily seen in older individuals, primarily in those with other forms of underlying heart disease. AFL can also be caused by conditions such as thyroid disease and sleep apnea. Lifestyle factors such as substance abuse, chronic use of certain medications, or chronic consumption of large amounts of caffeine are also thought to contribute to the development of AFL. Similar to some of the other PSVTs already discussed, treatments for AFL often include cardioversion, medications, and catheter ablation. Particularly to help reduce the potential for the formation of emboli, patients with chronic or frequent episodes of AFL may be put on blood thinners.

a. Impuls travels antegradely through AV node but then retrogradely reenters the atria through accessory pathway. It continues to spin around in the circuit producing a very rapid and regular rhythm

b. Impulse travels antegradely through accessory pathway but then retrogradely reenters the atria through AV node. It continues to spin around in the circuit producing a very rapid and regular rhythm

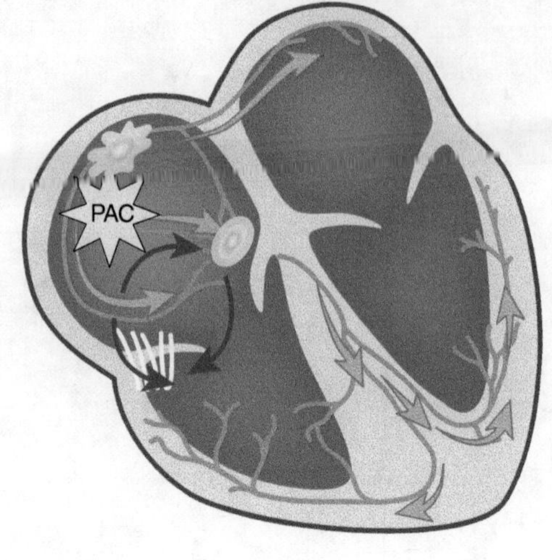

PAC

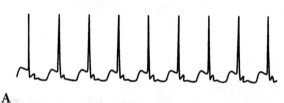

A

B

FIGURE 12.16 **A**, orthodromic AVRT. The electrical impulse proceeds anterogradely through AV Node and then loops around retrogradely through accessory pathway. **B**, antidromic AVRT. The electrical impulse proceeds anterogradely through the accessory pathway and then loops around retrogradely through AV Node.

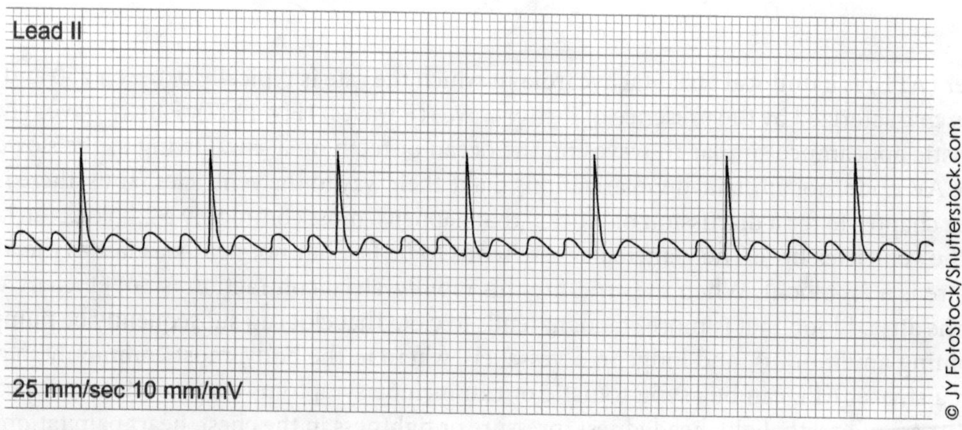

FIGURE 12.17 Atrial flutter is characterized by f-waves or flutter waves on the baseline and either a regular or an irregular ventricular rhythm (regular here).

Atrial Fibrillation

AF is the most common heart arrhythmia in the United States, affecting more than 2 million Americans, although some estimates put the number at as high as 6 million. Atrial fibrillation is attributable to very fast, chaotic firing of multiple sites in the atria. It appears as a wavy, chaotic baseline with QRS complexes appearing intermittently (Fig. 12.18). Although the atrial impulses typically fire at a rate somewhere between 400 and 600 times per minute, only some of those make their way to the ventricles, producing a ventricular rate typically between 100 and 200 beats per minute. And the ventricular rhythm is said to be "irregularly irregular," because the AV node is intermittently refractory in AF. The atrial depolarizations are so chaotic that the atria essentially quiver and do not contract as a unit to produce an atrial kick. Similarly to AFL, AF results in blood pooling in the atria, and the largest risk from AF is stroke. Causes and treatments for AF are nearly identical to those previously discussed for AFL. Patients may even go back and forth between episodes of AF and AFL. Most AF patients are put on anticoagulants, as AF increases stroke risk by fivefold.

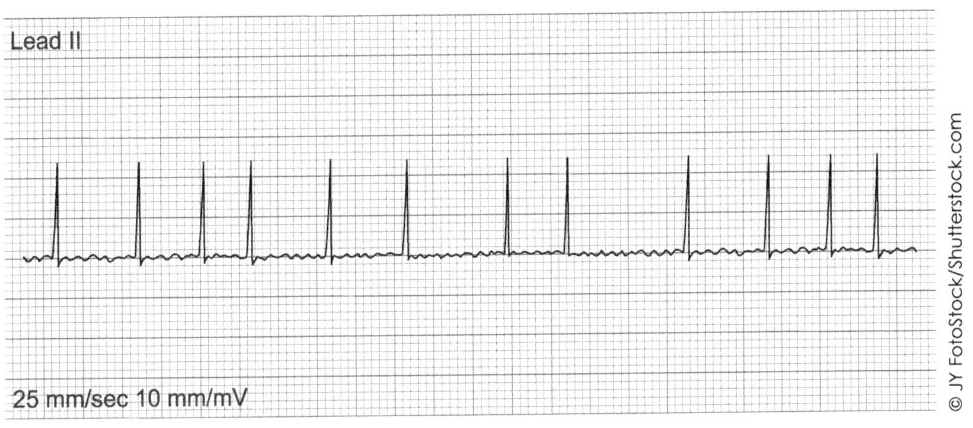

FIGURE 12.18 Atrial fibrillation is characterized by a very erratic baseline with no clearly discernible P waves and typically a very irregular ventricular rhythm, often called irregularly irregular.

Chapter Questions

1. Why does the P' wave take on different shapes, with different origination points within the atria? Similarly, why might the PRI' be of a different length than the sinus PRI?
2. Why do P waves usually appear retrograde in AVNRT and AVRT?
3. Why does the delta wave in WPW disappear when an episode of AVRT occurs?

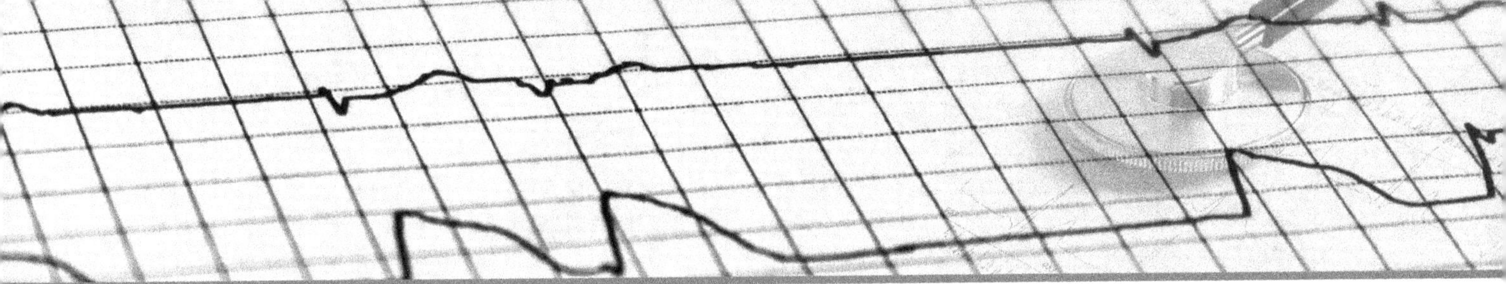

CHAPTER 13

Atrioventricular Heart Blocks

Atrioventricular heart blocks can be benign as in athletes or children, but in others the presence of these blocks is pathologic and can have several causes, including ischemia, infarction, fibrosis, and drugs.

CONTENT OUTLINE

- First-Degree AV Block
- Second-Degree AV Block
- Third Degree (Complete) Heart Block
- Atrioventricular (AV) Dissociation
- Chapter Questions

Atrioventricular (AV) conduction disturbance, or the more commonly used term, *heart block*, is the failure to normally propagate cardiac electrical signals through the AV node. Recall that the AV node holds the electrical signal for a brief period before spreading it through the junction and then down the bundle branches to the ventricles. With AV blocks, as with bundle branch blocks (presented in Chapter 8), the conduction delay is abnormally long (in some instances, there is a failure to conduct) and should be kept distinct from delays. Table 13.1 presents the classification scheme for heart blocks.

TABLE 13.1 AV Heart Blocks

Degree	*AV Conduction Pattern*
First-Degree Block	Uniformly prolonged PR interval
Second-Degree Block	Intermittent conduction failure Mobitz Type I (Wenckebach): Progressive PR elongation Mobitz Type II: Sudden conduction failure
Third-Degree Block	No atrioventricular conduction

The following examples indicate an important point, namely, that *absence of conduction is not the same thing as block*. First, consider what is occurring in atrial flutter. In the face of very high atrial depolarization rates, the refractory period of the AV node protects the ventricles from receiving every impulse generated by the atria. Second, in some instances there is no opportunity for conduction through the AV node to occur. For example, in an accelerated idioventricular rhythm control of pacing activity is seized from the sinus node. When this happens, the lower pacemaker can remain dissociated from the higher pacer (sinoatrial [SA] node) for several cycles, with P waves trailing the QRS complexes. Unless there is spontaneous reversion out of this newly established pacer, there is no chance of the SA node regaining its pacing function. Therefore, each P wave remains unconducted to the ventricles. This situation is properly referred to as *dissociation*, but not block.

In all forms of AV block, the conduction ratio is an important consideration to remember. The ratio of the rate of atrial firing to ventricular firing has physiologic consequences. For example, the clinical course is far better for a patient in the case of a 4:1 conduction ratio with an atrial rate of 300 as opposed to a 4:1 ratio with an atrial rate of 80. *Can you deduce the physiologic reason why this is so?*

First-Degree AV Block

Recall that the normal PR interval is between 0.12 and 0.2 s in duration. *Can you recall an important hemodynamic consequence of the normal delay in conducting a nerve impulse through the AV node?* First-degree heart block increases the normal delay at the AV node to longer than 0.2 s. This longer-than-normal delay in impulse conduction is also a permanent feature, meaning that the longer-than-normal PR interval is the same for each cardiac cycle and there are no dropped QRS complexes. First-degree heart block is primarily asymptomatic; the only negative cardiac functional consequences from a prolonged PR interval is that it can result in decreased cardiac output owing to a slow ventricular rate. Figure 13.1 presents an electrocardiogram (ECG) showing first-degree heart block.

First-degree heart block occurs primarily in situations of increased parasympathetic tone, as occurs fairly commonly in aerobically trained athletes. *Why might this be the case in these athletes?* For a clue, think about the response of the autonomic nervous system with aerobic conditioning and how this affects heart rate and perhaps the PR interval. Now think about the hemodynamic consequences question just posed.

First-degree heart block is also found in individuals on medications with negative chronotropic effects such as β-blockers and digitalis. Other associative causes include the following: ischemic heart disease, rheumatic heart disease, focal fibrosis, and hypokalemia. Mild PR interval prolongation can even be a normal variant occurring with physiologic sinus bradycardia during rest or sleep. First-degree heart block never requires treatment, unless it is to treat symptoms of reduced cardiac output.

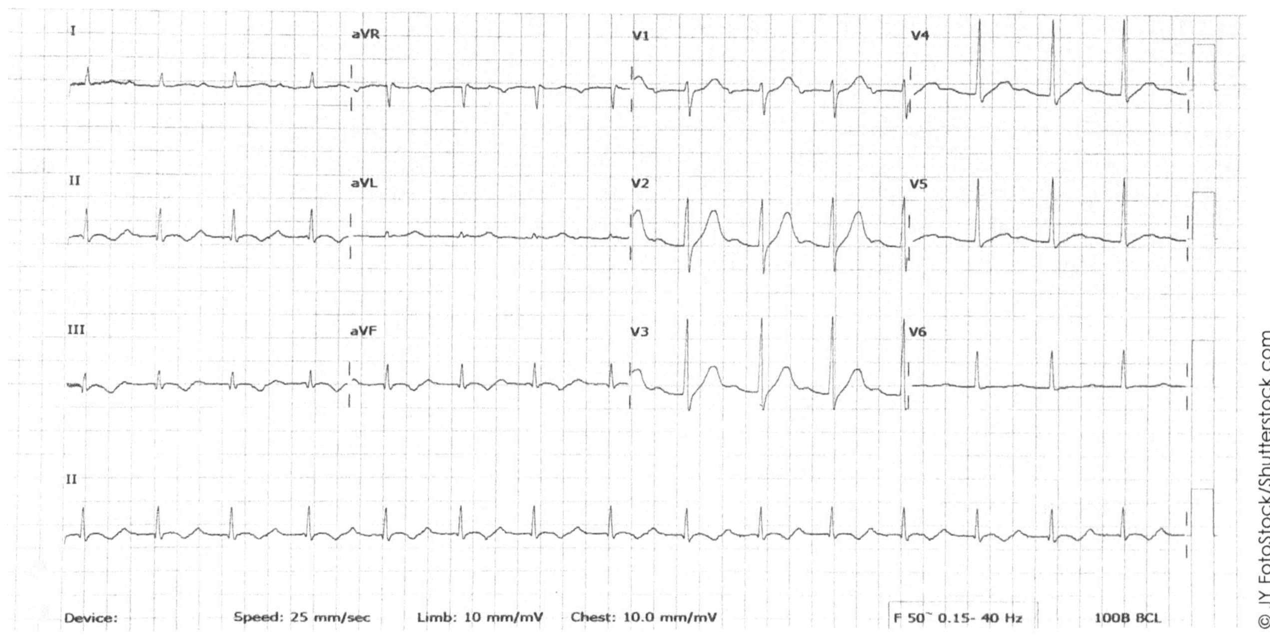

FIGURE 13.1 12-lead ECG showing first-degree heart block with a PR interval of 7- to 8-mm boxes

Second-Degree AV Block

Second-degree heart block is more complicated because there are two types, each of which leads to dropped ventricular beats. These dropped beats manifested on the ECG as isolated P waves without an associated QRS complex establish that second-degree heart block is present.

Second-degree heart block has two types: Mobitz type I (Wenckebach) and Mobitz type II. Students are sometimes perplexed by these somewhat confusing names; however, the names are of historical importance, as is sometimes the case in the study of physiology. In 1899, Karel Frederik Wenckebach, a Dutch anatomist, observed dropped beats while taking jugular vein tracings in a patient. The observed dropped beats were preceded by constant AV conduction intervals. Later, in 1906, he observed the phenomenon once again. Twenty years after that, Woldemar Mobitz, a Russian–German physician, proposed two forms of second-degree heart block (Table 13.1). AV block therefore carries the names of these important early observers.

The type I Mobitz (Wenckebach) phenomenon is relatively benign; defined as a progressive lengthening of the PR interval (as opposed to a constant length of > 0.2 s seen in first-degree AV block) with an eventual dropped QRS complex (a P wave that is not followed by a ventricular response). The number of P waves occurring before the QRS complex is dropped varies. In many cases, just two or three P waves are seen. After the dropped ventricular beat, the PR interval returns to its shortest duration, although even then it may be longer than 0.2 s (the upper limit of normal for the PR interval). The sequence then repeats. As seen in Figure 13.2,

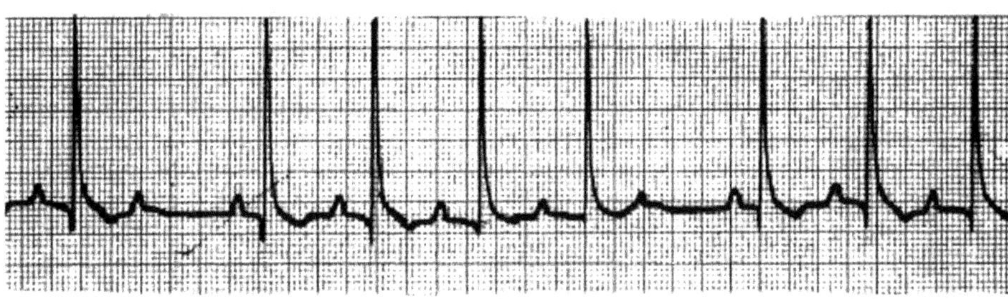

Second Degree AV Block Type I: Also Known as Mobitz I or Wenkebach

FIGURE 13.2 Mobitz type I 2° AV heart block (Wenckebach).

a clue to the interpretation of the Wenckebach phenomenon is the presence of grouping or clustering of ventricular beats (QRS complexes). These grouped beats are separated by a QRS pause that results from the dropped beat.

Electrically, Wenckebach heart block occurs high in the AV junction and may be transient. The progressive lengthening phenomenon occurs because each successive beat arrives earlier and earlier in the relative refractory period of the junction. This dictates a longer period of time to penetrate the junction and reach the ventricles. Wenckebach also occurs in many of the same settings as first-degree AV block and seldom progresses to complete heart block. As with type I AV block, specific treatment is not needed unless there is a slow ventricular rate resulting in a reduced cardiac output. A physiologic increase in vagal tone may also cause Mobitz type I AV block in athletes at rest.

Mobitz type II is the less common form of second-degree heart block. It is also much more serious than type I and is often associated with a bundle branch block pattern. In Mobitz type II, the site of the block is usually below the His bundle. Type II block is defined by the occurrence of dropped QRS complexes without a varying PR interval in the conducted beats. The key feature is the sudden appearance of a nonconducted sinus P wave without the progressive prolongation of the PR interval as seen in type I Mobitz (Fig. 13.3). The appearance of the dropped QRS complexes may occur randomly or in a set pattern. When patterned, they are named according to the number of P waves to QRS complexes present. For example, Mobitz type II with a 3:1 block is seen in Figure 13.4. In this case, we see three P waves for every QRS complex. A 2:1 block is indistinguishable from Mobitz type I, and, therefore, they are generally called second-degree AV blocks.

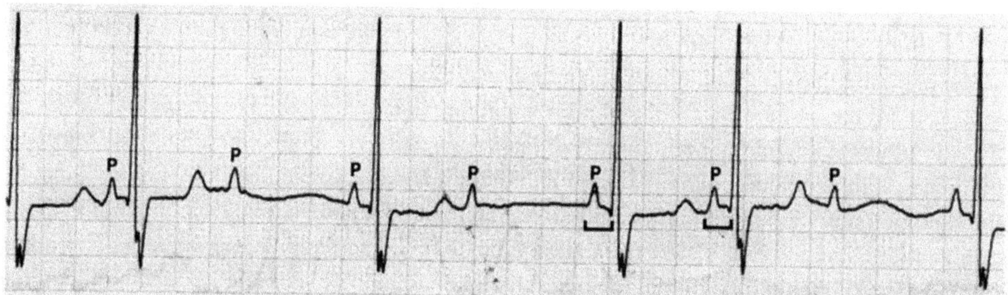

FIGURE 13.3 Mobitz type II 2° AV heart block. Notice the constant PR intervals (approximately 0.14 s) as opposed to the progressive lengthening in type I seen in Figure 13.2.

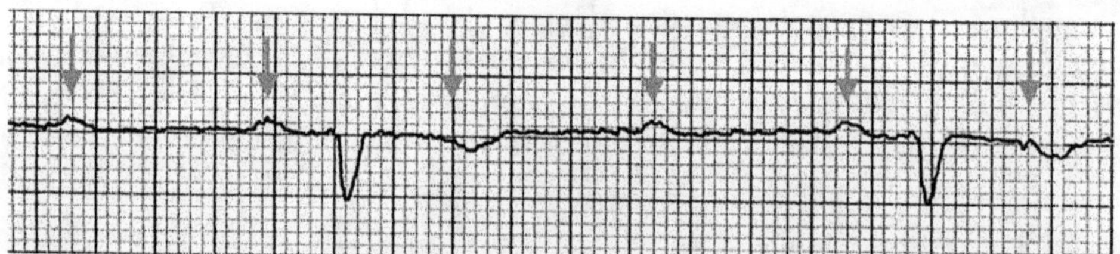

FIGURE 13.4 Fixed ratio 3:1 conduction pattern Mobitz type II second degree heart block. The atrial rate (arrows) is approximately 94 bpm. The ventricular rate rate is approximately 31 bpm. Every third P wave is almost entirely concealed within the T wave.

Mobitz type II is generally a sign of severe conduction system disease involving regions below the AV node (His-Purkinje system). Type II block often progresses to complete heart block, leading cardiologists to prescribe pacing as a remedy for Mobitz type II even prior to its eventual degeneration to complete heart block. Table 13.2 gives a side-by-side comparison of Mobitz I & II.

TABLE 13.2 Characteristics of Mobitz Type I and II AV Blocks

Characteristics	*Type I*	*Type II*
Pattern of block	Cycles of gradually increasing PR intervals followed by nonconducted P waves	Abrupt nonconducted P waves without preceding changes in the PR intervals
Location of Block	AV node	His bundle or bundle branches
Occurrence with acute MI	Inferior	Anterior
Risk of progression to complete heart block	Low	High
Indication for permanent pacemaker	Not usually	Usually

Third-Degree (Complete) Heart Block

When impulses are unable to pass the AV junction, complete heart block is present. First- and second-degree heart blocks are incomplete blocks because the AV junction conducts at least some stimuli to the ventricles. In complete heart block, the AV barrier is not penetrated at all, requiring the ventricles to be activated in a manner other than through the His-Purkinje system. This means that in complete heart block, the atria and ventricles are paced independently: the atria by the SA node or some lower pacer in the atria, and the ventricles by an escape pacemaker located somewhere below the point of the electrical block in the AV junction. This necessarily results in two distinct heart rates, one for the atria and the other for ventricles. The rate for each is dictated by the predominate rate of the controlling intrinsic pacer. Typically, therefore, the ventricular rate may be lower than 30 beats per minute or as high as 50 to 60 beats per minute, with the atrial rate usually faster (and usually within normal limits of 60 to 100 beats per minute when the atrial pacer is the sinus node).

Complete heart block is associated with the following conditions:

- Older individuals with chronic degenerative changes (sclerosis or fibrosis) in the heart's conduction system not related to myocardial infarction (MI)
- Complication of acute MI
  - Transient during acute inferior wall MI owing to common blood supply of inferior wall and AV junction—RCA—leading to temporary ischemia of the AV node. Usually does not require a temporary pacemaker unless hypotension is present or if episodes of tachyarrhythmia are occurring.
  - More serious with acute anterior wall MI, where there is generally more extensive myocardial damage—produces slow and unstable idioventricular escape rhythms—permanent pacing usually required.
- Digitalis intoxication
- Lyme disease
- Open heart surgery (particularly with aortic valve replacement)
- Bacterial endocarditis

Patients with complete heart block and slow ventricular rates are quite susceptible to fainting spells because of low cardiac output, a condition called **Stokes-Adams attacks**. Complete heart block is a very serious condition because escape rhythms may not occur, occur transiently, or occur but produce insufficient cardiac output. If no escape rhythm occurs, cardiac arrest is the prevailing condition.

Figure 13.5 shows an example of complete heart block. Remember that in complete heart block there is no AV conduction. This means that any QRS complexes present do not result as a direct consequence of prior atrial activity (the atrial pacer is not the ventricular pacer). Because of this distinction, it is important to remember that in complete heart block PR intervals are nonexistent. Instead, AV dissociation is established as a ventricular escape rhythm is created. In this scenario, the P waves present on the ECG strip appear to march through

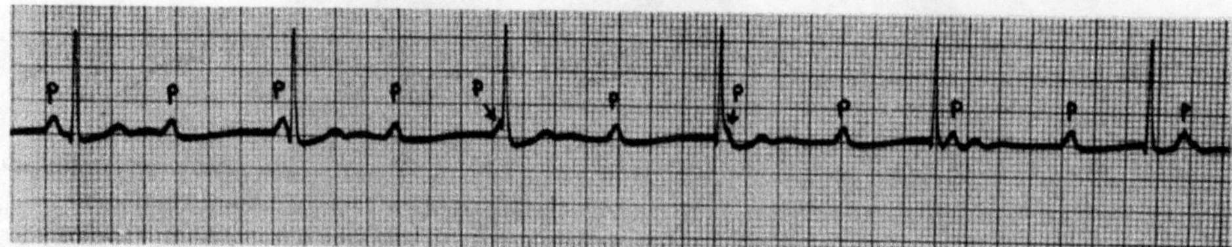

FIGURE 13.5 Complete heart block—AV dissociation with the atrial rate (90 beats per minute) independent of the ventricular rate (44 beats per minute)—showing the complete absence of AV conduction with *none* of the supraventricular impulses conducted to the ventricles. The perfusing rhythm is maintained by a junctional or ventricular escape rhythm. The strip shows a junctional escape rhythm.

the QRS rhythm (and vice versa). It is often said that in complete heart block, the atria and ventricles "each march to the beat of their own drum." Although some P waves and QRS complexes may appear to be associated, this is only a random occurrence because no connection is present. Thus, the lengths of the "apparent" PR intervals vary and have no pattern to them at all.

If no escape ventricular rhythm is generated during complete heart block, the situation is physiologically equivalent to asystole. Cardiopulmonary resuscitation is then required because there can be no cardiac output present and thus no blood pressure. Permanent pacing is always needed in this scenario. The following characteristics are important to distinguish the rhythm distinction inherent in complete heart block because the atria and ventricles are electrically disconnected:

- P waves are present with a regular atrial rate faster than the ventricular rate.
- QRS complexes (wide or normal width) are present with a slow, usually fixed, ventricular rate.
- P wave rhythm bears no relation to QRS rhythm, and, by definition, there are no PR intervals.

With complete heart block, the morphology of the QRS complexes depends in part on the location of the block in the AV junction. If the block is in the AV node, the ventricles are stimulated normally through the His-Purkinje system, resulting in narrow QRS complexes, unless the patient also has an underlying bundle branch block. With the electrical block below the node (within the His-Purkinje system or ventricular myocardium), the ventricles are paced by an idioventricular pacemaker. Idioventricular pacemakers produce wide QRS complexes (Fig. 13.5B). When the pace of an idioventricular pacemaker is fast, the resulting rhythm is referred to as an accelerated idioventricular rhythm (AIVR).

An AIVR was first described by Thomas Lewis in 1910 and is defined as an enhanced ectopic ventricular rhythm with at least three consecutive ventricular beats that are faster than the normal intrinsic ventricular escape rhythm (usually $\leq$ 40 beats per minute) but slower than ventricular tachycardia (at least 100–120 beats per minute). The differential diagnoses include slow ventricular tachycardia, complete heart block, junctional rhythm with aberrancy, supraventricular tachycardia with aberrancy, and slow antidromic atrioventricular reentry tachycardia. The rate of an AIVR distinguishes it from other rhythms of similar morphology. A rate $<$ 50 beats per minute is consistent with a ventricular escape rhythm, whereas a rate $>$ 110 beats per minute is consistent with ventricular tachycardia. The causes of AIVR include the following:

- Reperfusion phase of an acute MI (most common cause)
- Beta-sympathomimetics such as isoprenaline or adrenaline
- Digoxin toxicity, cocaine, and volatile anesthetics such as desflurane
- Electrolyte abnormalities
- Cardiomyopathy, congenital heart disease, myocarditis
- Return of spontaneous circulation (ROSC) following cardiac arrest
- Athletic heart

Clinically, patients with complete heart block involving wide QRS complexes are less stable than patients with narrow QRS complexes. The reason is that the intrinsic rate of ventricular pacing is slow and less consistent.

Atrioventricular (AV) Dissociation

AV dissociation is a misused term. In AV dissociation, the atria and the ventricles are under the control of separate pacemakers. There are four causes of this: (1) complete heart block, (2) slowing of the primary pacemaker, (3) acceleration of a subsidiary pacemaker, and (4) interference. Technically, AV dissociation is not an arrhythmia, but is the result of a mechanism causing independent beating of the upper and lower chambers.

Although complete heart block is a form of AV dissociation, AV dissociation is not a form of complete heart block. The terms are not synonymous because complete heart block is only one causative instance of AV dissociation. Complete heart block results in AV dissociation because the atria remain under the control of a sinus or atrial rhythm, whereas the ventricles are controlled by a junctional or ventricular escape rhythm. With complete heart block, atrial impulses cannot be conducted to the ventricles. In contrast, with AV dissociation, atrial impulses will be conducted to and stimulate the ventricles if nonrefractory tissue permits this. Capture beats, a hallmark of AV dissociation, are QRS complexes that occur prematurely relative to the rate of the lesser pacemaker. Capture beats often have morphologic features that are intermediate in configuration between QRS complexes that have been stimulated by atrial impulses and those that have been stimulated by ectopic foci (whether the focus is an accelerated one or an escape one). These complexes are referred to as fusion complexes. Because the occurrence of fusion implies capture of the ventricles from the supraventricular impulse, fusion complexes are also a hallmark of AV dissociation.

The sinus node is the primary pacemaker of the heart because it has the fastest rate of automaticity (recall this discussion from Chapter 1). However, cells in the AV junction and ventricles also possess automaticity, but with intrinsic rates slower than the sinus node: 40 to 60 beats per minute for junctional pacemaker cells and 20 to 40 beats per minute for ventricular pacemaker cells. These slower pacemakers are called *subsidiary* pacemakers because they are normally suppressed by the faster sinus node. However, if the sinus node (the primary pacemaker) slows enough, a junctional or ventricular pacemaker can emerge to take control of the ventricles. In this scenario, AV dissociation is present.

If a lower pacer (junctional or ventricular) fires at a greater rate than the sinus node, the subsidiary pacemaker can take over control of the ventricles while the sinus node remains in control of the atria. AV dissociation results as the acceleration of a subsidiary pacemaker rises above the rate of the sinus node.

Finally, anything interfering with the conduction of atrial impulses to the ventricles can result in AV dissociation. For example, AV dissociation can result from pauses produced by premature beats. These pauses present an opportunity for a subsidiary pacemaker to emerge and take charge of the ventricles.

Questions

1. Why is Mobitz type II considered a worsening clinical situation versus type I Mobitz.
2. Explain the mechanism in aerobic exercise training that may predispose adherents to type I heart block.

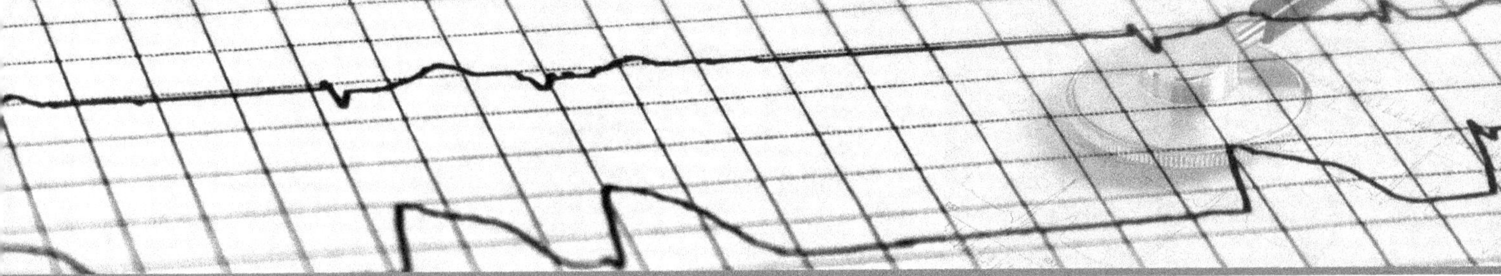

CHAPTER 14

ECG Differential Diagnoses

Differential diagnosis is the process of distinguishing between two or more disorders. Because different conditions may share similar symptoms, the process of differentiating between conditions is an invaluable and necessary practice by medical personnel.

CONTENT OUTLINE

- Wide QRS Complex
- Low-Voltage QRS Complexes
- Right Axis Deviation
- QT Prolongation
- Q Waves
- Tall V_1 R Wave
- ST Segment Elevations
- ST Segment Depressions
- T Wave Inversions
- Classes of Bradyarrhythmias
- Tall Positive T Waves
- Major Tachyarrhythmias
- Atrial Fibrillation
- Digitalis Toxicity
- Cardiac Arrest

This chapter provides a quick review of some of the major electrocardiogram (ECG) findings where a differential diagnosis/interpretation is necessary. The headings in the chapter outline are presented as boxes with bulleted points for easy reference. For each box, the title is the primary ECG finding, and the box content represents the various potential cause categories of the finding, that is, the differential diagnoses. This chapter is not meant to be exhaustive and is placed at the end of the text to spur extra reading and study by the student.

BOX 14.1: WIDE QRS COMPLEX (FIVE POTENTIAL DIFFERENTIAL DIAGNOSES)

- Intrinsic Intraventricular Delay: (1) LBBB & variants, (2) RBBB & variants, (3) Other potential patterns
- Extrinsic Intraventricular Delay: (1) Hyperkalemia, (2) Class I antiarrhythmic drugs
- Ventricular Beats: (1) Premature, (2) Escape, (3) Paced
- Ventricular Preexcitation (WPW patterns and variants)
- Electrocardiograph problem (using fast paper speeds unintentionally)

BOX 14.2: LOW VOLTAGE QRS COMPLEXES (NINE POTENTIAL DIFFERENTIAL DIAGNOSES)

- Artifact: unrecognized standardization of ECG at one-half usual gain (i.e., 1 mV = 5 mm)
- May be a normal variant but also seen in pregnancy and obesity
- **Pericardial tamponade** (usually with sinus tachycardia)
- **Pleural effusions**
- **Chronic obstructive pulmonary disease** (COPD)
- Extensive myocardial infarction
- **Myxedema** (usually with sinus bradycardia)
- **Cardiomyopathy** (dilation, usually with diffuse fibrosis)
- Left **pneumothorax** (midleft chest leads)

BOX 14.3: RIGHT AXIS DEVIATION (SIX POTENTIAL DIFFERENTIAL DIAGNOSES)

- Artifact: left–right arm electrode reversal (negative P wave and QRS complex in lead I)
- Normal variant
- Dextrocardia
- Right ventricular overload: (1) Acute: **pulmonary embolus**, (2) Chronic: COPD or any cause of right ventricular hypertrophy (e.g., pulmonic stenosis or primary pulmonary hypertension)
- Lateral wall myocardial infarction
- Left posterior hemiblock

BOX 14.4: QT PROLONGATION (NINE POTENTIAL DIFFERENTIAL DIAGNOSES)

- Acquired long QT syndrome
  1. Electrolyte abnormalities (**hypocalcemia**, hypokalemia, **hypomagnesemia**)
  2. Drugs: (1) Class I or III antiarrhythmic agents (e.g., quinidine, procainamide, disopyramide, sotalol, and amiodarone), (2) **Psychotropic agents** (e.g., phenothiazines, tricyclic antidepressants, tetracyclic agents, and haloperidol), (3) Other agents, including terfenadine, bepridil, certain antibiotics (e.g., erythromycin and pentamidine), probucol, and cisapride in high doses
  3. Myocardial ischemia or infarction (with deep T wave inversions)
  4. Cerebrovascular injury
  5. Bradyarrhythmias, especially high-grade AV heart block
  6. **Systemic hypothermia**
  7. Other conditions: liquid protein diets, starvation, **myocarditis**, arsenic poisoning

- Congenital long QT syndrome
  1. **Romano–Ward syndrome**
  2. **Jervell and Lange-Nielsen syndrome**

BOX 14.5: Q WAVES (FOUR POTENTIAL DIFFERENTIAL DIAGNOSES)

- Physiologic or positional factors: (1) Normal variant septal Q waves, (2) Normal variant Q waves in leads V_1, V_2, aVL, III, aVR, (3) Left pneumothorax or dextrocardia (loss of lateral R wave progression)
- Myocardial injury or infiltration: (1) Acute processes: myocardial ischemia or infarction, myocarditis, hyperkalemia, (2) Chronic processes: myocardial infarction, **idiopathic cardiomyopathy**, myocarditis, amyloid, tumor, sarcoid
- Ventricular hypertrophy or enlargement: (1) Left ventricular hypertrophy (poor R wave progression), (2) Right ventricular hypertrophy (reversed R wave progression) or poor R wave progression (particularly with chronic obstructive lung disease), (3) **Hypertrophic cardiomyopathy** (may simulate anterior, inferior, posterior, or lateral infarcts)
- Conduction abnormalities: (1) Left bundle branch block (poor R wave progression), (2) Wolff–Parkinson–White patterns

BOX 14.6: TALL V_1 R WAVE (FOUR POTENTIAL DIFFERENTIAL DIAGNOSES)

- Physiologic and positional factors: (1) Misplacement of chest leads, (2) Normal variant, (3) Displacement of heart toward right chest (**dextroversion**: congenital or acquired)
- Myocardial injury: (1) Posterior and/or lateral myocardial infarction, (2) **Duchenne muscular dystrophy**
- Ventricular enlargement: (1) Right ventricular hypertrophy (usually with right QRS deviation), (2) Hypertrophic cardiomyopathy
- Altered ventricular depolarization: (1) Right ventricular conduction abnormalities, (2) Wolff–Parkinson–White patterns (caused by posterior or lateral wall preexcitation)

BOX 14.7: ST SEGMENT ELEVATION (FIVE POTENTIAL DIFFERENTIAL DIAGNOSES)

- Myocardial ischemia or infarction: (1) Noninfarctional transmural ischemia (Prinzmetal's angina pattern), (2) Acute myocardial infarction, (3) Postmyocardial infarction (ventricular aneurysm pattern)
- Acute pericarditis
- Normal variant (early repolarization pattern)
- Left ventricular hypertrophy or left bundle branch block (lead V_1 and V_2 or V_3 only)
- Other conditions: (1) Myocardial injury (myocarditis, tumor invasion of ventricles, trauma to ventricles), (2) Hyperkalemia (leads V_1 and V_2 only), (3) Hypothermia (J wave or Osborne wave)

BOX 14.8: ST SEGMENT DEPRESSION (THREE POTENTIAL DIFFERENTIAL DIAGNOSES)

- Myocardial ischemia or infarction: (1) Acute subendocardial ischemia or non-Q wave myocardial infarction, (2) Reciprocal change with acute transmural ischemia
- Abnormal noncoronary patterns: (1) Left or right ventricular hypertrophy ("strain" pattern), (2) Secondary ST-T changes: left bundle branch block, right bundle branch block, Wolff–Parkinson–White preexcitation pattern, (3) Drugs (e.g., digitalis), (4) Metabolic conditions (e.g., hypokalemia), (5) Miscellaneous conditions (e.g., cardiomyopathy)
- Physiologic and normal variants: ST segment depressions usually less than 1 mm and seen especially with exertion or hyperventilation

BOX 14.9: T WAVE INVERSIONS (ELEVEN POTENTIAL DIFFERENTIAL DIAGNOSES)

- Primary T wave inversions: (1) Normal variants (e.g., juvenile T wave pattern), (2) Myocardial ischemia or infarction, (3) Left or right ventricular overload ("strain" pattern), (4) Cerebrovascular injury, (5) Postpacemaker T wave pattern, (6) Posttachycardia T wave pattern, (7) Miscellaneous conditions: cardiomyopathies, pericarditis, intermittent left bundle branch block, myocardial tumor
- Secondary T wave inversions: (1) Left bundle branch block, (2) Right bundle branch block, (3) Wolff–Parkinson–White preexcitation pattern, (4) Ventricular paced beats

BOX 14.10: CLASSES OF BRADYARRHYTHMIAS (FIVE POTENTIAL DIFFERENTIAL DIAGNOSES)

- Sinus bradycardia and its variants, including sinoatrial block
- Atrioventricular (AV) heart block or dissociation: (1) Second or Third-degree AV block, (2) Isorhythmic AV dissociation and related variants
- Junctional (AV nodal) escape rhythms
- Atrial fibrillation or flutter with a slow ventricular response
- Ventricular escape rhythms (idioventricular rhythms)

BOX 14.11: TALL POSITIVE T WAVES (NINE POTENTIAL DIFFERENTIAL DIAGNOSES)

- Ischemic causes: (1) Hyperacute phase of myocardial infarction, (2) Acute transient transmural ischemia (Prinzmetal's angina), (3) Chronic (evolving) phase of myocardial infarction (tall positive T waves reciprocal to primary deep T wave inversions)
- Nonischemic causes: (1) Normal variants (early repolarization patterns), (2) Hyperkalemia, (3) Cerebrovascular hemorrhage (more commonly, T wave inversions), (4) Left ventricular hypertrophy, (5) Left bundle branch block, (6) Acute pericarditis

BOX 14.12: MAJOR TACHYARRHYTHMIAS (SIX POTENTIAL DIFFERENTIAL DIAGNOSES)

- Narrow QRS complex: (1) Sinus tachycardia, (2) Paroxysmal supraventricular tachycardia (PSVT), a class of arrhythmias with three major mechanisms—atrial tachycardias, including single focus or multifocal (e.g., multifocal atrial tachycardia variants)—AV nodal reentrant tachycardia (AVNRT)—AV reentrant tachycardia (AVRT) involving a bypass tract, (3) Atrial flutter, (4) Atrial fibrillation
- Wide QRS complex: (1) Ventricular tachycardia (three or more consecutive premature ventricular complexes at a rate of 100 per minute), (2) Supraventricular tachycardia or atrial fibrillation or flutter, with *aberrant* ventricular conduction usually caused by either of the following: bundle branch block or atrioventricular bypass tract (Wolff–Parkinson–White preexcitation pattern)

BOX 14.13: ATRIAL FIBRILLATION (FIFTEEN POTENTIAL DIFFERENTIAL DIAGNOSES)

- Alcohol
- Autonomic factors: (1) Sympathetic (occurring during exercise or stress), (2) **Vagotonic** (occurring during sleep)
- Cardiothoracic surgery
- Cardiomyopathies or myocarditis
- Congenital heart disease
- Coronary artery disease
- Hypertensive heart disease
- Idiopathic ("lone" atrial fibrillation)
- Paroxysmal supraventricular tachycardias or the Wolff–Parkinson–White preexcitation syndrome
- Pericardial disease (usually chronic)
- Pulmonary disease (chronic obstructive pulmonary disease)
- Pulmonary emboli
- Sick sinus syndrome
- Thyrotoxicosis (hyperthyroidism)
- Valvular heart disease (particularly mitral valve disease)

BOX 14.14: DIGITALIS TOXICITY (SIX POTENTIAL DIFFERENTIAL DIAGNOSES)

- Bradycardia: (1) Sinus bradycardia, including sinoatrial block, (2) Junctional (nodal) escape rhythms, (3) Atrioventricular (AV) heart block, including the following Mobitz type I (Wenckebach) AV block and Complete heart block
- Tachycardia: (1) Accelerated Junctional Rhythm (nonparoxysmal junctional tachycardia), (2) Atrial Tachycardia with block, (3) Ventricular ectopy, including the following iterations—Ventricular Premature Beats, Monomorphic Ventricular Tachycardia, Bidirectional Tachycardia, and Ventricular fibrillation

BOX 14.15: ECG PATTERNS FOR CARDIAC ARREST (THREE POTENTIAL DIFFERENTIAL DIAGNOSES)

- Ventricular tachyarrhythmias: (1) Ventricular fibrillation, (2) Sustained ventricular tachycardia
- Ventricular standstill (brady-asystolic rhythms)
- **Electromechanical dissociation**

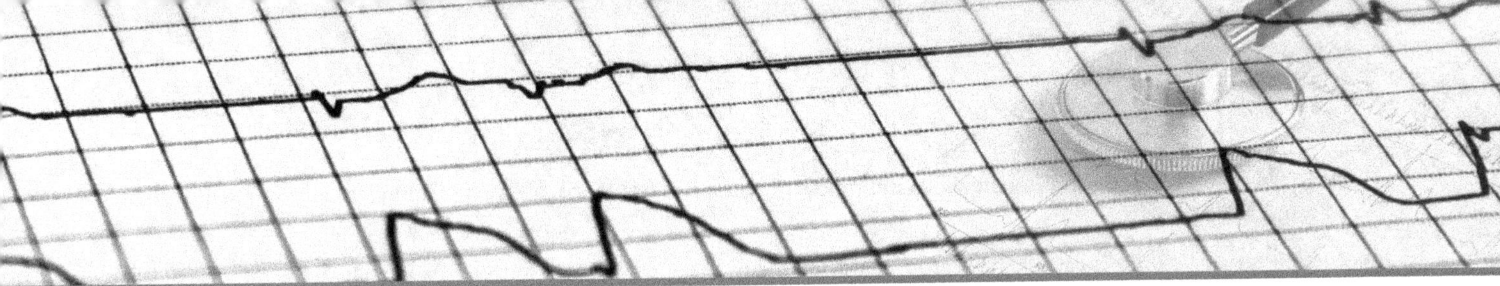

GLOSSARY

The chapter of the term's first occurrence is included in parentheses.

6-second method (5)—method of estimating heart rate when there is an irregular rhythm present. To use this method, locate a 6-second area on the ECG, count the number of QRS complexes within the 6-second area, then multiply that by 10 to get the heart rate.

1500 method (5)—method of calculating heart rate when a regular rhythm is present by counting the number of small boxes between consecutive R waves and dividing that into 1500 to get the heart rate.

AV reciprocating tachycardia (12)—a reentrant tachycardia in which signals enter a congenital accessory tract (usually occurring at a place other than at the atrioventral [AV] node) and starts looping back through the normal AV node pathway, producing a tachycardia. It is more likely to happen in childhood or during the teenage years.

AVNRT (10)—atrioventricular nodal reentry tachycardia (AVNRT) is the most common type of supraventricular tachycardia. An abnormally fast heartbeat that often starts and ends suddenly. Caused by a reentry circuit in or around the AV node. The circuit is formed by the creation of two pathways forming the reentrant circuit, namely the slow and fast pathways.

accelerated idioventricular rhythm (11)—a ventricular rhythm in which the rate is between 40 and 100 beats per minute.

accelerated junctional rhythm (12)—a rhythm in which all of the complexes arise from either within the atrioventricular node to the bundle of His and the rate is between 60 and 100 beats per minute

action potential (1)—rapid sequence of changes in electrical potential that take place across a cell membrane during depolarization and repolarization.

acute heart failure (2)—sudden and short-lasting diminution of pumping effectiveness of the heart attributable to damage, as happens, for instance, with myocardial infarction, leading to lowered cardiac output

acute transmural myocardial infarction (5)—a present or ongoing heart attack characterized by death of myocardial fibers; symptoms include chest pain, dyspnea, sweating, clammy skin, nausea, dizziness, shortness of breath, and so on.

afterload (1)—impedance to ejection of blood from the left ventricle.

agonal rhythm (11)—an idioventricular rhythm with a heart rate of less than 10 beats per minute.

agonist (2)—a drug that interacts with receptors to initiate a response

aneurysm (3)—occurs when part of an artery wall weakens, allowing it to balloon out or widen abnormally

antagonist (2)—a drug that interacts with receptors to block or inhibit a response

arrhythmia (2)—abnormal rhythm of the heart

artifact (5)—markings on the electrocardiogram that are not a result of the heart's electrical activity but rather a result of extraneous factors such as patient movement, electromagnetic interference of nearby electrical equipment, tense muscles, and so on.

atrial bigeminy (12)—premature atrial complexes alternate with sinus complexes; premature atrial complexes (PACs) appear every other complex

atrial couplets (12)—two unifocal atrial ectopic complexes firing in a row

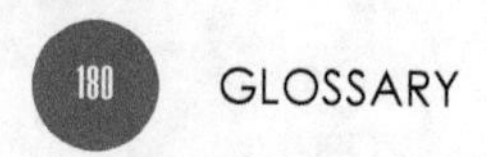

atrial fibrillation (12)—a condition in which multiple atrial impulses fire at an extremely fast rate, usually 400 to 600 times per minute

atrial flutter (12)—unifocal atrial tachycardia characterized by the appearance of flutter waves in which the rate is typically between 250 and 350 beats per minute

atrial quadrigeminy (12)—premature atrial complexes appear every fourth complex

atrial rate (5)—number of atrial depolarizations occurring per minute

atrial tachycardia (12)—a unifocal rhythm whose origin is within the atria but outside of the sinoatrial node and the rate is greater than 100 beats per minute

atrial trigeminy (12)—premature atrial complexes appear every third complex

atrioventricular blocks (5)—dysrhythmias that result from a partial or complete blockage of the signal from the AV node to the ventricles.

atrioventricular valves (1)—valves between the atria and ventricles (triscupid valve on right side and mitral valve on left side)

atropine (2)—an antimuscarinic drug that blocks cholinergic (acetylecholine) activity at effector organs

augmented voltage leads (5)—the unipolar limb leads aV_F, aV_L, and aV_R. Each uses one of the following limb electrodes (RA, LA, or LL) as its positive pole and a combination of the other two electrodes as the negative pole.

automaticity (1)—property of spontaneous impulse generation. Slow sodium channels are leaky and cause the polarity to spontaneously rise to threshold for action potential generation. The fastest of these cells, those in the SA node, set the pace for the heartbeat.

autorhythmicity (1)—natural rhythm of spontaneous depolarization. Those with the fastest rate of depolarization act as the heart's pacemaker.

bigeminy (11)—a cardiac rhythm in which every other cardiac beat is an abnormal one

bioavailability (2)—physiologic availability of a specific amount of a drug

biphasic deflection (5)—a waveform that contains parts that are above and below the baseline

bipolar limb leads (5)—the limb leads I, II, and III. Each uses one of the limb electrodes as its positive end and one as its negative end of the lead.

biventricular interdependence (9)—a phenomenon whereby the function of one ventricle is altered by changes in the filling of the other ventricle. This leads to an increase in the volume of one ventricle associated with a decreased volume in the opposite ventricle.

blocked PAC (12)—a premature atrial complex that does not result in ventricular depolarization; it is noted on the ECG as an early P wave without a subsequent QRS complex

bradycardic junctional rhythm (12)—a rhythm in which all of the complexes arise from either within the atrioventricular node to the bundle of His and the rate is less than 40 beats per minute

bundle branch (1)—specialized tissue in the heart that conducts depolarizations through the ventricles. The right and left ventricles have a bundle branch, called the right bundle branch and the left bundle branch, respectively.

bundle branch blocks (5)—blockage of the electrical signal through one of the bundle branches

bundle of His (1)—specialized tissue that conducts depolarizations from the atria to the ventricles

calibration mark (5)—markings present at either the beginning or the end of a 12-lead ECG printout that indicate the settings currently being used for the machine's calibration. Also known as a calibration signal.

calibration signal (5)—markings present at either the beginning or the end of a 12-lead ECG printout that indicate the settings currently being used for the machine's calibration. Also known as a calibration mark.

capacitance vessels (1)—in the circulatory system, the ability to "store" large amounts of blood. The veins are considered capacitance vessels owing to the large amount of blood that they contain. However, on the initiation of exercise, this "stored" blood can be rapidly mobilized to the working tissues (muscles) in the body.

cardiac cycle (1)—mechanical process whereby blood flows from the atria through the AV valves into the ventricles and out of the ventricles through the semilunar valves. Mechanical processes of the cardiac cycle correlate with the electrical activity observed on the ECG that indicate atrial and ventricular depolarization and repolarization.

cardiac output (1)—the volume of blood pumped from the heart each minute as the product of heart rate and stroke volume

cardiac skeleton (8)—the high-density single/homogeneous structure of connective tissue that forms and anchors the valves and influences the forces exerted by and through them

cardiomyopathy (14)—chronic disease of the heart muscle

catheter ablation (11)—a procedure during which either radio frequency energy or a laser is fed by catheter to the site of an irritable focus and used to terminate that irritable focus

central venous pressure (1)—pressure within the superior vena cava, reflecting the pressure under which the blood is returned to the right atrium. A high central venous pressure indicates circulatory overload as in congestive heart failure, and a low central venous pressure indicates reduced blood volume as in hemorrhage or fluid loss.

chamber enlargement (5)—generally used to indicate an increase in heart chamber size. Usually refers to the atria.

chest leads (5)—leads V_1, V_2, V_3, V_4, V_5, and V_6, also known as the ventral or precordial leads. These leads view the heart's electrical activity in the horizontal plane.

chordae tendinae (1)—collagenous strands that extend from the apical margin of papillary muscles of the heart and attach to atrioventricular valve cusps

chronic heart failure (2)—lower pumping effectiveness of the heart that the body has partially compensated with sympathetic reflexes, increasing pumping action and thus cardiac output

chronic obstructive pulmonary disease (14)—a chronic inflammatory lung disease that causes obstructed airflow from the lungs: symptoms include breathing difficulty, cough, mucus (sputum) production and wheezing

chronotropic (1)—chronotropic effects are those that change the heart rate.

class I antiarrhythmic drugs (14)—quinidine, disopyramide, procainamide, lidocaine, mexiletine, flecainide, and propafenone are all class I antiarrhythmic drugs used for the treatment of various atrial and ventricular arrhythmias

claudication (3)—pain caused by too little blood flow to your legs or arms

compliance (1)—the ability of a blood vessel wall to expand and contract passively with changes in pressure is an important function of large arteries and veins. At higher pressures and volumes, venous compliance (slope of the compliance curve) is similar to arterial compliance.

contractility (2)—force of contraction of the heart; the ability of a muscle to respond to a stimulus by shortening

coronal plane (5)—an imaginary line dividing the body into anterior and posterior halves. Also known as the frontal plane

couplet (11)—two abnormal myocardial complexes occurring in a row (the two premature beats may have identical morphologies as in a unifocal couplet or their morphologies may differ as in a multifocal couplet.

curare (2)—drug that blocks acetylcholine at the neuromuscular junction

cyanosis (3)—a bluish discoloration of the skin resulting from poor circulation or inadequate oxygenation of the blood

dark line method (5)—method of measuring heart rate when there is a regular rhythm in which one chooses an R wave that falls on a dark line on the ECG paper and then applies the following numbers to the subsequent dark lines: 300, 150, 100, 75, 60, 50, 44, 38, and so on until the next R wave is reached. Then the heart rate is estimated to be between the numbers that correspond to the dark lines that the second R wave falls between.

depolarization (1)—reversal of the resting membrane potential in excitable cells when stimulated or the tendency of a cell membrane to become positive with respect to the potential outside of the cell

dextroversion (14)—location of the heart in the right chest, the left ventricle remaining in the normal position on the left but lying anterior to the right ventricle

diaphoretic (9)—sweating

diastasis (1)—a relatively quiescent period of slow ventricular filling during the cardiac cycle; it occurs in middiastole, following the rapid filling phase and just prior to atrial systole.

diastole (1)—resting phase of the cardiac cycle

dromotropic (2)—influencing the conduction velocity of a nerve or muscle fiber

drug (2)—chemical that alters bodily function and may produce beneficial effects when taken in therapeutic doses

Duchenne muscular dystrophy (14)—a severe form of muscular dystrophy caused by a genetic defect and usually affecting boys

dyskinesis (2)—segmental cardiac wall motion abnormalities during systole

dyspnea (3)—difficult or labored breathing

dyssynchrony (8)—a difference in the timing, or lack of synchrony, of contractions in different ventricles in the heart. Large differences in timing of contractions can reduce cardiac efficiency and are correlated with heart failure.

ectopic (11)—from an abnormal place or position

edema (3)—excess of watery fluid collecting in the cavities or tissues of the body

Einthoven's triangle (5)—an imaginary equilateral triangle that is formed by lines that represent the three bipolar limb leads (leads I, II, and III)

ejection fraction (1)—a measurement of the percentage of blood leaving the ventricle each time it contracts

electrocardiogram (5)—a recording of the heart's electrical activity

electrocardiography (1)—refers to the recording of electrical changes that occur in the heart during the mechanical events of the cardiac cycle

electromechanical dissociation (14)—implies organized electrical depolarization of the heart without synchronous myocardial fiber shortening and, therefore, without cardiac output and blood pressure

electrodes (5)—conductive pads that are attached to the body's surface and then connected to an ECG machine by lead wires. They can sense changes in the heart's electrical activity.

embolus (12)—a mobile blood clot

end-diastolic volume (1)—the maximum volume of blood the ventricles achieve at the end of ventricular diastole. This is the amount of blood the heart has available to pump. If this volume increases, the cardiac output increases in a healthy heart.

endocardium (1)—smooth endothelial lining of the heart. This helps to reduce friction of blood flow and prevent clotting.

end-systolic volume (1)—the minimum volume remaining in the ventricle after its systole. If this volume increases, it means less blood has been pumped and the cardiac output is less.

enteral (2)—intestinal route of administering a drug

epicardium (1)—fibrous covering of the heart. This layer is the visceral layer of the fibrous pericardium.

equiphasic deflection (5)—a special subset of biphasic waveforms that contains equal parts of positive and negative deflections

exercise protocol (4)—the sequence of applying ergometric workloads to an individual in a timed and deliberate manner to elicit graded metabolic and physiologic responses

extreme axis deviation (6)—a heart whose mean electrical axis is located between 180° and -90°. This is an extremely unusual occurrence and always a result of either lead transposition or pathology.

first pass effect (2)—partial inactivation of a drug as a result of metabolic processes

flutter waves (12)—sawtooth-like or wavelike P waves

frontal plane (5)—an imaginary line dividing the body into anterior and posterior halves; also known as the coronal plane.

functional aerobic capacity (4)—the ability or power to perform necessary activities, especially of an endurance nature

gap junction (1)—a *gap* between adjacent cell membranes containing very fine latticelike connections that allow physiologic components to pass directly from cell to cell

half-life (2)—the time it takes for the plasma concentration of a drug to be reduced to 50% of its peak value

hexaxial reference system (5)—a diagram of the axes of the limb leads in the frontal plane. It is used primarily for the determination of the heart's mean electrical axis in the frontal plane.

horizontal plane (5)—an imaginary line dividing the body into superior and inferior halves; also known as the transverse or axial plane.

hyperkalemia (14)—high potassium levels

hypertrophic cardiomyopathy (14)—a disease in which the heart muscle becomes abnormally thick (hypertrophied)

hypocalcemia (14)—low calcium levels

hypokalemia (5)—low potassium levels

hypomagnesemia (14)—low magnesium levels

hypoproteinemic (2)—abnormal deficiency of protein in the blood

hypoxemia (7)—abnormally low concentration of oxygen in the blood

idiopathic cardiomyopathy (14)—cardiomyopathy of unknown or obscure cause

idioventricular rhythm (11)—a ventricular rhythm in which the rate is less than 40 beats per minute, usually between 20 and 40 beats per minute

inotropic (1)—inotropic effects are those that change the myocardial contractive force

instantaneous vectors (6)—the many small electrical currents in many different directions that are created by depolarizations within the heart

intercalated discs (1)—specialized junctions between the muscle fibers of the heart that allow depolarization to occur rapidly from fiber to fiber and throughout the heart

interpolated PVC (11)—a PVC that occurs without disrupting the normal underlying cardiac rhythm

irregularly irregular rhythm (10)—a rhythm in which the heartbeats are spaced irregularly but with no discernible pattern

irregular rhythm (5)—when there are varying distances between successive R waves on the ECG; RR intervals are significantly different from each other, and is usually defined as greater than a 2 small box difference in length between the longest and shortest RR interval

isoelectric (4)—the baseline of the ECG

isoproterenol (2)—a sympathomimetic beta-receptor stimulant like epinephrine, but it does not cause vasoconstriction

isorhythmic AV dissociation (14)—synchronized dissociation; while the atria and ventricles are beating independently of each other, they beat at the same rate.

isovolumic contraction (1)—time period at the beginning of systole. The ventricles are contracting against closed AV and semilunar valves.

isovolumic relaxation (1)—time period when the ventricles are rapidly relaxing during ventricular repolarization while the AV and semilunar valves are closed.

J point (5)—point at which the QRS complex ends and the ST segment begins. This point is often used as the point from which to measure ST segment elevation or depression.

J-60 point (5)—a point 60 ms after the J point. This point has been suggested to be more accurate for measuring ST segment elevation or depression than the J point.

J-80 point (5)—a point 80 ms after the J point. This point has been suggested to be more accurate for measuring ST segment elevation or depression than the J point.

Jervell and Lange-Nielsen syndrome (14)—a rare inherited disorder characterized by deafness present at birth (congenital) occurring in association with abnormalities affecting the electrical system of the heart. The severity of cardiac symptoms associated with JLNS varies from person to person.

junctional rhythm (5)—ectopic rhythm originating somewhere between the AV node and the AV bundle. The rate is between 40 and 60 beats per minute.

junctional tachycardia (12)—a rhythm in which all of the complexes arise from somewhere from the atrioventricular node to the bundle of His and the rate is greater than 100 beats per minute

lead (5)—consists of a positive and a negative end, either two electrodes of opposing polarity, or a single positive electrode and a fixed reference point

lead I (5)—one of the bipolar limb leads. It uses the left arm electrode as the positive pole and the right arm as the negative pole.

lead II (5)—one of the bipolar limb leads. It uses the left leg electrode as the positive pole and the right arm as the negative pole.

lead III (5)—one of the bipolar limb leads. It uses the left leg electrode as the positive pole and the left arm as the negative pole.

lead aV_F (5)—one of the unipolar limb leads. It uses the left leg electrode as the positive pole and a combination of the left arm and right arm electrodes as the negative pole.

lead aV_L (5)—one of the unipolar limb leads. It uses the left arm electrode as the positive pole and a combination of the left leg and right arm electrodes as the negative pole.

lead aV_R (5)—one of the unipolar limb leads. It uses the right arm electrode as the positive pole and a combination of the left arm and left leg electrodes as the negative pole.

lead V_1 (5)—one of the chest leads. It uses the V_1 electrode as the positive pole and a point in the center of the heart, usually said to be positioned at the AV node, as the negative pole.

lead V_2 (5)—one of the chest leads. It uses the V_2 electrode as the positive pole and a point in the center of the heart, usually said to be positioned at the AV node, as the negative pole.

lead V_3 (5)—one of the chest leads. It uses the V_3 electrode as the positive pole and a point in the center of the heart, usually said to be positioned at the AV node, as the negative pole.

lead V_4 (5)—one of the chest leads. It uses the V_4 electrode as the positive pole and a point in the center of the heart, usually said to be positioned at the AV node, as the negative pole.

lead V_5 (5)—one of the chest leads. It uses the V_5 electrode as the positive pole and a point in the center of the heart, usually said to be positioned at the AV node, as the negative pole.

lead V_6 (5)—one of the chest leads. It uses the V_6 electrode as the positive pole and a point in the center of the heart, usually said to be positioned at the AV node, as the negative pole.

left axis deviation (6)—a heart whose mean electrical axis is located between 0° and −90°. There are several pathologic and nonpathologic causes of LAD.

left ventricular hypertrophy (5)—a heart condition in which there is increased muscle mass of the left ventricle. It most commonly occurs as a pathological condition but can also occur in the athletic heart.

limb leads (5)—the six leads created by the limb electrodes, leads I, II, III, aV_F, aV_R, and aV_L

long QT syndrome (11)—a condition that occurs when the QT interval is longer than normal, which can be an inherited mutation or caused by certain drugs or electrolyte imbalance. It increases your risk for Torsades de Pointes.

mean electrical axis (6)—the direction and magnitude of the average of all of the instantaneous vectors within the ventricles

mitral regurgitation (1)—backflow of blood from the left ventricle into the atria. This occurs owing to the inability of the mitral valve to completely close after blood has flowed into the ventricles from the atria.

monomorphic (11)—consisting of one shape

multifocal (11)—originating from two or more foci or sites within the heart

multifocal atrial tachycardia (12)—a rhythm in which there are multiple ectopic atrial sites firing from beat to beat and the rate is greater than 100 beats per minute

myocardial infarction (5)—condition characterized by death of cardiac tissue, most commonly caused by prolonged myocardial ischemia

myocarditis (14)—inflammation of the heart muscle

myocardium (1)—muscular wall of the heart

myocytes (7)—isolated cardiac muscle cells

myxedema (14)—swelling of the skin and underlying tissues giving a waxy consistency, typical of patients with underactive thyroid glands

necrosis (9)—the death of body tissue. It occurs when too little blood flows to the tissue. This can be from injury, radiation, or chemicals. Necrosis cannot be reversed.

negative deflection (5)—an ECG deflection below the isoelectric line

nonsustained atrial tachycardia (12)—runs of three or more to up to 30 seconds of unifocal atrial complexes firing at a rate of greater than 100 beats per minute

nonsustained ventricular tachycardia (11)—beats of a ventricular origin occurring in succession at a rate of greater than 100 beats per minute and lasting anywhere from 3 complexes in a row up to 30 seconds in duration

normal axis (5)—the normal quadrant in which the heart's mean electrical activity in the frontal plane is located. On a circle, it is the lower right-hand quadrant, which, when looking at the patient's heart is downward and to the left. Normal axis is usually considered to extend to + 15° beyond the normal quadrant's boundaries. In this text the normal axis is considered to be 0° to 90°.

normal sinus rhythm (5)—the heart is said to be in normal sinus rhythm when all aspects of the ECG are within normal limits.

orthostatic hypotension (3)—a decrease in systolic blood pressure of 20 mmHg or a decrease in diastolic blood pressure of 10 mmHg within three minutes of standing when compared with blood pressure from the sitting or supine position

oscilloscope (5)—a device used for showing changes in electrical voltage, which is then displayed on a monitor

P axis (6)—the direction and magnitude of the average of all of the instantaneous vectors within the atria

P mitrale (7)—broad, notched P waves in lead II and sometimes other leads of the electrocardiogram with a prominent late negative component to the P wave in lead V_1, presumed to be characteristic of mitral valvular disease

P pulmonale (7)—an electrocardiographic syndrome marked by tall, narrow, peaked P waves in lead II and sometimes other leads of the electrocardiogram, presumed to be characteristic of cor pulmonale

P wave (5)—the first ECG deflection produced by atrial depolarization

PAC with aberrant conduction (12)—a premature atrial complex that reaches the ventricles but proceeds through the ventricles in an unorganized fashion instead of through the normal His-Purkinje system; it appears on the ECG as an early complex that appears very similar to a PVC except that it is preceded by a P wave.

PR interval (5)—the distance from the beginning of the P wave to the beginning of the QRS complex. It encompasses both the P wave and the PR segment. Thus, it includes the electrical events associated with atrial systole.

PR segment (5)—the distance from the end of the P wave to the beginning of the QRS complex. It is normally isoelectric because the atrial fibers are typically in phase 2 during this time period. Most of the atrial kick occurs during this time. The PR segment is the area of the ECG most commonly used to determine the position of the isoelectric line.

palpitation (3)—unpleasant sensations of irregular and/or forceful beating of the heart

papillary muscle (1)—a column of myocardium projecting into the ventricular cavity that is continuous with the ventricular wall and attached to the chordae tendinae of the atrioventricular valves

parasympatholytics (2)—drugs that inhibit cholinergic receptors of the autonomic nervous system

parasympathomimetics (2)—drugs that stimulate cholinergic receptors of the autonomic nervous system

parenteral (2)—route of administration of a drug through means other than the intestinal route

paroxysmal (12)—appearing suddenly

pericardial tamponade (14)—A life-threatening situation in which there is such a large amount of fluid (usually blood) inside the pericardial sac around the heart that it interferes with the performance of the heart

pericarditis (5)—inflammation of the pericardium of the heart

pharmacodynamics (2)—mechanism by which a drug achieves its effect within the body

pharmacokinetics (2)—movement of a drug within the body

pharmacology (2)—science dealing with the interactions between living systems and molecules

phenoxybenzamine (2)—a drug that blocks adrenergic activity at the alpha receptors

pleural effusion (14)—the build-up of excess fluid between the layers of the pleura outside the lungs

pneumothorax (14)—the presence of air or gas in the cavity between the lungs and the chest wall, causing collapse of the lung

polymorphic (11)—consisting of two or more different shapes

polypharmacy (2)—excessive and unnecessary use of medication, especially in elderly individuals, where many hospital admissions are medication related

positive deflection (5)—an ECG deflection above the isoelectric line

preload (1)—workload imposed on the ventricles just prior to contraction

premature atrial complexes (5)—early depolarizations that arise from an area within the atria other than the sinoatrial node

premature junctional complex (12)—early depolarizations that arise from an area anywhere from the atrioventricular node to the bundle of His

premature ventricular complex (11)—early depolarizations of ventricular origin, they usually disrupt the normal cardiac rhythm.

pressure-loaded exercise (1)—the nature of resistance exercise creates high afterload states in which mean arterial pressure and/or total peripheral resistance is increased in the face of modest cardiac outputs.

pressure overload (2)—demand placed on muscle, especially heart muscle, in response to high blood pressure or stenotic valves. May result over time in cardiac hypertrophy and, eventually, heart failure.

prolapse (3)—a condition is which valve leaflets bulge upward into the left atrium in the case of the mitral valve or the right atrium in the case of the tricuspid valve

propranolol (2)—drug that blocks the beta-adrenergic receptors

psychotropic agents (14)—any medication capable of affecting the mind, emotions, and behavior

pulmonary embolus (14)—a sudden blockage in a lung artery. The cause is usually a blood clot in the leg called deep vein thrombosis.

QRS complex (5)—a series of typically three deflections on the ECG that occur as a result of ventricular depolarization

QT interval (5)—the distance from the beginning of the QRS complex to the end of the T wave. It includes the QRS complex, ST segment, and T wave. As such, it includes all of the electrical events associated with ventricular systole.

quadrigeminy (11)—a cardiac rhythm in which every fourth beat is an abnormal one

RR interval (5)—the distance between two consecutive R waves on the ECG. It is used to determine regularity of rhythm and heart rate.

R on T phenomenon (11)—when a premature ventricular complex (PVC) occurs during the T wave of the complex preceding it

rate calculator (5)—a chart of heart rate values that can be held up to the ECG to quickly determine a subject's heart rate

rate pressure product (1)—also known as the double product. Used in cardiology and exercise physiology to determine the myocardial workload, RPP is equal to heart rate times the systolic blood pressure.

refractory (1)—inability of tissue to depolarize

regularly irregular rhythm (10)—a rhythm is regularly irregular if it has regularity to the pattern of the irregular occurring complexes.

regular rhythm (5)—when there is an equal distance between successive R waves on the ECG. Thus, RR intervals are not significantly different from each other, and is usually defined as less than a 2 small box difference in length between the longest and shortest RR interval.

reperfusion dysrhythmia (11)—disturbances in the cardiac rhythm that occur subsequent to restoration of blood flow to a previously ischemic area

repolarization (1)—reestablishment of polarity, especially the return of cell membrane potential to resting potential after depolarization

retrograde P wave (12)—a P wave that appears after the QRS complex, usually appearing within the ST segment

rhythm strip (5)—a longer strip of one or more leads printed at the bottom of a 12-lead ECG printout. Typically, the rhythm strip shows an entire 12-second view of that lead(s).

right axis deviation (6)—a heart whose mean electrical axis is located between 90° and 180°. There are several pathologic and nonpathologic causes of RAD.

Romano–Ward syndrome (14)—a condition that causes a disruption of the heart's normal rhythm (arrhythmia). This disorder is a form of long QT syndrome, which is a heart condition that causes the heart (cardiac) muscle to take longer than usual to repolarize between beats.

ST segment (5)—the distance from the end of the QRS complex to the beginning of the T wave. It should normally be flat and isoelectric. Most of the ejection of blood from the ventricles occurs during this time.

ST segment depression (5)—an ST segment that is significantly below the isoelectric line

ST segment elevation (5)—an ST segment that is significantly above the isoelectric line

semilunar valves (1)—valves between the right ventricle and pulmonary artery and between the left ventricle and aorta

sensitivity (4)—percentage of individuals with disease who have an abnormal test

specificity (4)—percentage of individuals free of disease who have a normal test

Stokes–Adams attacks (13)—sudden collapse into unconsciousness owing to a disorder of heart rhythm in which there is a slow or absent pulse, resulting in syncope (fainting) with or without convulsions.

stroke volume (1)—amount of blood ejected by ventricle in one cardiac cycle

subendocardium (9)—the layer of heart tissue lying between, and joins, the endocardium and the myocardium. It consists of a layer of loose fibrous tissue, containing the vessels and nerves of the conducting system of the heart. The Purkinje fibers are located in this layer.

supraventricular arrhythmias (12)—arrhythmias in the heart that have their origination point above the ventricles but outside of the sinoatrial (SA) node

supraventricular tachycardias (12)—includes all tachycardias whose origin is above the ventricles but outside of the sinoatrial node

sustained atrial tachycardia (12)—greater than 30 seconds in duration of unifocal atrial complexes firing at a rate of greater than 100 beats per minute

sustained ventricular tachycardia (11)—beats of a ventricular origin occurring in succession at a rate of greater than 30 seconds in duration of unifocal ventricular complexes firing than 100 beats per minute and lasting for at least 30 seconds

sympatholytics (2)—drugs that inhibit adrenergic receptors of the autonomic nervous system

sympathomimetics (2)—drugs that stimulate adrenergic receptors of the autonomic nervous system

syncope (2)—temporary loss of consciousness owing to generalized cerebral ischemia

syncytium (1)—a network of electrically connected cardiac muscle cells creating a functional unit of contraction. The wave of contraction that allows the heart to work as a unit, called a functional syncytium, begins with the pacemaker cells.

systemic hypothermia (14)—core body temperature below 35°C

systole (1)—phase of the cardiac cycle when the myocardium is contracting.

T wave (5)—normally, the last deflection of each heart complex, which occurs because of ventricular repolarization. It should occur in the same direction as the QRS complex and is normally asymmetrical with a steeper downslope than upslope.

TP interval (5)—the distance from the end of the T wave to the beginning of the P wave of the following complex. During this time, both the atria and the ventricles are in diastole.

tachyarrhythmias (2)—irregular heart rhythms producing rates greater than 100 beats per minute

target heart rate (5)—the minimum heart rate necessary to reach the level of exertion required for cardiovascular fitness. It is specific to the person's age, gender, and physical fitness.

threshold potential (1)—the critical level to which a membrane potential must be depolarized to initiate an action potential

torsades de pointes (5)—a form of polymorphic ventricular tachycardia in which the QRS complexes are of varying shapes, heights, and widths and appear to twist around the isoelectric axis.

total peripheral resistance (1)—total force in the vascular system in opposition to blood flow.

toxicity (2)—the degree to which a substance (a toxin or poison) can harm humans or animals.

transverse plane (5)—an imaginary line dividing the body into superior and inferior halves. Also known as the horizontal or axial plane.

trigeminy (11)—a cardiac rhythm in which every third beat is an abnormal one

U wave (5)—a last, small, rounded wave that is sometimes present after the T wave. It is thought to occur owing to the last stages of ventricular repolarization, such as of either the Purkinje fibers or papillary muscles.

unifocal (11)—originating from a single focus or site within the heart

unipolar limb leads (5)—the augmented voltage limb leads aV_F, aV_L, and aV_R. Each uses one of the limb electrodes (RA, LA, LL) as its positive pole and a combination of the other two electrodes as the negative pole.

vagotonic (14)—excessive excitability of the vagus nerve resulting typically in vasomotor instability, constipation, and sweating

vasoconstriction (1)—narrowing of the blood vessels resulting from contracting the muscular wall of vessels; usually evoked by impulses in sympathetic nerve fibers.

vasodilation (1)—widening of blood vessels resulting from smooth muscle relaxation in the vessel walls

ventricular arrhythmias (11)—abnormal heart rhythms originating within the ventricles

ventricular fibrillation (5)—a condition in which multiple sites within the ventricles fire rapidly and chaotically. It is a form of cardiac arrest. This rhythm is ineffective in creating cardiac output; therefore, the patient is unconscious and pulseless.

ventricular rate (5)—number of ventricular depolarizations occurring per minute.

ventricular tachycardia (11)—ventricular rhythms in which the rate is greater than 100 beats per minute.

volume-loaded exercise (1)—class of exercise characterized by graded levels of cardiac output in response to incremental exercise. Blood pressure increases are moderate. The stimulus for cardiac physiological and structural (increased internal diameter of the left ventricle) adaptations is periodic (endurance exercise training) high preload states.

volume overload (7)—refers to the state of one of the chambers of the heart in which too much blood volume exists within it for the chamber to function efficiently. Ventricular volume overload is approximately equivalent to an excessively high preload and is a cause of cardiac failure.

wandering atrial pacemaker (12)—a rhythm in which there are multiple ectopic atrial sites firing from beat to beat and the rate is less than 100 beats per minute

CPSIA information can be obtained
at www.ICGtesting.com
Printed in the USA
JSHW051945050722
27703JS00003B/22